CURRENT
PHYSICAL THERAPY

Current Therapy Series

CURRENT
PHYSICAL THERAPY

MALCOLM PEAT, PH.D.

Professor and Director
Associate Dean (Rehabilitation)
School of Rehabilitation Therapy
Faculty of Medicine
Queen's University
Kingston, Ontario

1988

B.C. Decker Inc • Toronto • Philadelphia

Publisher

B.C. Decker Inc
3228 South Service Road
Burlington, Ontario   L7N 3H8

B.C. Decker Inc
320 Walnut Street
Suite 400
Philadelphia, Pennsylvania   19106

Sales and Distribution

United States and Possessions	**The C.V. Mosby Company** 11830 Westline Industrial Drive Saint Louis, Missouri 63146
Canada	**The C.V. Mosby Company, Ltd.** 5240 Finch Avenue East, Unit No. 1 Scarborough, Ontario M1S 5P2
United Kingdom, Europe and the Middle East	**Blackwell Scientific Publications, Ltd.** Osney Mead, Oxford OX2 OEL, England
Australia	**Harcourt Brace Jovanovich** 30–52 Smidmore Street Marrickville, N.S.W. 2204 Australia
Japan	**Igaku-Shoin Ltd.** Tokyo International P.O. Box 5063 1–28–36 Hongo, Bunkyo-ku, Tokyo 113, Japan
Asia	**Info-Med Ltd.** 802–3 Ruttonjee House 11 Duddell Street Central Hong Kong
South Africa	**Libriger Book Distributors** Warehouse Number 8 "Die Ou Looiery" Tannery Road Hamilton, Bloemfontein 9300
South America (non-stock list representative only)	**Inter-Book Marketing Services** Rua das Palmeriras, 32 Apto. 701 222–70 Rio de Janeiro RJ, Brazil

Current Physical Therapy   ISBN 1–55664–025–0

Library of Congress catalog card number: 87-72381

10 9 8 7 6 5 4 3 2 1

CONTRIBUTORS

CATHERINE ANDERSON, B.Sc., B.H.Sc. (PT)

Senior Physiotherapist, Intensive Care Unit, Victoria Hospital, London, Ontario, Canada
Inspiratory Muscle Training: An Adjunct to Weaning

SUSAN M. ATTERMEIER, M.A., L.P.T.

Assistant Professor, Division of Physical Therapy, University of North Carolina School of Medicine; Section Head, Physical Therapy, Clinical Center for the Study of Development and Learning, University of North Carolina, Chapel Hill, North Carolina
Rood Approach: An Evaluation

TADEJ BAJD, D.Sc., Dip. Eng.

Associate Professor, Faculty of Electrical Engineering, Edvard Kardelj University, Ljubljana, Yugoslavia
Four-Channel Electric Stimulator: An Ambulatory Aid for Spinal Cord Injured Patients

HANS W. BLASER, R.P.T., M.C.P.A.

Course Instructor, School of Physiotherapy, Queen's University; Director of Physiotherapy, St. Mary's of the Lake Hospital, Kingston, Ontario, Canada
Massage: Current Application

WILLIAM F. BOYCE, B.A., B.Sc. (PT), M.Sc.

Clinical Instructor, School of Rehabilitation Therapy, Queen's University; Physiotherapy Research Coordinator, Hotel Dieu Hospital, Kingston, Ontario, Canada
Power Wheelchair Training for Handicapped Children

JUDITH A. BRADLEY, B.S.c., P.T., M.C.S.P.

Clinical Consultant, Private Practice, Ganges, British Columbia, Canada; Instructor, Acupuncture Foundation of Canada, Toronto, Ontario and Instructor, Upledger Institute, Palm Beach Gardens, Florida
Acupuncture, Acupressure, and Trigger Point Therapy
Cranial Osteopathy and Craniosacral Therapy

PEGGY CLOUGH, B.S., M.S.

Supervisor, Physical Therapy Division, The University of Michigan Hospitals, Ann Arbor, Michigan
Respiratory Care for the Spinal Cord Injured Patient

JOYCE CONATY, B.Sc.

Physiotherapist, Addiction Research Foundation, Toronto, Ontario, Canada
Management of Substance Abuse

DAVID F. M. COONEY, M.Sc., P.T., C.P.O.

Senior Vice President, Beverly Hills Prosthetics-Orthotics, Inc., Beverly Hills, California
Gait Training of the Lower Extremity Amputee

LINDA M. COUSINS, B.Sc. (PT)

Guest Lecturer, Program in Physical Therapy, Faculty of Applied Health Sciences, University of Western Ontario; Staff Physiotherapist, Cardiopulmonary Division Department of Physiotherapy, University Hospital, London, Ontario, Canada
Assessment: The Basis of Chest Physical Therapy
Blood Gas Analysis
Physical Therapy in Critical Care
Preoperative and Postoperative Chest Care

PATRICIA J. CROSS, Dip. P. & O.T., B.Sc. (PT), M.C.P.A.

Clinical Instructor, School of Rehabilitation Therapy, Queen's University; Director of Physiotherapy, St. Mary's of the Lake Hospital, Kingston, Ontario, Canada
Stroke Management: Brunnstrom Approach
Motor Relearning

CLARICE M. DOLIBER, M.S., R.P.T.

Clinical Supervisor, Physical Therapy Department, Braintree Hospital, Braintree, Massachusetts
Role of the Physical Therapist in Pain Treatment Centers

BRIAN R. DURWARD, M.Sc., M.C.S.P.

Lecturer in Physiotherapy, Queen Margaret College, Edinburgh, Scotland
Physical Management of the Unconscious Head-Injured Patient

JENNIFER INGLIS ELLIS, Dip. P.T., M.A.P.A., M.C.P.A.

Staff Physiotherapist, Rheumatic Diseases Unit and Hemophilia Program, Kingston General Hospital, Kingston, Ontario, Canada
Rheumatoid Arthritis in the General Hospital Setting
Physical Therapy in Hemophilia

MAREL FIELDING, M.C.S.P.

Lecturer (Hon.), Department of Physical Therapy, Faculty of Applied Health Sciences, University of Western Ontario; Manager, Physiotherapy Services, University Hospital, London, Ontario, Canada
Physical Therapy in Chronic Airway Limitation
Techniques for Pulmonary Physical Therapy
Conventional Chest Care Techniques: Breathing Exercises, Postural Drainage, Percussion, and Spirometry

RANDALL GEE, B.A., P.T.

Project Coordinator, Regional Workers' Compensation Department, Kaiser Permanente, Oakland; Inpatient Coordinator of Physical Therapy, Kaiser Permanente Medical Center, San Francisco, California
Physical Therapy in Patients with Acquired Immunodeficiency Syndrome

JACQUELINE HARVEY, M.C.S.P.

Staff Physiotherapist, Montreal General Hospital, Montreal, Quebec, Canada
Heat and Ice in Musculoskeletal Disorders

KEITH C. HAYES, Ph.D.

Associate Professor, Department of Physical Medicine and Rehabilitation, University of Western Ontario; Director of Research, Parkwood Hospital, London, Ontario, Canada
Management of Spasticity
Balance Disorders

ELIZABETH C. HENLEY, B.P.T., M.Cl.Sc.

Lecturer, School of Physiotherapy, Cumberland College of Health Sciences, Lidcombe, New South Wales, Australia; Formerly Attending Staff, Department of Physiotherapy, University Hospital, London, Ontario, Canada
Isometric Exercise

DIANA HOLMES HOPKINS-ROSSEEL, B.Sc. (PT)

Lecturer, School of Rehabilitation, Queen's University; Senior Cardiopulmonary Therapist, Hotel Dieu Hospital, Kingston, Ontario, Canada
Pulmonary Physical Therapy: A Treatment Approach
Exercise in Cardiac Rehabilitation

SHAYNA HORNSTEIN, B.Sc.P.T.

Clinical Coordinator of Programs, Neil Squire Foundation, Vancouver, British Columbia, Canada
Ventilatory Muscle Training

MARILYN F. HUMPHREY, B.Sc. (PT)

Senior Physiotherapist, Regional Rehabilitation Unit, Parkwood Hospital, London, Ontario, Canada
Adult Hemiplegia: Rood Approach

OSÅ LITTRUP JACKSON, Ph.D., P.T.

Chairman, Department of Kinesiological Science and Director and Associate Professor, Physical Therapy Program, Oakland University, Rochester, Minnesota; Adjunct Assistant Professor, University of Pittsburgh School of Health Sciences, Pittsburgh, Pennsylvania
Motivating Older Persons

HELEN A. JOHNSON, B.Sc. (PT)

Program in Physical Therapy, Faculty of Applied Health Sciences, University of Western Ontario; Staff Physiotherapist, Neurosciences Unit, University Hospital, London, Ontario, Canada
Chest Physical Therapy and the Neurologic Patient
Preoperative and Postoperative Chest Care

JOHN B. JOHNSON, B.A., Dip. P.T.

Director of Physiotherapy, Hotel Dieu Hospital, Kingston, Ontario, Canada
Flexor Tendon Repair

KATHERINE A. JOHNSON, B.M.R. (PT)

Senior Physiotherapist, Clinical Studies, Department of Physiotherapy, St. Boniface General Hospital, Winnipeg, Manitoba, Canada
Low Frequency Currents: Electrical Stimulation of Muscle

NANCY S. MICK JONES, B.Sc. (PT), M.Sc.

Research Assistant, Department of Physical Therapy, University of Western Ontario; Chief Physiotherapist, Occupational Health Center, University Hospital, London, Ontario, Canada
Sacroiliac Pain
Management of the Geriatric Patient

DONNA L. KASABIAN, P.T.

Staff Physical Therapist, La Calle Physical Therapy and Associates, Carmichael; Staff Physical Therapist, Kaiser Permanente Medical Center, San Francisco, California
Physical Therapy in Patients with Acquired Immunodeficiency Syndrome

ALOJZ KRALJ, D.Sc., Dip. Eng.

Professor, Faculty of Electrical Engineering, Edvard Kardelj University, Ljubljana, Yugoslavia
Four-Channel Electric Stimulator: An Ambulatory Aid for Spinal Cord Injured Patients

LORETTA L. LANGIS, B.Sc.P.T.

Senior Physiotherapist, Medical–Surgical Unit, University Hospital, London, Ontario, Canada
Inspiratory Muscle Training: An Adjunct to Weaning

BRENDA M. LOVERIDGE, B.P.T., M.Sc., Ph.D.

Associate Professor, Division of Physical Therapy, School of Medical Rehabilitation, University of Manitoba Faculty of Medicine, Winnipeg, Manitoba, Canada
Ventilatory Muscle Training
Breathing Patterns in Chronic Obstructive Pulmonary Disease

JOYCE L. MacKINNON, Ed.D., M.P.T.

Associate Professor and Director, Division of Physical Therapy, University of New England, Biddeford, Maine
Current Application of Ultraviolet Light

DAVID J. MAGEE, B.A., Dip. P.T., B.P.T., M.Sc., Ph.D.

Professor and Chairman, Department of Physical Therapy, School of Rehabilitation Medicine, University of Alberta, Edmonton, Alberta, Canada
Orthopaedic Manual Therapy: Cyriax Approach
Orthopaedic Manual Therapy: Kaltenborn Approach
Orthopaedic Manual Therapy: Maitland Approach
Orthopaedic Manual Therapy: Mennell Approach

ANNE L. McDERMOTT, B.S., L.P.T.

Physical Therapist, Harmarville Rehabilitation Center, Pittsburgh, Pennsylvania
Functional Electrical Stimulation in Spinal Cord Injury

JENNIFER McEWEN-HILL, B.Sc. (PT)

Senior Physiotherapist, Rehabilitation/Rheumatic Disease Unit, University Hospital, London, Ontario, Canada
Rehabilitation in Spinal Cord Injury

ANN L. McKEEMAN-MARCOTTE, M.Cl.Sc (PT)

Senior Physiotherapist, Ottawa Children's Treatment Center; Ottawa, Ontario, Canada
Management of Spasticity
Balance Disorders

MARY ELLEN McLEAN, B.Sc. (PT)

Staff Physiotherapist, Parkwood Hospital, London, Ontario, Canada
Adult Hemiplegia: Rood Approach

NANCY BUCHHOLZ MOODIE, B.Sc.P.T.

Assistant Manager, Physical Therapy Department, St. Joseph's Health Center, London, Ontario, Canada
Functional Approach to Multiple Sclerosis

LINDA S. MOORE, B.Sc.P.T.

Physiotherapist, The Orthopaedic and Arthritic Hospital, Toronto, Ontario, Canada
Clinical Applications of Postoperative Transcutaneous Electrical Nerve Stimulation

ROBERTA A. NEWTON, P.T., Ph.D.

Associate Professor, Department of Physical Therapy, Medical College of Virginia, Richmond, Virginia
Interferential Current Stimulation in Recurrent Jaw Pain

MARY ORTI, P.T.

Physiotherapist, Rheumatic Diseases Unit, Kingston General Hospital, Kingston, Ontario, Canada
Rheumatoid Arthritis in the General Hospital Setting

BARRIE PICKLES, B.P.T., M.S.

Professor, Schools of Rehabilitation Therapy and Physical and Health Education, Queen's University, Kingston, Ontario, Canada
Osteoporosis and Exercise
Preventive Role of the Physical Therapist in the Management of Osteoporosis
Role of the Physical Therapist in the Management of Osteoporotic Fractures

MONIQUE PRENDERGAST, B.Sc., P.T.

Senior Physical Therapist, Rehabilitation and Long-Term Care Unit, Physical Therapy Department, St. Joseph's Health Center, London, Ontario, Canada
Functional Approach to Multiple Sclerosis

SANDY RENNIE, M.Sc., B.P.T.

Assistant Professor, Department of Physical Therapy, University of Alberta, Edmonton, Alberta, Canada
Interferential Current Therapy
Diadynamic Current Therapy

KATHERINE TRIST RICHARDSON, B.Sc., P.T.

Physiotherapist, The Orthopaedic and Arthritic Hospital, Toronto, Ontario, Canada
Clinical Applications of Postoperative Transcutaneous Electrical Nerve Stimulation

LORNA SAGORSKY, B.Sc.

Senior Physiotherapist, Addiction Research Foundation, Toronto, Ontario, Canada
Management of Substance Abuse

DEBRA R. SEBURN, B.S.R.

Clinical Instructor, University of Western Ontario; Physiotherapist, University Hospital, London, Ontario, Canada
Importance of Mobility in Chest Care

CHRISTOPHER J. SNOW, B.P.T., M.Sc.

Lecturer, Division of Physical Therapy, University of Manitoba; Service Head, Clinical Studies, Physiotherapy Department, St. Boniface General Hospital, Winnipeg, Manitoba, Canada
Ultrasonic Therapy

DALE STASZEWSKI, B.Sc. (PT)

Staff Physiotherapist, Montreal General Hospital,
Montreal, Quebec, Canada
Heat and Ice in Musculoskeletal Disorders

CAROL STUART-BUTTLE, M.S., P.T.

Senior Physical Therapist, Pennsylvania Hospital,
Philadelphia, Pennsylvania
Physical Therapy in a Psychiatric Hospital

ROBERT W. SYDENHAM, B.Sc., D.P.T., M.C.P.A.,
M.A.P.T.A., R.P.T.

Director of the URSA Foundation, Seattle, Washington;
Member, Canadian Orthopaedic Manipulative
Physiotherapists and Proprietor, Academy Place Physical
Therapy Ltd., Edmonton, Alberta, Canada
*Muscle Energy: An Approach to the Evaluation and
Treatment of Somatic Dysfunction*

G. ELIZABETH TATA, B.P.T., M.Cl.Sc.

Honorary Lecturer, Program in Physical Therapy,
University of Western Ontario; Clinical/Research
Physiotherapist, University Hospital,
London, Ontario, Canada
*Principles of Electromyographic Feedback and Its Clinical
Application in Stroke Rehabilitation*

KATHY TAYLOR, M.S., P.T.

Staff Physical Therapist, Department of Physical Therapy,
Medical College of Virginia, Richmond, Virginia
Interferential Current Stimulation in Recurrent Jaw Pain

JANE TOOT, Ph.D., P.T.

Associate Professor and Chairperson, Department of
Physical Therapy, Northeastern University,
Boston, Massachusetts
Physical Therapy in Hospice

GEORGE I. TURNBULL, B.P.T., M.A., M.C.S.P.,
Dip. T.P.

Associate Professor, School of Physiotherapy, Dalhousie
University, Halifax, Nova Scotia, Canada
Facilitation Techniques

ANTHONY A. VANDERVOORT, Ph.D.

Assistant Professor, Department of Physical Therapy,
Faculty of Applied Health Sciences, University of Western
Ontario, London, Ontario, Canada
Maintenance of Mobility in the Elderly
Management of the Geriatric Patient

ROY P. WALMSLEY, M.Sc.

Professor and Head, Program in Physical Therapy, School
of Rehabilitation Therapy, Queen's University,
Kingston, Ontario, Canada
Acustimulation in Musculoskeletal Disorders

MARY E. WHEELWRIGHT, B.Sc. (PT)

Director, Department of Physiotherapy, Dufferin Area
Hospital, Orangeville, Ontario
Hemiplegia: Bobath Approach

DEBORAH A. WILLEMS, B.Sc. (PT)

Senior Physiotherapist, Geriatric Unit, Department of
Physiotherapy, Parkwood Hospital,
London, Ontario, Canada
Hemiplegia: Bobath Approach

MARILYN J. WRIGHT, B.Sc.P.T.

Clinical Lecturer, Queen's University Faculty of Medicine;
Senior Pediatric Physiotherapist, Child Development
Center, Hotel Dieu Hospital, Kingston, Ontario, Canada
Bivalved Casts for Neurologically Involved Children

RIKI YAMADA, Dip. P. & O.T., M.C.P.A.

Senior Physiotherapist, York County Hospital,
Newmarket, Ontario, Canada
McKenzie Approach for Low Back Pain

PREFACE

The intent of *Current Physical Therapy* is to provide a description of management strategy for a variety of disorders currently treated by physical therapists. The text does not attempt to review etiology and pathophysiology, but concentrates on the more practical matters of treatment.

In recent years the scope of practice in physical therapy has expanded considerably, and advances in the basic and clinical sciences have stimulated the continuing development of the profession. A view of current practice, however, cannot describe fixed or static situations in clinical management, so that here only a circumscribed view of a developing science and its clinical application is given. *Current Physical Therapy* includes sections dealing with major aspects of clinical practice: cardiopulmonary, musculoskeletal, and neurologic, and two sections that concentrate on pain management and the application of selected electrophysiologic agents. The final section, Developing Practice, is an indication of some new directions in physical therapy.

Current Physical Therapy draws on the individual clinical experience of physical therapists, each of whom describes his or her particular methodology in one aspect of practice. Each chapter is a personal, current, and clinical point of view, not a summary of alternative techniques. The authors are all involved in the area of therapy they describe.

I am grateful to the contributors who have produced uniformly interesting up-to-date articles. Special appreciation is offered to Mary Mansor of B.C. Decker, Inc. for her guidance and unfailing support. Finally, I would like to express my special thanks to Enid Peat for advice and comment and for many hours of invaluable assistance.

Malcolm Peat, Ph.D.

CONTENTS

NEUROLOGIC PHYSICAL THERAPY

ELECTROPHYSIOLOGIC AGENTS

PAIN MANAGEMENT

DEVELOPING PRACTICE

CARDIOPULMONARY PHYSICAL THERAPY

ASSESSMENT: THE BASIS OF CHEST PHYSICAL THERAPY

LINDA M. COUSINS, B.Sc. (PT)

As in all other areas of physical therapy when dealing with the cardiopulmonary patient assess is of paramount importance. Assessment should include an appropriate history, an accurate and complete physical examination, and knowledgeable use of diagnostic test results. Each stage of the assessment should be directed to formulating a probable diagnosis and to determining the amount of detail required at further stages of the assessment.

HISTORY

A baseline knowledge of the patient's overall medical condition and history, in addition to specific information regarding cardiac and pulmonary problems, should be obtained from the medical chart and from patient questioning. Important areas to include in the history taking are as follows:

1. Relevant medical history and current complaint
2. Social history
3. Family history
4. History of respiratory and cardiac problems
5. Shortness of breath (SOB)—dyspnea
6. Cough and sputum production
7. Smoking history
8. Occupational history
9. Chest pain
10. Previous surgery.

Relevant medical history and the complaint that has led the patient to seek medical help can be obtained from the medical chart, and patient questioning should focus only on areas that need clarification. It is important to note particulars that may affect treatment selection or the patient's ability to carry out treatment requirements. These include chronic illnesses, previous or current neurologic conditions, and reasons for and type of surgery if a surgical patient. Social history can also be obtained from the chart and

should take into account marital status and physical home situation, which could affect the patient's ability to cope at home. Family history can also be important, especially in regard to cancer or cardiac disease.

Any specific history relating to the patient's cardiopulmonary status should be obtained by direct patient questioning, as it is interesting how often the information received may vary, depending on which member of the health care team is asking the questions. When asking about history of cardiac or pulmonary problems, it is helpful to be specific and to inform the patient about some of the conditions in which you are interested. For instance, a chronic chest patient may not perceive his or her condition as a "problem," but does indicate that he or she has had emphysema for 20 years and has had pneumonia six times in the last 10 years. Thus, a more helpful approach is to ask if the patient has had asthma, bronchitis, emphysema, or pneumonia, or to ask if they ever had a heart attack, high blood pressure, or heart failure. If history of any of these is reported, it is important to determine when the condition occurred and whether medical treatment was received.

Questions about dyspnea should determine whether it occurs at rest or with exertion, if with exertion at what level, and what provides relief. The patient should also be asked about orthopnea (inability to lie flat without SOB) and paroxysmal nocturnal dyspnea (SOB that wakes them from sleep), which may indicate cardiac disease.

History of cough should determine frequency and timing of cough (e.g., only in the morning, throughout the day, after a cigarette) and production of sputum. Sputum should be described by amount, color, consistency, and absence or presence of hemoptysis. Recent changes in amount or color are also important for the chronic chest patient.

Smoking history should determine both the number of cigarettes smoked each day and the number of years the patient has smoked; this allows determination of pack years (packs per day times years smoked), which is a more objective measure of smoking history. If the patient has quit smoking it should be determined when they quit and why. The latter may provide some information about patient attitudes towards health teaching and potential compliance with it.

Occupational history can provide useful information if the patient has had prolonged exposure to coal dust, silica dust, asbestos fibers, solvent fumes, grain dust, or other irritants that may have led to chronic chest changes. Questioning about chest pain should include the type of pain, what brings it on or causes it to exacerbate, and what provides relief. Other pain, such as back or shoulder pain, may also provide helpful clues. If the patient has had previous thoracic or major abdominal surgery, it is useful to know the type of surgery and whether any postoperative respiratory complications occurred. With the information obtained from the chart and from patient questioning one can begin to formulate an idea of what diagnosis and what problems to expect, and what amount of assessment is necessary.

CURRENT SUBJECTIVE STATUS

Each time a patient is seen, whether on initial assessment or on subsequent visits, it is important to formulate a picture of their current status, based on the patient's subjective reports. It is helpful to ask a general question such as, "how are you feeling?", to begin this process. Questions should be asked about dyspnea (i.e., "how is your breathing?"), about cough and sputum production, and about pain and its relief, particularly with surgical patients. This information gives an indication of the patient's status and helps determine the direction of the assessment.

PHYSICAL EXAMINATION

The traditional and most useful organization of the cardiopulmonary system comprises, in order, inspection, palpation, percussion, and auscultation (IPPA). Within the IPPA format, there are other assessment techniques within each part of the basic assessment, and these should be addressed dependent on whether the assessment is initial or secondary and on the particular patient. Figure 1 illustrates this principle, showing basic elements in the center and additional elements on either side.

Inspection

The essential elements in the inspection are respiratory rate, rhythm, depth and pattern of breathing. A general observation of the patient and his or her environment precedes inspection, taking into consideration ventilatory assistance, supplemental oxygen and its means of delivery, chest tubes, nasogastric tubes, intravenous lines, monitoring devices, dressings, and bedside documentation of the patient's vital signs and fluid balance; each may affect or give information regarding the patient's cardiopulmonary system.

Resting respiratory rate should be observed without the patient's awareness, for example, while making preliminary introductions or while reviewing the bedside information. Respiratory rate should be taken over 10 to 15 seconds unless it is very slow or irregular, in which case it should be taken for a full minute. Normal rates should range from 12 to 18 breaths per minute.

Rhythm can be regular or irregular. Irregular rhythm should be described and length of apneic periods noted. The irregularity may be Cheyne-Stokes breathing that may be associated with congestive heart failure, increased intracranial pressure and drug overdoses—where rate and depth follow a repeated pattern of gradual increase to a maximum and subsequent decrease to an apneic period. Alternatively, Biot's respirations are "irregularly irregular" and are usually seen with neurologic abnormalities. It is often more helpful simply to describe the rhythm than to attempt to label it.

Depth should be described using a continuum of terms such as shallow, moderately shallow, moderate, normal, or increased. Depth of breathing can be altered by pain, neurological status, hypoxia, fever, and metabolic abnormalities. Breathing pattern should be described as primarily upper chest, lower chest, abdominal excursion, or a combination of these.

Chest wall shape should also be evaluated on initial assessment. Normal chest shape is elliptical with the lateral diameter greater than the anteroposterior diameter. Variations from this should be noted.

Beyond these basic areas, further areas of inspection may be addressed, depending on the history and subjective findings. Alterations in chest shape, such as increased anteroposterior diameter, barrel chest (a generalized rounding of the chest cage with prominence of the sternum), pectus excavatum (depressed sternum), and pectus carinatum (protruding sternum), should be observed. Also to be noted are abnormalities in spinal curvature, such as kyphoscoliosis, asymmetry in levels of scapulae, and flaring of the lower ribs.

Use of accessory muscles of respiration such as the sternocleidomastoids, trapezius, latissimus dorsi, and paravertebrals should be noted; use should be described as mild, moderate, or marked in degree. Indrawing of intercostal spaces, the suprasternal notch, supraclavicular areas, or the lower chest wall should be noted. It should be observed whether indrawing occurs on inspiration or expiration, the location of the indrawing, and the degree whether minimal, moderate, or marked.

Cyanosis, a bluish discoloration of the skin, may be best observed in the mucous membranes of the lips or nares or on the underside of the tongue. This discoloration may not always be an accurate indication of hypoxia as adequate hemoglobin levels are necessary for cyanosis to be present. Cyanosis of nailbeds and digits is not usually helpful as it is often caused by peripheral arteriolar vasoconstriction. Pursed lip breathing, flaring of the nares, finger clubbing, and paradoxical abdominal breathing should also be noted if present.

An assessment of the patient's cough, obtained by asking them to cough or by observing any spontaneous coughs that occur, can be included here. The cough should be described by its depth (shallow, moderate, deep) or its strength (weak, moderate, strong) and its productiveness. Sputum, if produced, should be observed and described by color and consistency. Audible wheezes or secretions may also be heard, as well as stridor—a crowing sound produced by laryngeal spasm or edema, or by tracheal stenosis.

Palpation

Two basic items should always be included in palpation: expansion and flexibility. Expansion is the movement of the chest wall that the patient can produce. Lateral costal expansion should be assessed in all patients as this is most likely to be altered. Assessment is done by placing the hands on the chest wall with the thumbs at the xiphoid notch and the fingers resting along the anterolateral chest just below the nipples or breasts. Amount and symmetry of movement is noted. Upper and lower (posterior) chest movement can also be palpated using other hand positions.

Flexibility describes the compressibility of the chest wall by external force. The hands are placed on the chest wall in varying positions and gentle compression is applied. Flexibility should be described using a continuum of terms such as slightly decreased, decreased, moderate, moderately rigid, and rigid.

Other areas of palpation if indicated by preceding assessment findings may be included. Tracheal position can be palpated in the suprasternal area to indicate mediastinal shifts. This indication is not usually found unless a marked shift is present, such as with massive pleural effusion or intrathoracic tumor. Amount of abdominal tone may provide useful information as it affects both inspiratory and expiratory abilities. Abdominal tone can be described as flaccid, decreased, normal, or increased. If present, subcutaneous emphysema can be palpated and produces a crackling, bubbly feeling under the skin. It is usually present over the lateral or anterior chest wall and the neck, but may extend to the face, upper arms, abdominal wall, and upper thighs in severe cases.

In some patients, tactile fremitus should also be assessed. The ulnar border of the dominant hand is placed horizontally against the chest wall, and the patient is asked to say "ninety-nine" or a similar phrase. The vibration transmitted through to the hand is felt and described as being decreased, normal, or increased. For comparison the hand is moved from side to side and moved over the chest wall to assess all areas. Alterations in density of the underlying lung tissue or in amount of fluid or presence of air in the pleural space lead to changes in tactile fremitus. Increased density of underlying tissue, such as with consolidation, causes increased fremitus, whereas fluid or air in the pleural space, as in pleural effusion or pneumothorax, causes decreased fremitus.

Percussion

As indicated in Figure 1, percussion is not necessary in every assessment. It is an assessment technique that may be used to help develop a diagnosis, particularly when other assessment techniques have not provided sufficient information. Percussion is carried out by placing the middle phalanx of the second digit of the nondominant hand in firm contact with the chest wall parallel to the ribs and by striking the phalanx with the tip of the second digit of the dominant hand. The resonance produced by this action is described as normal, decreased or dull, or increased or hyperresonant. Percussion note should be compared side to side and all areas of the chest should be covered. Alterations in underlying lung tissue or fluid or air in the pleural space causes changes in the percussion note. A decrease or dullness in the percussion note is found with pleural effusion, consolidation, large areas of atelectasis, or fibrosis. An increased or hyperresonant percussion note is found over a pneumothorax, areas of emphysema, or a large cavity

Auscultation

Auscultation should be the last part of the assessment, not the first and only as happens if assessment is quick and cursory. Based on previous parts of the assessment, auscultation should clarify diagnosis and problems being identified. Auscultation should be carried out with the stethoscope in firm contact with the chest wall. Three basic locations should always be auscultated: anterior upper lobes over the mid-anterior chest wall; right middle lobe and lingula anterolateral to the nipple line; and lower lobes posterolateral or posterior. Auscultation should be done on both resting respiration and deep breaths, but this is usually only feasible with chronic chest patients since with most postoperative or acute medical patients resting respirations do not provide useful findings

Breath sounds and adventitia are the two things that should be assessed during auscultation. Breath

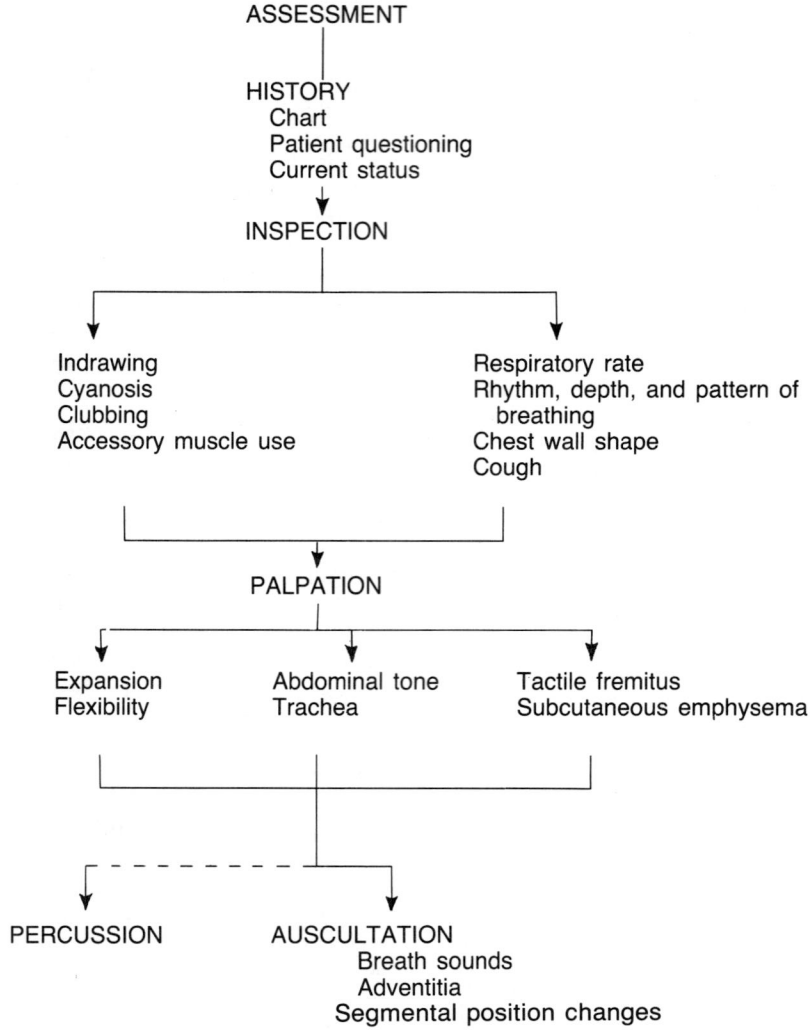

Figure 1 Assessment of the patient presenting with cardiopulmonary problems.

sounds are produced by turbulent air flow through the first few generations of bronchi and are transmitted to the chest wall by the lung tissue. Changes in air flow, in density of the transmitting lung tissue, or in fluid or air in the pleural space cause alterations in breath sounds. Breath sounds should be described by quality, and intensity or quantity.

Quality refers to whether breath sounds are normal (vesicular), bronchial, or of some intermediate type (bronchovesicular). In normal breath sounds, all of inspiration and up to the first third of expiration are heard as a soft rustling sound. In bronchial breath sounds, all of inspiration and all of expiration are heard, with a silent gap between them. They are of a hollow, echo-like type as if one were listening down a pipe. Bronchial breath sounds are produced when lung tissue density is increased, such as with consolidation

or large areas of atelectasis. They are also found at the upper limit of a large pleural effusion. These are normally found over the trachea and may be found in the normal patient over the right anteromedial chest or in the auscultatory triangles between the scapulae because of decreased chest wall impedance or proximity of the large bronchi to the chest wall. Intermediate or bronchovesicular breath sounds are those where expiration is increased but not of true bronchial quality; they represent intermediate degrees of pathology.

Quantity or intensity of breath sounds describes the loudness of the breath sounds. They should be described as decreased, normal, or increased. Decreased breath sounds may be found with pleural effusion or pneumothorax, where the sound transmission is blocked, with atelectasis, or occasionally with early stages of consolidation where air flow is decreased. Increased breath sounds may be found in consolidation or other pathologies that may produce bronchial breath sounds.

Adventitia should be described as crackles or wheezes. Crackles are discontinuous, explosive, nonmusical sounds. They should be classified by timing in the ventilatory cycle, quality (fine, medium, coarse), and number (few, diffuse). It is postulated that fine to medium crackles may be produced by rapid equalization of gas pressures when airways suddenly become patent. Medium to coarse crackles are thought to be produced by the action of air flow through or by secretions. Crackles may indicate a number of different sources including pulmonary edema, atelectasis, pulmonary fibrosis, secretions, and upper airway secretions.

Fine end-inspiratory crackles can be found in the dependent zones in pulmonary edema and shift with position changes. They may also be found in atelectasis, particularly following treatment. Fine inspiratory and expiratory crackles, which do not change with position or treatment, are found in pulmonary fibrosis. Medium to coarse crackles are those found with secretions—the most coarse crackles or upper airway sounds indicating secretions in the largest airways.

Wheezes are continuous musical sounds that may be monophonic or polyphonic. They should be described in terms of timing and pitch. Current theory states that wheezes are produced by vibration or by airway walls, and a partial obstruction by a similar mechanism to that which produces notes in a reed instrument. Wheezes may also be created by a number of situations including bronchospasm, pulmonary edema, secretions, or incomplete airway occlusion.

Coarse, monophonic wheezes indicate secretions in a large airway and usually clear with coughing. A coarse monophonic wheeze that does not clear may be due to a tumor or another obstruction. Scattered, polyphonic wheezes on expiration usually indicate bronchospasm. Scattered monophonic wheezes may also be found in pulmonary edema. It is important to note that absence of wheezing in an asthmatic attack may indicate severe bronchospasm such that almost no air is flowing. Another adventitious sound is a pleural rub—a creaking, squeaky sound caused by the movement of the two layers of pleurae on each other when they are roughened by inflammation or developing adhesions.

If obvious abnormalities are noted, or previous assessment findings indicate potential problem areas, a more detailed auscultation can be carried out over each lung segment, and differences with position change can be noted. Voice sounds can also be assessed during auscultation if it is necessary to clarify the diagnosis further. Speech is normally transmitted as a low-pitched mumble. Alterations in density increase or decrease the transmission of voice sounds. Voice sounds decrease with pleural effusion or pneumothorax, except at the upper limit of an effusion, where the phenomenon of egophony is heard. Here the higher-pitch vowels are transmitted more clearly, but with a change in character to a nasal bleating sound where "a" sounds like "ee." Voice sounds increase (bronchophony) over consolidation or large areas of atelectasis. Whispering pectoriloquy, where usually nontransmitted whispered sounds are audible, also occurs with the same pathologies.

OTHER DATA

After obtaining all of the information from the history and physical examination, the therapist has other available sources of data. These sources include: arterial or capillary blood gas tests, pulmonary function tests, and chest x-ray examinations. Interpreted reports of pulmonary function tests and x-ray examinations are available, although if they are unavailable the therapist should be able to interpret them on a basic level. These interpretations are beyond the scope of our discussion and resources are available to assist with this. The analysis of blood gas tests is discussed in a separate chapter.

The final stage of the assessment should be a review of all of the information obtained, from which a working diagnosis and a problem list is developed and then used to determine treatment techniques and frequency. Assessment should continue during each treatment and at each subsequent visit. This should eventually lead to the decision to discharge the patient from treatment either because the problem has been resolved, the patient is able to manage alone, or a problem has been identified in which physical therapy has no role.

SUGGESTED READING

Cherniak R, Cherniak L, Naimark A. Respiration in health and disease. 2nd ed. Philadelphia: WB Saunders, 1972.
Forgacs P. The functional basis of pulmonary sounds. Chest 1973; 73(3):399–408.
Squires LB. Fundamentals of radiology. 3rd ed. Cambridge, MA: Harvard University Press, 1982.
West JB. Respiratory physiology—the essentials. 3rd ed. Baltimore: Williams & Wilkins, 1985.

BLOOD GAS ANALYSIS

LINDA M. COUSINS, B.Sc. (PT)

In clinical practice, arterial or capillary blood gas results are often available, but are also often misused or ignored. These values can provide important information in guiding treatment decisions and perhaps most importantly in helping to define those patients for whom physical therapy intervention is not indicated and for whom consequences could be serious.

Analysis of blood gas results should not focus solely on oxygen levels and is really an assessment of the acid-base balance of the body. In order to understand what these values mean, it is necessary to review some basic chemistry and physiology.

CHEMISTRY

Beginning with some definitions, recall that an acid is any substance that can release hydrogen ions (H^+), whereas an alkali or base is any substance that can accept hydrogen ions. The acidity or alkalinity of a solution is determined by its H^+ concentration. Hydrogen ion concentration is very small (0.000001 mol per liter) and so is expressed as pH, the negative logarithm of the actual concentration.

Also, recall that any gas exerts a pressure, whether it is free in the atmosphere, confined in a container (e.g., the lungs), or dissolved in a liquid (e.g., plasma). When two or more gases are mixed together, each gas exerts a pressure as if it were the only gas present. This is known as its partial pressure and is usually measured in millimeters of mercury (mm Hg). Oxygen and carbon dioxide concentrations in the blood are expressed as their partial pressures (Po_2 and Pco_2).

The values of pH, Po_2, and Pco_2 are normally measured by a blood gas analyzer from a sample of arterial or "arterialized" capillary blood. Other values that make up a complete set of blood gases include the bicarbonate (HCO_3^-) level, which is usually a calculated value and is expressed in milliequivalents per liter, and sometimes base excess (BE) or base deficit. This is a standardized measure of deviation from normal standard HCO_3^-, i.e., the HCO_3^- concentration measured in equilibrium with a gas with a Pco_2 of 40 mm Hg at 37° C, which is expressed as a positive or negative numerical value.

PHYSIOLOGY

Acid-Base

Normal acid-base balance in the body maintains a pH of between 7.35 and 7.45, which is the extracellular pH at which cells can function. This level is attained by balancing the generation of hydrogen ions with their elimination or buffering. Hydrogen ions are released by acids produced by tissue breakdown and normal metabolism. Hydrogen ions are also yielded from carbonic acid that results from the chemical reaction of metabolically produced CO_2 with water ($H_2O + CO_2 \leftrightarrows H_2CO_3 \leftrightarrows H^+ + HCO_3^-$). Bicarbonate ions are also produced in this reaction.

Elimination of volatile CO_2 from the lungs is the primary mechanism for maintaining normal pH. Changes in ventilation alter the amount of CO_2 that is eliminated. The renal system also plays an important part in acid-base balance through selective excretion or retention of H^+ and HCO_3^-. Various buffers that remove hydrogen ions from solution are found throughout the body. Phosphate and ammonia levels in the urine are controlled by the kidneys. Hemoglobin and other proteins also act as buffers.

Whenever an imbalance in acid-base status occurs, the pH shifts from normal, and the body is in a state of acidosis (pH $\leq$ 7.35) or alkalosis (pH $\geq$ 7.45). This can be caused by metabolic or respiratory disturbances. Normal arterial blood gas values are shown in Table 1. Elevations in HCO_3^- lead to an increase in pH, whereas elevations in Pco_2 lead to a decrease in pH. Disturbances come from a variety of sources: some metabolic causes are listed in Table 2; respiratory causes are listed in Table 3. Respiratory disturbances are ultimately a result of either alveolar hypoventilation with retention of CO_2 or alveolar hyperventilation with increased elimination of CO_2. Compensation for a particular disturbance occurs in the other systems involved in acid-base balance. In respiratory abnormality, compensation occurs via changes in renal and other buffering systems, and takes 24 to 48 hours. In metabolic disturbance, compensation occurs in minutes to hours via the respiratory system, and then gradually by other buffer systems. Compensation brings pH back to within normal limits, and is reflected in changes in HCO_3^- and Pco_2.

Oxygenation

Arterial oxygenation is determined by numerous factors including ventilation, perfusion, and diffu-

TABLE 1   Normal Arterial Blood Gas Values

Po_2	80 to 100 mm Hg
Pco_2	35 to 45 mm Hg
pH	7.35 to 7.45
HCO_3^-	22 to 26 mEq per liter
BE	-3 to $+3$

sion. Anything that alters one of these factors can cause abnormal oxygenation. Some of the things that may decrease ventilation are (1) acute or chronic airway obstruction, (2) acute or chronic restrictive disease, (3) decreased central drive. Physical therapy can have an effect on many of these. Causes of altered perfusion include (1) decreased or increased cardiac output or cardiac failure, (2) decreased blood volume, (3) decreased hemoglobin, (4) pulmonary embolism. Causes of altered diffusion include (1) emphysema, large atelectasis (decreased diffusion area), (2) fibrosis, asbestosis (increased diffusion surface thickness).

Room air has a fraction of inspired oxygen (FIO_2) of 0.21, that is it contains 21 percent oxygen. Normal Po_2 values are 80–100 mm Hg, but should be proportionally higher with supplemental oxygen. A guideline for expected Po_2 can be obtained by dividing Po_2 by FIO_2. The result should be at least 200 ($Po_2 \div FIO_2 \geq 200$).

ANALYSIS

Once these basics are understood, it is relatively easy to analyze blood gas values provided and to apply the information to treatment decisions. The steps to follow are summarized in Table 4.

The first step is to determine whether pH is normal, acidotic, or alkalotic. Once pH is determined, decide whether the abnormality is metabolic or respiratory in origin. Next, determine the state of com-

TABLE 2   Metabolic Causes of Acid-Base Disturbances

Acidosis
  Diabetic ketosis
  Shock (i.e., anaerobic metabolism)
  Lactic acidosis
  Ingestion acids
  Methyl alcohol poisoning
  Ethyl alcohol overdose
  Renal failure
  Peritonitis
  Diarrhea

Alkalosis
  $NaHCO_3$ overdose
  Vomiting
  Small bowel drainage
  Potassium or chloride deficiency
  Gastric lavage without chloride replacement
  Mercurial diuretic therapy (rarely used)

TABLE 3   Respiratory Causes of Acid-Base Disturbances

Acidosis
  CNS depression (drugs, increased ICP)
  Chronic lung disease
  Acute lung disease
  Anatomic deformities
  Pain

Alkalosis
  Anxiety
  Hysteria
  Fever
  Hypoxia
  CNS damage

pensation. In an uncompensated disturbance, pH is abnormal and HCO_3^- or Pco_2 have not begun to change to reflect compensation. With partial compensation, pH returns to normal and there are changes in HCO_3^- or Pco_2. With full compensation, pH is normal and both HCO_3^- and Pco_2 are abnormal. Finally, look at the clinical picture and decide whether or not physical therapy is indicated. With a respiratory disturbance, treatment will almost always be indicated, whereas with a metabolic disturbance inappropriate treatment could be detrimental to the patient by counteracting a compensatory mechanism.

Oxygenation should be considered at this point in the analysis. If Po_2 is below normal, it is important that it be compared to premorbid and preoperative values, if possible. Oxygenation may need to be assessed in another way. Since most oxygen is combined with hemoglobin for transport, oxygen saturation (i.e., hemoglobin saturation) may be a more helpful measurement. Oxygen saturation can be measured from arterial blood samples or by an oximeter, which measures it using an attachment on the ear lobe or fingertip. Normal saturation is from 90 to 100 percent, which indicates that almost all of the available hemoglobin is carrying a maximum amount of oxygen. In this situation, ventilation is not the limiting factor to oxygenation, and physical therapy treatment may not be indicated. Saturations between 85 and 89 percent indicate mild hypoxia, which may not be clinically evident. Moderate to severe degrees of hypoxia are indicated by saturations ranging from 89 to 35 percent, with saturation below 70 percent indicating a situation requiring immediate intervention.

TABLE 4   Analysis of Blood Gases

Is pH normal, acidotic or alkalotic?
Is it of metabolic or respiratory origin?
Is it uncompensated, partially compensated, or fully compensated?
What is the clinical situation, including oxygenation?

Some examples, with treatment suggestions, serve to illustrate the method of analysis using these steps:

Example 1: Mr. M, a 95-year-old male, admitted to hospital this morning after a 5-day history of nausea and vomiting

Po_2 85, Pco_2 37, pH 7.55, HCO_3^- 40, BE +14

Analysis: 1. pH is alkalotic ($\geq$ 7.45)
2. Metabolic origin (HCO_3^- increased and Pco_2 normal)
3. Uncompensated (Pco_2 normal)
4. No physical therapy intervention.

Example 2: Mr. R, a 65-year-old male, 50 pack year smoker, two days post-op small bowel resection

Po_2 65, Pco_2 60, pH 7.30, HCO_3^- 32, BE +4

Analysis: 1. pH is acidotic ($\leq$ 7.35)
2. Respiratory origin (Pco_2 increased, which decreased pH)
3. Partial compensation (HCO_3^- increased, pH still abnormal)
4. Oxygenation is also low (PO_2 < 80); physical therapy intervention to assist with secretion mobilization and increasing ventilation; ensure adequate analygesia.

Example 3: Miss A, a 23-year-old female, involved in a motor vehicle accident last night with multiple orthopaedic injuries, temperature 39.2° C

Po_2 98, Pco_2 25, pH 7.50, HCO_3^- 16, BE − 7

Analysis: 1. pH is alkalotic
2. respiratory origin
3. partial compensation
4. physical therapy intervention to decrease respiratory rate and to encourage relaxation; ensure adequate analgesia; oxygenation is not a concern.

Example 4: Mrs. C, a 46-year-old female, in hospital for control of her diabetes

Po_2 83, Pco_2 30, pH 7.32, HCO_3^- 15, BE −10

Analysis: 1. pH is acidotic
2. metabolic origin
3. partial compensation
4. physical therapy intervention not indicated; hyperventilaton is compensatory; monitor for ventilatory fatigue resulting from maintained high minute ventilation, currently not a problem as oxygenation is adequate.

Example 5: Mr. Q, 58-year-old man, renal failure, receiving O_2 40 percent by mask

Po_2 68, Pco_2 50, pH 7.46, HCO_3^- 35, BE +9

Analysis: 1. pH is alkalotic
2. metabolic origin
3. almost total compensation
4. physical therapy intervention to optimize ventilation by increasing depth and decreasing rate to improve oxygenation ($Po_2 \div FiO_2$ = 170) and to prevent atelectasis due to shallow pattern.

By making use of blood gas results to assess acid-base balance and oxygenation, the clinician is able to make more accurate treatment decisions regarding the cardiopulmonary patient. This is particularly valuable in those patients where injudicious physical therapy intervention could worsen a metabolic-based problem by reversing compensatory mechanisms.

SUGGESTED READING

Any chemistry and/or physiology text

MacLeod J, ed. Davidson's principle and practice of medicine. 12th ed. New York: Churchill & Livingstone, 1977:164.

Oh TE, ed. Intensive care manual. 2nd ed. Stoneham, MA: Butterworths, 1981.

West JB. Respiratory physiology—the essentials. 3rd ed. Baltimore: Willimas & Wilkins, 1985.

PHYSICAL THERAPY IN CRITICAL CARE

LINDA M. COUSINS, B.Sc. (PT)

The provision of physical therapy in a critical care setting, particularly chest physical therapy, is of both great importance and value. In the minds of many clinicians it is also an area fraught with great anxiety. The critically ill patient usually has not only a respiratory condition of great concern, which requires immediate attention, but also may have severe cardiac and other systems involvement, which complicates the picture and increases the severity of the situation. In the intensive care setting, a wide variety of patients may be encountered; these range from cardiovascular and thoracic surgery patients to neurosurgery patients, patients with multiple trauma, or patients who are septic following abdominal surgery or during a prolonged illness. In this sense critical care physical therapy is a great challenge since it requires not only a thorough knowledge of cardiopulmonary physiology and pathology, but also a reasonable understanding of numerous other systems and medical and surgical problems.

However, from the point of view of dealing with respiratory problems, physical therapy in an intensive care unit is little different than in any other setting. In spite of some minor variations and alterations, assessment skills and techniques remain the same. The treatment techniques come from the same repertoire used with any patient with similar problems; some techniques are obviously inappropriate and particular precautions have to be taken and specific parameters monitored more closely. The following pages present an approach to treating the critically ill patient who requires physical therapy intervention.

TREATMENT APPROACHES

A number of approaches are possible in dealing with the critically ill patient. The first may be to avoid physical therapy treatment altogether because of the perceived risks associated with cardiac or respiratory instability. Avoidance may be appropriate if the severity of pulmonary pathology or the effectiveness of treatment does not outweigh either the difficulties of carrying out treatment or the potential for creating further instability.

For instance, in adult respiratory distress syndrome (ARDS), where there is significant refractory hypoxemia because of severe hemorrhagic pulmonary edema (caused by increased pulmonary capillary permeability), physical therapy intervention is unlikely to be of any benefit and could have harmful effects by increasing fluid movement into the alveoli or by increasing metabolic demands by requiring active movements from the patient. Here educated monitoring of the patient's status, until the underlying pathology is treated and hypoxemia begins to improve, is the best treatment option.

A second approach is to use the traditional techniques of postural drainage with manual percussion and vibration. This approach is used in many centers, but is fraught with difficulties associated with accurate and effective positioning for drainage because of monitoring lines, traction and drainage tubes. In addition, there are contraindications to the head-down position with elevated intracranial pressure and cardiac disease, which are found in many critically ill patients.

A third alternative is the use of the mechanical vibrator. This technique has proven effective in mobilizing secretions and in improving arterial oxygenation in critically ill patients, with minimal side effects and few contraindications.

A final approach is the use of various manual treatment techniques as described by Waldemar Kolaczkowski and Delva Bethune, and as outlined in *Techniques for Pulmonary Physical Therapy*.

CURRENT APPROACH

At University Hospital, London, Ontario, physical therapy in the Intensive Care Unit (ICU) deals with a varied patient population. About one-third of the patients treated are cardiovascular surgery patients who have difficulty weaning from ventilation postoperatively. Medical or surgical patients who have developed septic shock or respiratory failure are also admitted for care. Smaller percentages consist of neurologic patients requiring ventilatory assistance (e.g., Guillain-Barré) and multiple trauma patients (a trauma unit exists at another center in the city). Although each of these groups presents its own particular set of problems and precautions, the general approach remains the same throughout.

Assessment

The principles and techniques of assessment remain the same in the critically ill patient as for any other patient. However, some areas of the assessment are no longer available or as useful in the patient who is intubated and mechanically ventilated. Respiratory rate, rhythm and depth are set parameters with fully controlled ventilation. Expansion is not assessed in the ventilated patient. It is not possible to use techniques such as tactile fremitus or voice sounds. Percussion and auscultation may be difficult, and position changes, to clarify certain findings, may be difficult or impossible.

When evaluating auscultation findings, be aware of abnormal sounds produced by water in the ventilator tubing (a bubbling sound similar to upper airway sounds), by airflow through the ventilator circuit when high levels of positive end expiratory pressure are used (a coarse wheeze usually also audible at the bedside without the stethoscope), or by air leaking past the cuff of the endotracheal tube.

Because of the decreased usefulness of some assessment techniques or findings, it is most important to make knowledgeable use of chest x-ray examination findings, and blood gas results when evaluating the chest status.

Treatment Techniques

A combination of the use of the mechanical vibrator and a selection of manual techniques is the suggested protocol. Usual treatment of a patient who is mechanically ventilated consists of the use of the vibrator over areas of pathology (e.g., atelectasis, pulmonary infiltrates, pneumonia) found on chest x-ray film or from assessment findings (e.g., areas of increased or decreased breath sounds), and a combination of manual treatment techniques.

The vibrator is moved over the surface anatomy corresponding to each area of pathology for a period of 15 to 20 minutes; it is held in one location for 30 seconds to 1 minute. Firm pressure is used, and the patient may be in any position. This technique is particularly useful in those patients where postural drainage positions are contraindicated or where position changes are difficult or impossible because of traction and other lines and drains.

Secretion mobilization from small airways and relaxation of the chest wall are the effects of mechanical vibration. Secretion mobilization decreases the development of, or leads to the resolution of, atelectasis and prevents further secretion retention and development of pneumonia. Both lead to improvement in ventilation and to better matching of ventilation to perfusion, thereby leading to an improvement in oxygenation. Chest wall relaxation results in more even distribution of ventilation and, ultimately, leads to improved oxygenation. There have also been observations of improvement in cardiac output and other hemodynamic indices following mechanical vibration chest physical therapy. This technique is currently being studied in one or more centers in Canada.

The manual techniques chosen may be those such as squeezing, shaking, bouncing, applying chest wall pressure on the contralateral side, and sternochondral mobilizations. Some of the manual techniques (squeezing, shaking) may have an effect on secretion mobilization from larger airways. Squeezing, shaking, or bouncing may alter chest wall mechanics and lead to better regional distribution of ventilation. All of the techniques should help to maintain chest wall flexibility, which decreases quickly with prolonged ventilation and decreased use of respiratory muscles.

If secretions are evident, these techniques are followed by manual hyperinflation (bagging) and suctioning. Physical therapy care also includes passive or active range of motion and progressive mobilization of the patient by sitting at the bedside (dangling) or by getting up to a chair. The *Importance of Mobility in Chest Care* discusses this subject in detail.

Assessment of results of treatment are based on changes in clinical assessment findings, such as auscultation findings and chest wall flexibility, and most accurately by improvement in chest x-ray examination findings and blood gas results.

In the long-term ventilated patient, in whom acute lung pathology is no longer a concern, physical therapy intervention may be required to assist with weaning from the ventilator. Inspiratory muscle training is one means of assisting with weaning and is described in *Inspiratory Muscle Training: An Adjunct to Weaning*.

The critical care patient who is intubated but breathing spontaneously or is on intermittent mandatory ventilation receives a treatment regime similar to that of the fully ventilated patient. Manual techniques are coordinated with respirations and consist of manual pressures, squeezing, shaking, bouncing, posterior lifts, and abdominal bouncing. These techniques also result in improvement in depth of breathing, particularly lateral costal or lower chest-diaphragmatic action, and also lead to a concurrent decreased rate of breathing. Increased depth improves ventilation and decreases the risk of development of atelectasis or secretion retention. Lower rate decreases work of breathing; this is a very important consideration in the impending respiratory failure or weaning patient.

The nonintubated patient is treated in a similar manner, but, in addition, is instructed in regular deep breathing and coughing, and in hourly use of the incentive spirometer (unless contraindicated by asthma, severe bullous emphysema, or neurologic status [e.g., subarachnoid hemorrhage]).

Treatment is usually provided once or twice daily, depending on the severity and the extent of lung pathology. Nursing personnel are instructed in the use of the mechanical vibrator once or twice in the evening, in follow through with deep breathing and coughing, and in hourly use of the incentive spirometer. If an acute lobar collapse occurs, treatment may be provided every 2 to 3 hours for the first few hours to facilitate rapid resolution. However, improved blood gases and obvious clearing on chest x-ray film are often found after only one treatment.

Special Considerations

In dealing with the critical care patient population, particular conditions and situations require extra caution and knowledge of potentially harmful results or side effects. The patient with ARDS has been mentioned earlier. Similar precautions are necessary with patients in whom pulmonary edema is the primary pulmonary pathology. In addition to the fact that physiotherapy has no positive effect on pulmonary edema there is a chance that it may in fact cause deterioration and further hypoxia. This is the case particularly in spontaneously breathing patients where deep breathing and incentive spirometry increases negative intra-alveolar pressure.

Patients with hemodynamic instability, reflected in low or labile blood pressure or low cardiac indices, require close monitoring. Position changes may lead to significant drops in blood pressure. Exertion, such as with active exercise or coughing, may also create serious alterations in blood pressure or cardiac output. Cardiac arrhythmias may also be exacerbated by position change, activity, or coughing.

The intra-aortic balloon pump is used for support of cardiac function in patients unable to maintain adequate cardiac output with inotropic support following cardiac surgery or myocardial infarction. The pump cycles from the output of surface electrocardiograph (ECG) leads, and therefore, is interfered with by the use of the mechanical vibrator. The interference picked up by the ECG causes the pump to fail to function at assist ratios of 1:1 and 1:2, thus contraindicating its use. Manual treatment techniques may also cause interference by disturbing the electrodes. These techniques are also often made difficult by numerous monitoring wires, chest tubes, and intravenous lines, in addition to dressings and the often accompanying delayed closure of the sternotomy.

Patients with severe gastrointestinal (GI) bleeding may be admitted to ICU for monitoring and fluid resuscitation. As well as problems with hemodynamic instability, the hemorrhage can be exacerbated by the use of the mechanical vibrator; in particular, upper GI bleeding worsens with mechanical vibrator treatment. Therefore, wait until there has been no evidence of fresh blood from the nasogastric tube for 36 hours before treatment. Esophageal varices seem to be especially susceptible to transmitted vibration, and patients with varices should not be treated using the mechanical vibrator.

Disseminated intravascular coagulopathy or other coagulopathies, which often occur in critically ill patients, lead to a risk of pulmonary bleeding. Use of the mechanical vibrator with these patients should be cautioned and should be discontinued if there are signs of hemoptysis greater than that attributable to airway trauma with suctioning.

Patients with elevated intracranial pressure (ICP) also require additional caution. The use of the mechanical vibrator and most manual techniques have not been observed to increase ICP, but it may be increased by position change or by coughing. If an ICP monitor is in place, levels should be closely watched to ensure that they return to acceptable levels following transient increases. If no monitor is in place, level of consciousness should be closely attended to during the treatment.

The treatment techniques discussed may occasionally be ineffective in patients with excessively tenacious secretions. In these patients, percussion and the use of modified postural drainage positions, if not contraindicated, may have to be added to the treatment protocol. Flexible fiberoptic bronchoscopy may be a last resort if physical therapy intervention is unsuccessful.

Physical therapy treatment of the critical care patient is essentially the same as with any other patient. Assessment has to be modified somewhat with the ventilated patient, and precautions have to be taken with certain patient types. The use of the mechanical vibrator and a variety of manual treatment techniques is an effective approach to mobilizing secretions and improving ventilation and chest wall flexibility in the critically ill patient.

SUGGESTED READING

Bethune DD. The neurophysiological facilitation of respiration in the unconscious adult. Physiother Can 1975; 27(5):241–245.

Holody B, Goldberg HS. The effect of mechanical vibration physiotherapy on arterial oxygenation in acutely ill patients with atelectasis or pneumonia. Am Rev Respir Dis 1981; 124:372–375.

Kolaczkowski WL. Chronic obstructive pulmonary disease: a practical review of treatment techniques. Physiother Can 1977; 29(4):198–202.

MacKenzie CF, ed. Chest Physiotherapy in the Intensive Care Unit. Baltimore: Williams & Wilkins, 1981.

Oh TE, ed. Intensive care manual. 2nd ed. Stoneham, MA: Butterworths, 1981.

PHYSICAL THERAPY IN CHRONIC AIRWAY LIMITATION

MAREL FIELDING, M.C.S.P.

Physical therapy can provide comfort and help for the patient afflicted with chronic airway limitation, whether this is a result of asthma, bronchitis, emphysema, or some of the less well known conditions, such as bronchiectasis, amotile cilia, sarcoidosis, or adult respiratory distress syndrome (ARDS).

It is important to reiterate the necessity for the physical therapist and the physician to work closely together. The physical therapist should be familiar with the drugs that the patient is taking. The effects and side effects of these drugs may affect the patient's ability to comply with physical therapy.

At University Hospital, London, Ontario, the largest portion of the physical therapist's caseload is the so-called "end stage" acute on chronic. Patients with already compromised lung function are admitted with an acute infection; these people often have blood gas analysis findings that the text books tell us are incompatible with life; however, with treatment many survive and are referred to physical therapy for assistance in clearing secretions and for rehabilitation.

For many years, physical therapy has been considered by some respirologists to be of little benefit in treating patients with chronic airways limitation, more specifically, in treating chronic bronchitis, emphysema, and asthma. This is possibly due to a misconception on the part of respirologists and physical therapists as to what physical therapy can be expected to accomplish. If realistic limitations and expectations are set, the contribution of physical therapy to the continuing care of patients with chronic airway limitation is valuable.

One must first accept that physical therapy cannot effect a cure any more than medicine can. As in all rehabilitation our contribution is to assist the patient in making the best possible use of whatever residual function he or she has.

An analogy can be drawn with the patient who is unable to walk because his leg is broken—he eventually returns to at least near normal—compared with the patient who cannot walk because he has neurologic damage to the muscles that control walking—

he will never walk normally, but he can be assisted to function either with braces or walking aids or with even a wheelchair. The same is true of the chest patient; an acute bout of bronchitis upsets the ability to breathe effectively, but, with correct treatment, breathing does return to normal. However, the patient with chronic bronchitis or emphysema will probably never have totally normal respiratory function, but can be assisted by a skilled cardiopulmonary physical therapist to live as fully as possible within the limitations of his handicap.

The expectations of all concerned must be realistic. My experience is mainly with the so-called acute on chronic (i.e., the patient who has end stage respiratory failure who is admitted to hospital with an acute exacerbation). Care for patients with chronic airway limitations can be divided into two main headings: chest care and mobility.

CHEST CARE

Chest care includes a thorough assessment of the breathing pattern. The physical therapist needs to look at all of the following aspects of breathing:

- Head and neck posture
- Posture of mouth (i.e., open or closed)
- Rate and rhythm of breathing
- Noisy or silent breathing
- Lips pursed or slack
- Shape and contours of the rib cage
- Flexibility of the rib cage
- Movement of the ribs and abdominal wall with each breath
- Skin colour—lips, face, body, nails
- Dryness of skin
- Finger clubbing
- Ability to cough to clear secretions
- Texture, amount and color of expectorant.

Pulmonary function test results, blood gas analysis and radiologic examinations may be reviewed, but it is my experience that they do not alter significantly with physical therapy.

Once a thorough evaluation has been completed, the physical therapist should decide which abnormalities detected are contributing to respiratory distress and which are most likely to respond to physical therapy intervention.

Chest Wall Stiffness

If the patient has a rigid chest wall, the need for weakened muscles to fight against it can be reduced by mobilizing the costochondral and costovertebral joints. Mobilization can be accomplished by manual therapy techniques and also by some trunk rotation. This is effective with the patient in sidelying, one of the therapist's hands fixing the pelvis, and the patient assisted to roll the upper part of his trunk forwards and backwards—breathing can be incorporated with this activity: the patient is instructed to breathe in as he is rolled backwards and to breathe out as he is rolled forwards. Shoulder and scapular mobilizing is also useful. Mobilizing can also be done by placing the hands over the lateral aspects of the lower ribs and squeezing and or shaking with the expiratory phase of breathing.

Difficulties Related to Secretions

If the patient is having difficulty coughing to clear secretions then it is useful to coordinate treatment with respiratory therapy so that mechanical vibration or other manual techniques can be given while the patient is receiving bronchodilator drugs by inhalation.

Immediately following the drug therapy, the patient is encouraged to cough. As the patient coughs, firm support to the rib cage or the abdominal wall or both often enables the patient to generate enough force to expectorate. This technique is most effective with the patient sitting on the side of the bed with arms resting on a bedside tray-table.

Coughing often leaves the patient short of breath. Some manual pressure to the rib cage, mechanical vibration or massage to the chest wall facilitates the return of normal respiratory rate and rhythm.

Breathing Pattern

Attempts to alter breathing patterns by asking the patient to perform specific breathing exercises has been found to be ineffective. However, sometimes a more normal breathing pattern can be facilitated by altering head and neck posture. This is done by placing a soft ball or equivalent behind the patient's back at the level of the scapula as he or she sits in a straight chair (Fig. 1). The mechanism for this is not clear but the patient is observed to reduce cervical lordosis, close the mouth, lower the elevation of the shoulders and breathe at a slower deeper rate with the reintroduction of the occasional deep breath or sigh.

A more normal breathing pattern can also be accomplished by suggesting that, while sitting relaxed, the patient make a conscientious effort to keep the tongue in the roof of the mouth. Some patients do this well, thereby resulting in a return to breathing with a closed mouth; however, for others it is ineffective as it adds to their respiratory distress.

Pursed Lip Breathing

Some patients suffering from a chronic chest condition develop a pattern of breathing described as

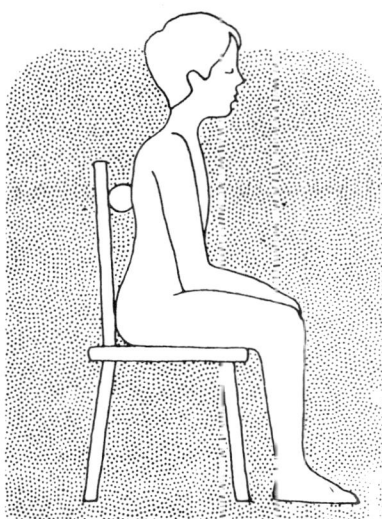

Figure 1 Posterior cocontractions using a ball.

pursed-lip breathing. These are usually the so-called "pink puffers" i.e., those patients who attempt to maintain normal blood gas levels by expiring carbon dioxide by whatever means they can. For some patients, pursing lips during expiratory phase of breathing prevents premature airway collapse and allows a greater volume of air to be expelled. Most patients who benefit from this method of breathing develop it on their own. However, it is worthwhile attempting to teach it to the patient who is retaining carbon dioxide, but if not successful after two or three times it is unlikely that pursed-lip breathing will be a useful technique for that particular patient.

Head Down Position

For many years physical therapists have used the head down position to drain secretions posturally from the chest. Even with patients who can tolerate the position, I have not found that postural drainage is my treatment of choice in aiding expectoration. However, I have found some interesting effects of the head down position, which may contribute to some of the benefits attributed to this technique.

Patients with a markedly increased respiratory rate, for example 40 breaths per minute (bpm) will reduce their rate to a near normal rate when tilted head down approximately 10 to 16 degrees. Other effects also have been observed including the following:

- A "pinking" up of bluish tinged lips and face
- An increase in the blood oxygen saturation as measured by ear oxymetry
- A general relaxation of neck and shoulder muscles

- An apparent increase in the depth of respiration determined by observing the chest wall movement.

Many suggestions have been made regarding these changes. Of further interest is the fact that once the patient is returned to the normal upright position, all the changes revert to their previous level (i.e., respiratory rate immediately increases, but not to pretreatment level; however, it will return to the pretreatment level in a very short time).

Breathlessness Positions

Patients usually assume the position in which they can breathe best. There may be some variations that they have not discovered that the physical therapist can suggest.

For extreme shortness of breath, sitting upright with hands on knees, elbows extended and shoulders pushed upwards is the most common position chosen by the patient. Do not try to alter this immediately. Once some chest care has been tried, i.e., manual pressure or mechanical vibration, the patient may be able to move to a more relaxed position.

Positions that will ease breathlessness are as follows:

1. Sitting on side of bed with feet resting on a stool. Place the bed table (or similar) in front of patient with a pillow on the table. The patient can rest his arms over the pillow;
2. As 1, but put two or three pillows on the table so that the patient can rest his head on them;
3. Sitting in a high-backed chair or rocking chair with pillows behind the patient's back to maintain an erect trunk;
4. Sitting astride a chair, facing the back of the chair. A pillow over the back of the chair provides a cushion for the patient to rest his head;
5. Leaning against a wall, knees slightly bent, hands resting on knees;
6. Sitting crosslegged on a bed or on the floor.

NOTE: 4 and 5 are not possible for most elderly patients who do not have enough range of motion in their hip and knee joints.

MOBILITY

The degree to which assistance with mobility is required varies greatly depending on severity of chest disease and extent of previous exercise. I use two approaches.

Isotonic Exercise

The first approach consists of some generalized low intensity isotonic exercises for the lower extremities, such things as hip and knee flexion, knee extension over a quads roll, and foot and ankle exercises. Emphasize the need to avoid straining and breath holding. The prescription is little and often. Repeating each exercise four to six times five or six times a day has a better effect than 20 to 30 repetitions once a day. The patient is much more likely, and probably more able, to comply with the "little and often" regime.

Ambulation

The second approach is an assessment of the patient's ability to ambulate and the development of a program to increase this ability. This development can range from simple movement from bed to chair, to walking to the bathroom, to walking in the halls, and eventually to walking increasing distances outside. Many patients are unable to progress to any distance; others require supplemental oxygen when moving about. I encourage walking since the patient perceives this as a useful activity.

The patient is told to set his or her own pace, going slower rather than faster than able, to try to keep shoulders and trunk relaxed, to rest as often as needed, and especially to avoid breath holding. I also encourage daily exercise. In winter when the temperature drops below 0° C, the patient is told to walk indoors—up and down a hallway—or, if able, to drive to a shopping mall and to walk there.

The physical therapist's role in the care of the patient with airway limitation can be very effective in assisting the patient to cope with the disease. As with all physical therapy intervention, a thorough assessment and analysis of the problems the patient is encountering is the key to success. Also there is a need to develop some understanding of the best method of approach. It is difficult for the patient to be sociable and to respond to questions in other than monosyllables when short of breath. Talk slowly, ask questions that do not require too many words to answer, do not make demands of the patient, but be reassuring, and have a calm and relaxed approach, thus, the patient is more likely to benefit from intervention.

TECHNIQUES FOR PULMONARY PHYSICAL THERAPY

MAREL FIELDING, M.C.S.P.

The following chart has been developed as a result of 8 years of working with patients who have disorders of the cardiopulmonary system. Some of the techniques have been learned from other physical therapists working with chest patients. In many cases, they have been adapted or modified, and those included are described as they are used on the medical surgical unit at University Hospital, London, Ontario.

Many of the techniques have similar expected outcomes. We have found the variety of techniques useful as they give the physical therapist a greater degree of flexibility in selecting the techniques that will achieve the desired results.

The benefits of having various techniques at the disposal of the physical therapist include the following: being able to take into account each patient's response to treatment; being able to progress, as some techniques are more vigorous than others; being able to relieve boredom of a patient who requires chest care for many days or even weeks. Compliance can often be enhanced by introducing a new technique.

TABLE 1 Techniques Used by a Physical Therapist for Pulmonary Care

Technique	Indications	Contraindications or Restrictions	Precautions	Expected Results	Methods
Manual pressure type 1	Decreased chest wall motion Decreased flexibility Shallow breathing pattern Tension/panic Pathology of underlying lung tissue	Heavy bandages	Chest tubes Rib fractures	Relaxation Deeper, slower breathing pattern	Patient positioned comfortably (supine, sidelying, sitting). Place hand over appropriate area of lower or upper rib cage. Firm contact with mild pressure to the area is applied. Hold for however long it takes to achieve results—usually 30 sec to 2 min.
Manual pressure type 2	Tension/panic Excessive use of upper chest Shallow rapid breathing pattern	Fractured clavicle	Swan Ganz or central venous pressure lines Rib fractures	Relaxation Deeper, slower breathing pattern with abdominal swelling on inspiration	Place hands over upper part of chest anteriorly and apply mild/moderate pressure. Hold for 30 to 60 sec.
Squeezing	Shallow breathing Tension Chest wall stiffness Secretions	Unstable sternum postoperatively	Rib fractures Thoracic incisions	Relaxation Deeper breathing Increase chest wall movement or flexibility Mobilize secretions	Patient positioned comfortably. Place hands over area of chest wall. lateral costal upper chest Increasing amounts of pressure are applied over ribs during expiration in a medial-caudal direction.
Shaking/vibrations	Tension Secretions Decreased breath sounds	Flail chest	Extreme shortness of breath Pain Osteoporosis	Relaxation Mobilize secretions Metastatic lesions in rib cage Increased air entry	Position hands as for "squeezing." Shake chest as patient breathes out. The number of shakes and the vigor used are dependent on length of the expiratory phase, degree of rigidity or fragility of the chest wall, as well as individual tolerance of treatment.
Post lifts	Shallow breathing Poor bed mobility; posture		Fractured vertebrae	Increased air entry to post basal section Improved posture	Patient in supine lying. Place hands under patient's lower chest wall (posteriorly). As the patient inspires, lift up the lower ribs

Springing	Decreased breath sounds, Splinting	Patient unable or unwilling to cooperate	Fractured ribs, Thoracic incisions, Poor cooperation	Increased breath sounds; Reexpansion of collapsed areas, Increased excursion of chest cough, Mobilize secretion	Patient in supine lying. Position hands as for manual pressures. As the patient inspires, resist the movement of the rib cage. When you feel the patient is pushing into your hands, release the resistance suddenly. NB Most effective the first time. Rib springing can also be done at the end of expiration
Rotation	Stiffness of trunk—post surgical, chronic chest	Fractured ribs, Fractured vertebrae, Delayed closure abdominal wound	Fractured vertebrae	Increased chest and trunk mobility, Deeper breaths	Patient in side lying. Place one hand on patient's iliac crest, the other hand on patient's shoulder. As the patient breathes in, rotate trunk backwards by pulling on upper trunk, hold hips still. Rotate forwards with expiration.
Bouncing	Shallow breathing pattern	Fractured vertebrae, Obese chest	Chest tubes, Incisions, Fractured ribs	Deeper breathing	Hold hand with fingers extended over area of chest to be treated and bounce lightly on and off the chest wall. (A similar action to bouncing a ball)
Clapping	Secretions, Consolidation/atelectasis	Intolerance	Fractured ribs or Fractured vertebrae, Incision-thorax	Mobilize secretions	Use one cupped hand to lightly percuss the chest wall corresponding to the area of underlying lung pathology.
Incentive spirometry	Atelectasis, Decreased breath sounds, Decreased inspiratory effort	Emphysema, Congestive heart failure (especially left ventricular failure), Pulmonary edema		Reexpand atelectasis, Increased breath sounds	Set spirometer at estimated level for patient. Instruct patient to place mouth piece between lips making a tight seal. Inhale quickly to raise ball to the top. Adjust setting to maximum level for the patient. Instruct the patient to repeat 10 times per hour while awake.

TABLE 1 (Continued)

Technique	Indications	Contraindications or Restrictions	Precautions	Expected Results	Methods
Mechanical vibration	Shallow breathing pattern Tension Retained secretions Atelectasis	Recent gastrointestinal Bleed patient on intra-aortic balloon pump at 1:1 or 1:2 ratio Recent esophagectomy Thoracic aortic aneurysms and repairs of same		Relaxation Deeper, slower breathing pattern Expectoration of secretions	Apply mechanical vibrator to chest wall using firm pressure, maintain for 30-60 seconds and then move to adjacent spot. Gradually move vibrator over area of chest to be treated—total treatment time between 15-60 min. Treatment area of chest wall corresponds to area of affected lung.
Breathing exercises	Shallow breathing, no incentive spirometer available or patient unable to use	Patient unwilling or unable to cooperate		Temporary deep breaths	Ask patient to take slow relaxed breaths, breathing in through the nose and out through the mouth. May add a 3 sec breath hold at full inspiration before expiration.
Positioning	Post surgical	Delayed closure abdominal/hip surgery	Drainage tubes, intravenous lines	Increased breath sounds Increased cough Decreased incidence of deep vein thrombosis Clearing secretions Increased bed mobility	Method is dependent on condition. Postoperatively, have patient lying on alternate sides and supine for 2 hr each. With atelectasis, have patient lie with affected side up.
Positioning shortness of breath positions	Respiratory distress as with chronic airway limitation or congestive heart failure	Compliance of patient	Fractures	Relaxation Improved breathing pattern	Method is dependent on (patient's) condition and preference, e.g., In congestive heart failure (corpulmonale) sit high in bed or raise head of bed to comfortable level. In chronic airway limitation sit on side of bed with arms resting on bed table. Sit astride a chair facing back with arms resting on back of chair (pillow may also be used to rest head on).

Technique	Indications	Contraindications	Precautions	Objectives	Technique
(continued from previous page)					Stand leaning back against wall, rest hands on knees.
Splinted/ assisted coughing	Decreased cough Increased pain Retained secretions		Drainage tubes Intravenous lines	More effective productive cough	Postoperative Place hand over incision site with/without a blanket to support incision as patient coughs. Medical chest Support abdomen, lower rib cage, or sternum with hands to assist cough. Spinal cord injury Use an abdominal thrust to assist cough.
Cocontractions Abdominal	Poor abdominal tone Tension/panic Lack of/poor cooperation Shallow breathing	Young children Abdominal distension	Abdominal distension Moribund patient	Relaxation Deeper breathing Increased abdominal tone	Patient in supine Place one hand over lateral aspect of lower rib cage and one on pelvis—apply light pressure until response occurs
Posterior	Shallow breathing Excessive use of accessory muscles Poor posture			Improved breathing pattern Increased extensor tone Relaxation of accessory muscles	Patient sitting over side of bed Place one hand over thoracic spine between scapula, apply pressure. May also be done with patient in side lying or supine.
Perioral stimulation	Shallow breathing pattern Tension Decreased level of consciousness or unconscious patient Decreased ability to swallow		Tubes in mouth or nose	Mouth closure, swallowing, or sucking Occasional deep breath or sighs Relaxation	Place index finger on patient's top lip and apply light pressure.
Massage	Tension—physical and mental		Intolerance Bandages Incisions Fractures	Relaxation Deeper breathing pattern	Do effleurage and gentle kneading over lower rib cage, back pectorals, and trapezius
Postural drainage	Copious secretions (i.e., bronchiectasis)	Intolerance Nasogastric tube Brain surgery Congestive heart failure		Increased clearing of secretions	Position patient so that gravity can assist with drainage of secretions from bronchi.

TABLE 1 (Continued)

Technique	Indications	Contraindications or Restrictions	Precautions	Expected Results	Methods
Relaxation	Tension Chronic asthma			Deeper breathing pattern	Use any familiar relaxation technique, e.g., contract/relax muscle groups where tension is detected.
Increase exercise tolerance	Decreased exercise tolerance Debility and shortness of breath with activity	Cardiac conditions Too short of breath Condition too unstable	Monitor shortness of breath	Increased ability to perform activities of daily living	Design program appropriate to condition. Isotonic exercises for lower extremities. Walking program.
Ambulation	Shallow breath with no acute pathology Residual atelectasis Also used as test with chronic obstructive lung disease	Joint or orthopaedic problems	Muscle weakness	Maintain/improve chest status and circulation	Post cardiovascular surgery Monitor pulse before and after walking Postoperative or illness Monitor general status of patient Chronic obstructive lung disease 12-min walk test Patient walks at own speed with as many rests as wishes for 12 minutes—measure distance walked.

CONVENTIONAL CHEST CARE TECHNIQUES: BREATHING EXERCISES, POSTURAL DRAINAGE, PERCUSSION, AND SPIROMETRY

MAREL FIELDING, M.C.S.P.

In other chapters of this book, many different techniques for treating the problems detected in evaluations of pulmonary problems have been described. What are often referred to as the more conventional or traditional techniques are also employed in patient care.

Breathing Exercises

For many many years, physical therapists have instructed patients in breathing exercise. Sometimes belts, towels, or weights have been employed with claims that these aid lateral costal expansion or diaphragmatic breathing.

Breathing involves movement of many joints, and contraction and relaxation of many muscles. It is a complex movement that happens most of the time without conscious thought.

Asking the patient to control his or her breathing can be useful in certain situations. The patient is instructed to breathe slowly in through the nose and out through the mouth letting him breathe at his own rate and rhythm to begin with. Then, depending on the desired effect, various maneuvers can be added.

For the tense patient, slow relaxed breathing is used. Instruct the patient to "breathe in slowly, pause, now breathe out." This has a calming effect and gives the physical therapist an opportunity to observe color and posture of the patient. Once the patient is relaxed then the physical therapist places his or her hands on the rib cage. As the patient breathes in and out, evaluate the flexibility of the rib cage and chest movement at each phase of respiration. Avoid expressions such as take a deep breath, or a big breath, but rather suggest that he breathe slowly, at his own pace in through the nose and relax and let the breath out easily through the mouth.

If breathing is shallow, some manual pressure can be introduced to try to encourage a deeper breath.

Asking the postoperative patient to hold full inspiration for a second or two also helps to produce a deeper, more relaxed breathing pattern.

The emphasis is on breathing as a single activity with no particular emphasis on any one area of the chest. Patients tend to revert to their usual pattern of breathing as soon as they cease to think about their breathing.

A variation in breathing, where the patient is instructed to expel the air forcibly, either in a single burst or in several short bursts, has been found to be useful in aiding expectoration. The patient is asked to breathe in the normal way and then to breathe out in short, sharp bursts—often described as "huffing" as the patient makes an "h" sound in his throat.

Postural Drainage

In earlier years, postural drainage—especially when accompanied by percussion—was one of the mainstays of physical therapy for the chest patient. At University Hospital, London, Ontario, many of the patients that are referred for treatment are not able to tolerate this treatment. Alternative techniques were developed and good results were achieved. Therefore, it seemed reasonable to use these alternate techniques with all patients. Many studies have been done and many reports written that prove the effectiveness of postural drainage and just as many that point out the hazards with or without percussion. This makes it difficult to draw a conclusion based on the results reported in the literature.

At University Hospital we have found postural drainage to be of limited use as a technique; however, positioning is used with good results. If there is a problem in the right lung, having the patient lie on his or her left side facilitates treatment, and the combination of turning to alternate sides has produced positive results.

Percussion

For the majority of patients, regular two-handed percussion tends not to be the treatment of choice. Patients become tense and either hold their breath or breathe very shallowly. Since breath holding and shallow breathing do not facilitate the expulsion of excess secretions, alternative techniques need to be sought. (NB there are some patients with chronic chest conditions who have accommodated to percussion and are able to relax and breathe normally during percussion. For these patients the technique is helpful)

There are two variations of percussion that we find useful.

Type 1 Percussion at full inspiration

This is done by asking the patient to take a breath in and to hold the breath; by percussing the chest wall with one hand for one or two strokes; and by instructing the patient to breathe out. The patient will sharply inhale or gasp, thereby producing a cough that causes expectoration of mucus. Adding some shaking or vibration of the chest wall during the expiratory phase of breathing also assists in removal of secretions.

Type 2 Single-handed percussion

This is done by lightly percussing the chest wall with one hand for 3 to 5 minutes. Observed effects include increased breath sounds on auscultation and productive cough. This method of percussion does not produce the tension and breath holding that the more vigorous two-handed percussion produces.

Spirometry

Several years ago, incentive spirometery was introduced as an adjunct to postoperative physical therapy. When deciding which patients might benefit from using a spirometer, the physical therapist should take into consideration general medical condition, and ability and willingness to use the device.

The spirometer in use at University Hospital has a single ball and the readings on the variable resistance vary from 145 cc to 1,800 cc.

The patient is instructed to place the mouthpiece in his mouth and to make a tight seal with his lips. He then inhales and attempts to raise the ball to the top of the tube. The physical therapist assesses the appropriate level of resistance. The patient is then instructed to use the incentive spirometer once per hour while awake; attempting to raise the ball 6 to 10 times.

The advantages this device provides include a concrete reminder for the patient to do his breathing exercises; a goal (incentive) to reach in attempting to raise the ball and/or increase the resistance; an increased compliance with breathing-exercise routines; and a reduction in "splinting" of the chest movement as the patient concentrates on raising the ball.

Patients with a tracheostomy have successfully used an incentive spirometer with an adaptation to the mouthpiece.

Disadvantages associated with the device are that some patients are unable to maintain a seal over the mouthpiece and experience increased anxiety when attempting to do it; some patients are able to inspire greater volumes than the device is set for; and a few patients have stated annoyance at being asked to use what they see as a "toy."

CHEST PHYSICAL THERAPY AND THE NEUROLOGIC PATIENT

HELEN A. JOHNSON, B.Sc. (PT)

Chest care is an integral part of the physical therapy management of many neurologic and neurosurgical patients. Diseases of the central and peripheral nervous systems can alter the respiratory system in a multitude of ways and can provide many challenges to understanding the condition.

NEURAL CONTROL OF BREATHING

Control of breathing is known to comprise a combination of neural and humeral factors and is still not fully understood. The intricacies of pathways and receptors involved is beyond the scope of this book; however, Table 1 provides a simplified illustration of the levels of neural control of respiration and the most common diseases that can alter these mechanisms.

Voluntary control of breathing occurs via the cerebral cortex and the corticospinal tracts. Voluntary control includes the ability to hold a breath, to hyperventilate voluntarily, and to perform the integrated responses involved in speaking or singing. Patients with significant cortical damage may exhibit Cheyne-Stokes respirations or monotonous shallow breathing that quickly results in atelectasis. Some patients are disoriented or confused and unable to cooperate with instructions.

The centers responsible for generation and maintenance of rhythmic respiration are located in the pons and the medulla. Lesions in various areas of the brain stem may result in hyperventilation or irregular and ataxic patterns of breathing, which can result in the complications of atelectasis and pneumonia.

The cranial nerves and spinal motor neurons are the next level of integration in the neural control of breathing. Patients with lesions affecting these areas present with difficulties in swallowing and coughing and consequently, in protecting the airway. Other phenomena include Ondine's curse and hypo- or hypertonia of the respiratory muscles or pharynx. Significant chest pathology, such as atelectasis and pneumonia, can develop due to airway obstruction, aspiration, and secretion retention.

The final pathways in the control of breathing consist of the peripheral nerves to the muscles of respiration. Afferent input from the lungs and from various receptors provides feedback to all the previously described levels. Diseases in the peripheral nervous system can result in paresis or paralysis of the intercostals, accessory muscles, and diaphragm. Thus, the patient's ability to move air in and out of the lungs, and to cough is directly impaired, thereby risking atelectasis and pneumonia.

CHEST CARE

The most vital part of physical therapy management is the continuous assessment of the patient as a whole. In neurologic patients, the chest assessment begins as with other chest problems (see chapter on *Assessment: The Basis of Chest Physical Therapy*). In addition, note should be made of level of consciousness, orientation, and ability to follow commands. Presence of neurologic deficits affecting sensory and motor function should be documented, and usually treatment for these is ongoing. This includes oral motor function and ability to protect the airway. Some signs of difficulty in this area are drooping of the mouth, deviation of the tongue, drooling, pocketing of food, diminished gag and cough, dysarthria and harsh vocal quality. Other motor deficits or restrictions on activity may affect ability to move within, and out of bed, thus increasing the risk of chest complications.

In conjunction with laboratory and radiological data, the assessment allows the therapist to form a physical diagnosis of present chest status and concurrent risk factors. Management can then focus on treatment and prevention.

Patients with significant cortical or brain stem damage may require measures to improve the depth and pattern of respiration. Neurophysiologic facilitation techniques, such as perioral stimulation, abdominal cocontractions, manual pressures, posterior lifts and intercostal stretches, can be particularly effective especially in patients with diminished level of consciousness and inability to cooperate with treatment. Altered patterns of breathing (Fig. 1) caused by brain damage, such as Cheyne-Stokes respirations (series of waxing and waning breaths interspersed with periods of apnea) or Biot's respirations (periodic breathing with breaths of varying depths with unequal pauses in between), remain unaffected by any type of physical therapy intervention. With Ondine's curse, where automatic control of breathing is impaired with normal voluntary control, a diaphragmatic pacer may be used,

TABLE 1   Consequences of Altered Neural Control of Breathing

Conditions	Problems	Chest Complications

Cerebrum
  Head injury
  Stroke
  Encephalitis
  Meningitis
  Subdural hemorrhage
  Subarachnoid hemorrhage
  Tumor
  Multiple sclerosis
	Decreased level of
	  consciousness
	Cheyne-Stokes respirations
	Lack of sigh if ventilated
		Atelectasis—pneumonia
		Aspiration pneumonia

Brain stem
  Stroke
    pontine lesion
    basilar artery occlusion
  Tumor
  Multiple sclerosis
  Subarachnoid hemorrhage
	Apneustic breathing
	Central neurogenic
	  hyperventilation
	
	Ataxic breathing
	Biot's respirations
		Atelectasis—pneumonia

Spinal motor neurons cranial nerves
  Polio
  Multiple sclerosis
  Amyotrophic lateral sclerosis
  Spinal cord lesions
	Swallowing difficulties
	Poor cough
	Altered tone of pharynx
	Altered tone of respiratory
	  muscles
	Ondine's curse
		Aspiration pneumonia
		Secretion retention—pneumonia
		Poor oral muscle tone—airway
		  obstruction
		Atelectasis
		Spastic diaphragm
		Sleep apnea

Peripheral nerves muscles of
  respiration
  Guillain Barré
  Amyotrophic lateral sclerosis
  Multiple sclerosis
  Spinal cord lesion
	Decreased muscle strength
	Poor cough
		Reduced movement of air in and out
		Atelectasis—pneumonia

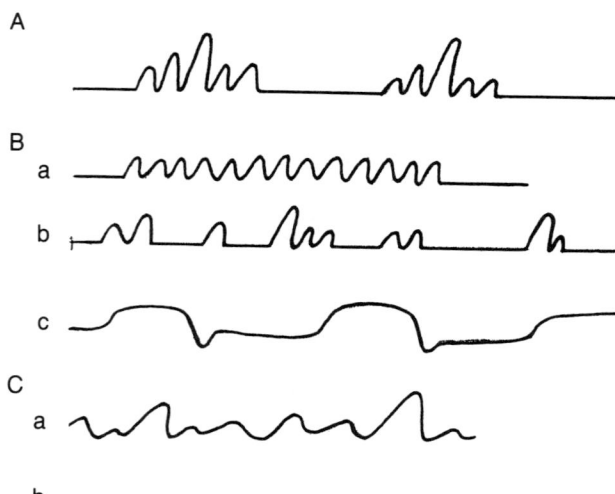

Figure 1   Altered respiratory patterns. *A*, Cerebrum: Cheyne-Stokes respiration. *B*, Midbrain-pons: (a) central neurogenic hyperventilation; (b) Biot's respirations; (c) apneustic respirations. *C*, Medulla: (a) ataxic respiration; (b) apnea.

and a tracheostomy is sometimes performed to reduce the amount of resistance to breathing as much as possible.

Other important physical therapy measures include regular change of position in bed (incorporating side lying and prone lying as appropriate); manual techniques, such as massage, squeezing, bouncing, and shaking (see chapter on *Techniques for Pulmonary Physical Therapy*) to maintain chest wall mobility and to assist in mobilization of secretions; mechanical vibration, and suctioning.

In patients with cranial nerve involvement affecting oral motor function and airway protection, physical therapy management should include assessment of the ability to swallow, in conjunction with speech and occupational therapy if possible. At University Hospital, in London, Ontario, a "swallowing team" consisting of a speech therapist, an occupational therapist, a physical therapist and a radiologist may be consulted to assess swallowing and to assist the medical team in choosing the most appropriate form of feeding and care. After preliminary assessments, including a complete oral-motor evaluation by the speech therapist, a modified barium swallow study may be undertaken. This procedure entails various consistencies of barium-laced foods and fluoroscopic analysis of the patient during swallowing. After the study, specific recommendations can be made as to which consistencies of food are dangerous for the patient and might lead to aspiration. In addition, corrective procedures or devices can be recommended, such as cricopharyngeal myotomy or palatal lift. Intervention required for aspiring patients may include positioning, manual techniques and mechanical vibration to mobilize secretions, assisted coughing, and suction. Patient and family education regarding steps to take in case of choking may be indicated where swallowing is of continued concern. Home suction units may be required to assist with clearance of secretions, and home care physical therapists can instruct patient and family in their use. Instruction in deep breathing and incentive spirometry is used when appropriate to prevent atelectasis.

Patients with poor mouth closure have difficulty with techniques such as incentive spirometry and pulmonary function testing because of inability to produce enough resistance with the mouth. Low oral motor tone can also lead to difficulties with airway obstruction, particularly during sleep. Devices such as palatal lifts can be beneficial in some cases.

Lesions in spinal motor neurons can also be associated with altered tone of the respiratory muscles, particularly the diaphragm. Movement of the diaphragm can be demonstrated by lateral chest x-ray examinations, Respitrace recordings, and fluoroscopy to differentiate between spastic and paralyzed diaphragms. With a spastic diaphragm, the patient has little control for deep breaths, but may trigger enough contractions to maintain adequate minute volumes. A paralytic diaphragm is often the more serious condition, as the patient may not produce enough force to maintain adequate respiration, especially if accompanied by intercostal respiratory muscle weakness as in amyotrophic lateral sclerosis (ALS).

Patients with peripheral lesions affecting the muscles of respiration have difficulties with coughing, and with moving air in and out of the lungs. In some patients, the strength of the respiratory muscles can be improved through inspiratory muscle training. Resistive inspiratory muscle trainers may also be useful in the maintenance of respiratory muscle strength in ALS, if begun prior to its deterioration; however, to date there is little documentation to support this. Other deep breathing techniques, such as incentive spirometry, can also be effective in decreasing atelectasis. Manual techniques, including squeezing, posterior lifts, and stretching, are important in the maintenance of chest wall mobility, especially in patients in whom muscle strength is expected to recover (e.g., Guillain-Barré syndrome). Positioning (including prone, sidelying, and head down positions), manual support, and use of suction to assist coughing may be required. If indicated, many of these techniques can be taught to family when the patient is returning home.

PRECAUTIONS SPECIFIC TO THE NEUROSURGICAL PATIENT

Subarachoid Hemorrhage (SAH)

Many patients suffering from subarachnoid hemorrhage have a cerebral aneurysm or arteriovenous malformation (AVM) that has ruptured. Usually the patient is placed on SAH routine, which involves measures to keep stimulation and, consequently, changes in blood pressure to a minimum, in order to reduce chances of rebleeding. The routine, developed at University Hospital in London, Ontario, involves placing the patient on strict bed rest in a darkened room, with limited noise and visitors. Assistance is provided for all activities, including turning and eating. Physical therapy is usually only consulted in cases of acute chest pathology which may delay surgery to clip the aneurysm. Gentle manual techniques (such as manual pressures, squeezing, bouncing) and mechanical vibration can be used. Observation of monitored patients has shown that these modalities do not cause increases in either blood pressure or intracranial pressure. However, incentive spirometry and forced coughing are avoided as these are thought to cause sharp increases in blood pressure and, consequently, in intracranial pressure. Suctioning is used only when absolutely necessary, and only after consultation with the physician. Once the patient has undergone successful clipping or resection of the aneurysm or AVM, any indicated chest care techniques can be used.

Increased Intracranial Pressure

Intracranial pressure can be elevated in patients with head trauma, tumors, hydrocephalus, and neurosurgical postoperative complications involving altered vascular pressures from vasospasm or SAH. If the pressure increase is severe enough, an intracranial pressure monitor is inserted to measure the actual pressure, in addition to allowing drainage of cerebrospinal fluid as required to relieve pressure. Normal intracranial pressure ranges from 5–15 mm Hg. Prolonged increases in intracranial pressure can be detrimental to the brain because of decreased cerebral perfusion. Thus, in management of these patients, physical therapists should be aware of techniques and situations which can increase blood pressure and intracranial pressure, including Valsalva's maneuver, coughing, and suctioning.

Chest care in neurologic and neurosurgical patients can be challenging and intriguing. Neural control of breathing can become impaired at many different levels, with varying consequences. In some cases, physical therapy intervention can directly alter these changes, whereas in others, treatment must be directed only at minimizing further potential complications. Many patients go home with a permanent deficit, and others with a continuously deteriorating status, which requires ingenuity and much family education and support; in many others, respiratory care is only part of the acute, early management, but of vital importance to the long-term prognosis. Understanding the intricacies of neural control of respiration in the context of each patient's condition allows the physical therapist to treat the patient with efficiency, effectiveness, and confidence.

SUGGESTED READING

Bethune DD. Neurological facilitation of respiration in the unconscious adult patient. Physiother Can 1975; 241–245.

Smith AR. Neurology and neurosurgery. In: Frownfelter DL, ed. Chest physical therapy and pulmonary rehabilitation. Chicago: Year Book, 1979:265.

Netter FH. Control and disorders of respiration in the CIBA collection of medical illustrations, Volume 7—The respiratory system. Summit, NJ: CIBA, 1979.

Guymer, AJ. Handling the patient with speech and swallowing problems. Physiother 1986; 72:276–280.

PULMONARY PHYSICAL THERAPY: A TREATMENT APPROACH

DIANA HOLMES HOPKINS-ROSSEEL, B.Sc. (PT)

Clinical practice of chest physical therapy (CPT) requires much more than appreciation of technical skills. Both in the literature and in the clinic, CPT is overwhelmingly described as treatment of respiratory disorders through use of deep breathing, coughing, postural drainage, percussion, and vibration. I feel that this grossly inaccurate myth must be dispelled.

The collective goal of the health care team is to help the patient attain the best possible state of health; this ranges from the complete recovery of patients with acute illnesses to an improved quality of life for patients with chronic disease. The goal of the chest physical therapist is the treatment *and* the prevention of respiratory disorders; specifically, atelectasis, pneumonia, and chronic obstructive pulmonary disease (COPD). Our treatments are designed to (1) maintain or improve the patient's ventilation, (2) maximize secretion clearance, (3) maximize exercise tolerance, and (4) improve patient mobility. If any one of these aims is neglected or ignored the patient's respiratory function can deteriorate. Therefore, CPT requires a holistic, comprehensive, and integrated approach to each individual patient. This chapter will outline the method by which these goals can be achieved.

PATIENT SELECTION

In an acute-care setting there are three patient groups that benefit significantly from CPT: surgical patients, medical patients, and patients with traumatic injuries.

Because of time limitations and financial constraints, only those patients, within the surgical group, who are at high risk of developing respiratory complications postoperatively are treated. Predisposing factors for developing respiratory complications are underlying chronic obstructive disease, obesity, cigarette smoking, advanced age (over 65 years), prolonged ventilation, tracheostomy and abnormal pulmonary function test results. Yet absence of these factors does not preclude development of respiratory difficulties. Other factors to consider are the location of the surgical incision since risk is greater in thoracic surgery than in lower abdominal surgery and is higher still in upper abdominal surgery; the neurologic and emotional status of the patient; and the nature of the surgery. Extensive procedure requires prolonged use of general anesthetics and results in greater postoperative pain. Pain can lead to ineffective breathing patterns and poorer ventilation, as can anxiety or any neurological impairment effecting the respiratory center of the brain or the motor function of the respiratory muscles.

The most significant group of medical patients requiring treatment is the one with COPD. Patients from this group not only exhibit increased mucous production and/or broncho-constriction and the tendency to develop chest wall rigidity, but also develop poor coping mechanisms.

Other potential CPT candidates are those individuals who have suffered traumatic injuries directly to the lungs (puncture or contusion) or the thorax (especially rib fractures). In addition, any injury causing neurologic damage, severe pain, or anxiety can affect respiratory function. There are also those patients whose injury or disease process involves an actual physical abnormality that limits respiratory function—for instance, a patient with a distended abdomen or a severe kyphoscoliosis.

Two questions arise when discussing patient selection. First, should palliative care patients be treated? This must be considered on an individual basis and is at the therapist's discretion. The question might better be rephrased: will the CPT treatment cause discomfort (very often it does not) and if so, do the benefits of treatment outweigh the discomfort? Certainly if the treatment results in the patient being able to breathe, talk, eat, and perform self care more easily then it may be justified. Second, should treatment be avoided with patients who are in acute distress? Aggressive manual maneuvers may not be indicated, but often other treatment techniques (to be discussed later) can improve ventilation in respiratory distress or prevent secondary respiratory deficits following other system involvement.

ASSESSMENT

The lungs do not function in isolation. The therapist must always be aware of other organ systems, the circulatory system, musculoskeletal function, and mental and emotional status. In addition, the therapist must understand how these other physical and psychological deficits might potentially affect respiratory function.

History

Before performing the actual clinical assessment the therapist attempts to determine not only respiratory and functional status prior to hospital admission, but also any past medical history of pulmonary disorders. Table 1 demonstrates an outline for a complete initial evaluation. If possible, the history should be gathered from three sources: (1) the patient, (2) any available family members and (3) the patient's medical chart. Strict reliance on medical records can lead to misinterpretation of findings or to missing conditions that may either contraindicate or require modifications to treatment (e.g., undocumented history of childhood asthma or a recent gradual decline in exercise tolerance).

Clinical Assessment

It is not within the scope of this report to review a clinical respiratory assessment in depth (see Table 1); however, there are a few salient points that deserve elaboration. Equally important to the hands-on examination is careful observation prior to examination. A methodical head-to-toe scan is made with an emphasis on the distinction between underlying COPD (clubbing, nicotine stained fingers, peripheral cyanosis, translucent skin, barrel chest and mild to moderate use of accessory muscles) and acute distress (nasal flaring, retraction or indraining, central cyanosis, diaphoresis and moderate to maximal use of accessory muscles).

The examination is easily structured into four parts: (1) inspection—taking observation one step further to the in-depth evaluation of breathing patterns; (2) palpation—touching the patient to determine both chest wall mobility and quality of underlying structures. This includes testing for tactile fremitus, which, if decreased, indicates fluid or air in the pleura or an obstruction causing atelectasis. An increase in intensity occurs with an increase in the density of the underlying parenchyma as occurs with a consolidation; (3) percussion—striking a single finger (usually the long finger), placed flat on the chest wall, with the tip of the opposite long finger in order to discover any al-

---

TABLE 1   Assessment of the Respiratory System

History of present illness
    Reason for seeking medical attention
    Chief complaints
    Date of onset
    Progression of illness
    Treatment to date

Past medical history
    Relevant to present complaints (especially respiratory)
    Previous injuries or operations

Medications sociodemographic data
    Occupation
    Marital status
    Living environment
    Functional status

Habits
    Smoking history
    Etoh abuse
    Substance abuse

Subjective
    Chief complaint
    Pain—site, radiation, nature, periodicity, duration, intensity, shortness of breath, shortness of breath on exertion, orthopnea, paroxysmal nocturnal dyspnea,
    Cough—frequency, amount of sputum produced

Objective
    Observation
        Head and neck eyes, mouth/mucosa.
        Chest,
        Abdomen,
        Extremities,
        Overall impression,
    Mental status

TABLE 1 Continued

Examination

Inspection
  Respiratory rate
  Mechanism of respiration (apical, lateral costal, diaphragmatic)
  Anterior-posterior diameter
  Nasal flaring, indrawing, use of accessory muscles,
  Clubbing
  Ratio I.E.
  Presence of incisions
Palpation
  Position of the trachea
  Presence of splinting
  Mobility of the thorax
  Sites of pain
  Tactile fremitus
  Skin temperature
  Presence of rib fractures, subcutaneous, emphysema
Percussion
  Record site and density
Auscultation
  All lung fields
  To detect depth of air entry and presence of adventitia
Functional status
  Range of motion (ROM)
  Ambulatory status (gait deviations, shortness of breath)
  Strength
  Endurance
Cough
  Strength, frequency, if productive, note volume, viscosity and color
  of sputum
  Arterial blood gas (ABG) results
  Sputum cytology
  Pulmonary function testing (PFT) values

Investigation findings
Chest x-ray examination results
Vital signs—respiratory rate, heart rate, blood pressure, temperature

teration in the density of the underlying area of lung (Table 2). Percussion, in association with tactile fremitus, can be very useful in determining the extent and nature of the respiratory disease, yet these tools are rarely used by physical therapists; (4) auscultation—the detection of breath sounds, both normal and abnormal (adventitia), by means of a stethoscope. Ability to perform auscultation is a critical skill in the assessment of respiratory function, but if relied on too heavily it can lead to misinterpretation of the disease process, which in turn can result in ineffective and occasionally detrimental treatment.

Laboratory Results and Investigation Findings

It is essential to combine clinical examination findings with the results of laboratory findings and other investigations as listed in Table 1. These results often confirm or refute the tentative diagnosis. To complete the assessment, a review of the patient's other

systems is incorporated. Only then can treatment goals be determined and an effective, comprehensive treatment plan be proposed.

Constant assessment of respiratory function is necessary because respiratory status can change rapidly. Ongoing observation and examination are essential to ensure both the safety of the patient and the effectiveness of treatment.

MODALITIES OF CARE

Although the standard CPT maneuvers mentioned in the introduction are still in use and are effective when used in the appropriate patient-care situation, there are many other valuable modalities of care available to chest physical therapists. These other modalities are effective when used in conjunction with standard treatment or independently to improve respiratory function; most important, they take into account the patient's total well being.

TABLE 2 Clinical Signs Associated with Commonly Occurring Acute Lung Pathology

Pathological Process	Inspection	Palpation	Percussion	Auscultation
Pneumothorax	$\searrow$ or $\downarrow$ movement: $C_T \downarrow P_{max} \uparrow P_{IF}$ $\uparrow$ if tension: otherwise may be N	Possible subcutaneous emphysema: tracheal deviation away from pneumothorax if tension	Hyperresonance over pneumothorax	Breath sounds $\downarrow$ or absent
Pulmonary edema	Movement N: frothy sputum in tracheal tube: C_T $\downarrow P_{max} N$ or $\nearrow$ $P_{IE} \uparrow$	If florid, palpable fluid in airways	Dullness	Crackles and wheezes
Atelectasis	$\downarrow$ movement: $\downarrow C_T P_{max} N$ or $\nearrow P_{IE} \uparrow$	Tracheal deviation towards lesion if complete upper lobe atelectasis	Dullness over area of collapse	Breath sounds $\downarrow$ or absent with major collapse; maybe bronchial breathing and crackles
Contusion	Bruising may be present: movement N or $\downarrow$: $C_T \downarrow \downarrow P_{max}$ N or $\nearrow$: $P_{IE} \uparrow$	May be tenderness and crepitus over fractured ribs	Dullness over contusion	Bronchial breathing wheezes if excessive bleeding
Aspiration	Movement N or $\downarrow$: $C_T N$ or $\downarrow$: $P_{max} N$ or $\nearrow$: $P_{IE} N$ or $\nearrow$	Crackles (rhonchi) may be palpable	Dullness may be present	Vesicular breathing, Crakles (rhonchi)
Pleural fluid	Movement $\downarrow$: $C_T N$ or $\downarrow$: P_{max} or $\uparrow$; $P_{IE} N$ or $\uparrow$ depending on quantity	No breath sounds palpable: Tracheal deviation away from fluid if voluminous	Stony dullness may clear on turning patient if fluid not loculated	Breath sounds absent; may be bronchial breathing above fluid
Pneumonia	Movement $\downarrow$: $\downarrow$ C_T: $P_{max} \nearrow$: P_{IE}	Pleural rub may be palpable	Dullness over consolidation	Early breath sounds $\downarrow$; bronchial breathing crackles and pleural rub
Fibrosis	Movement $\downarrow$: $\downarrow C_T$: $P_{max} \uparrow P_{IE} \uparrow$	Tracheal deviation towards fibrosis	Dullness over fibrosis	Breath sounds $\searrow$; bronchial breathing and crackles

SIGNS $\searrow$, slightly decreased; $\downarrow$, decreased; $\uparrow$, increased, $\nearrow$, slightly increased.
ABBREVIATIONS C_T, total lung/thorax compliance; P_{max}, maximum airway pressure; P_{IE}, end-inspiratory pressure; N, normal.

Education

Every patient benefits from some degree of education. Teaching the patient and his family the indications for and the importance of his treatment decreases anxiety and increases compliance. These are vital points to consider if maximum treatment benefit is to be realized and further complications avoided.

It is now recognized that the education of patients with COPD does not change the outcome of the disease, but may prolong the patient's life and will improve his or her quality of life. This teaching process must continue after discharge from hospital to encourage and assist with lifestyle changes, adaptations to the home environment, and improvement or maintenance of cardiovascular exercise tolerance. The greatest benefits from COPD teaching are realized if

diagnosis and treatment happen early. At present, most patients with COPD do not receive CPT treatment until their disease has progressed to the moderate or severe level. Given this situation, treatment becomes much more difficult: lung compliance decreases, muscles weaken, and cardiovascular endurance decreases. The patient develops feelings of hopelessness and poor coping mechanisms that must be unlearned before appropriate ones can be utilized effectively.

Surgical patients have the potential to recover to their premorbid respiratory status. The process begins preoperatively, thereby allowing the patient time to understand the rationale, to practice breathing routines, and to maximize ventilatory capabilities. This makes postoperative treatment easier and more effective, thus decreasing risk of postoperative respiratory complications.

Education includes the following: (1) treatment techniques utilized, (2) breathing exercises, (3) the nature of the illness (basic anatomy, physiology, and pathophysiology), (4) mobility and exercise tolerance exercises, (5) effective use of inhaled pharmacological agents, (6) effects of the environment and psychological status on the illness, and (7) effective coughing.

Relaxation Techniques

The patient responds to pain by tightening or "splinting" the surrounding muscles, and by breathing in a shallow manner at an increased rate. This response often leads to constriction and collapse of the distal airways and the entrapment of mucus. The result is often atelectasis or pneumonia. Anxiety can magnify these responses, thereby increasing the risks of respiratory complications. Simple relaxation, voluntary and reflexive, can alleviate these problems. Numerous relaxation techniques exist. A list includes simple vocal cueing, meditation, biofeedback, progressive muscular relaxation, distal contract-relax exercises, massage, gentle muscle stretching, and relaxation breathing exercises.

Breathing Retraining

Breathing retraining is more than deep breathing exercises. Dyspneic patients exhibit breathing patterns that are ineffective, consume large amounts of energy, and increase oxygen consumption. The purpose of breathing retraining is to reduce the work of breathing and to improve the ventilation and perfusion of the lungs. Some components of treatment are as follows:

1. Diaphragmatic breathing control—stresses slow abdominal diaphragmatic breaths to strengthen the diaphragm, improve oxygenation with increased depth of respiration and decreased accessory muscle use and to promote relaxation.

2. Lateral costal breathing—emphasizes the "bucket handle" action of the ribs, minimizies splinting, increases depth of respiration and assists in increased use of the diaphragm.

3. P-Flex muscle trainers—one method of strengthening the diaphragm during diaphragmatic breathing exercises.

4. Pursed lip breathing—exhalation through pursed lips lengthens the time of positive pressure in the airways allowing time for O_2 and CO_2 transport.

5. Positioning—maximizes relaxation, assists respiration with gravity, and provides maximum mechanical advantage for respiratory muscles.

6. Thoracic mobility—trunk or upper extremity range of motion increases the size of the thoracic cavity, thereby creating a negative intrathoracic pressure and allowing maximum air entry with less effort.

7. Incentive spirometry—apparatus given to encourage compliance with frequent, independent breathing exercises with maximum depth of respiration.

Massage

The goals of massage are twofold for relaxation and for an increase in chest wall mobility. The most widely used techniques are effleurage, stroking, deepkneading, chest wall pressures, and occasional frictions. Massage that is properly performed prior to treatment can greatly enhance the results of treatment in addition to promoting patient comfort and confidence.

Standard CPT Maneuvers

As previously stated, standard CPT maneuvers include postural drainage, percussions, vibrations, coughing, and suctioning. These techniques need not be painful or aggressive and can be modified for the safety of the complicated patient with multiple medical problems. Several different methods of coughing are taught by physical therapists. The methods enable surgical patients to cough effectively with minimal pain. Patients with chronic and sometimes uncontrolled coughs can employ these techniques to decrease the frequency and to improve the effectiveness of their coughs.

Mechanical Modalities

Mechanical vibrators and percussors are in wide use at present. These can be more comfortable than normal treatment, thus increasing patient tolerance during an extended treatment period. Mechanical modalities also function at a frequency that the literature* describes as more effective in decreasing the viscosity of the secretions, increasing the action of the cilia, and increasing the speed of secretion clearance.

Neurofacilitation Techniques (NFT)

NFTs were developed to provide chest care for the unconscious adult patient. These techniques facilitate and increase normal mechanical respiratory movement patterns by producing reflexive respiratory reactions. A discussion of the basis of these tech-

---

* Holody B, Goldberg HS. The effect of mechanical vibration physic-therapy on arterial oxygenation in acutely ill patients with ate ectasis or pneumonia. Am Rev Resp Dis 1981; 124:372–375.

niques is beyond the scope of this text. The procedures described include perioral stimulation, abdominal cocontractions, vertebral pressures, basal lifts, and intercostal stretches.

Mobility

Simple immobilization results in a decrease in total lung capacity, functional residual capacity, and residual lung capacity. This decrease is of course magnified after anesthesia or with underlying COPD.

One of the physical therapist's primary goals is to enable the patient to regain early mobility. After an acute illness or surgery, therapy treatment follows the distinct pattern of frequent repositioning in bed, progressing to a move out of bed and into a chair, followed by progressive, frequent ambulation. Close attention is paid to exercise tolerance. As the patient begins to recover, an appropriate aerobic exercise program is developed. (This is often an extension of the patient's ambulation program.) Early mobility not only helps to avoid progressive atelectasis but also helps to prevent the many adverse effects of bed rest, namely pulmonary emboli, venous stasis, thrombophlebitis and deep vein thromboses, and muscle atrophy.

Selecting the appropriate combination of treatment modalities is important; their correct sequential arrangement is also vital. For example, if airways are partially obstructed due to bronchospasm, attempts to inflate the distal airways or mobilize secretions in the distal airways are futile. Relieve the bronchospasm first, and then reevaluate the method of secretion clearance. This simple problem-solving approach is effective, but often not followed in the clinic.

The timing of the treatments is also crucial. An attempt should be made to coordinate treatments to coincide with the administration of bronchodilators. Treatments should also follow the administration of pain medications or muscle relaxants by 15 to 20 minutes. Treatments should occur when the patient is rested. They should be short in duration, held frequently, and include an early morning and late evening meeting.

ASSESSMENT OF THERAPEUTIC RESPONSE

Continual reassessment of respiratory disease is a preoccupation of the chest therapist. Chest physical therapists must constantly observe the patients for signs of improvement or deterioration. Laboratory and investigation results trace the medical progress of the disease. However, these results are not immediate and are often not readily available. In clinical terms, improvement would be evidenced by increased sputum production, decreased work of breathing and improved breathing pattern, improved ventilation to auscultation, stabilization of vital signs and an improvement in symptoms of dyspnea, pain, and anxiety. These changes may not be dramatic and often occur 20 to 30 minutes after a treatment.

The classical or traditional approach to chest physical therapy is one of aggressive manual techniques, postural drainage, deep breathing, and coughing in an effort to improve secretion clearance. With such a narrow focus the treatment results are understandably varied and often poor. The most logical and effective approach to take in the management of acute and chronic respiratory disorders is a holistic one that centers on an awareness not only of the treatment of these disorders, but also of their prevention and potential recurrence.

Physical therapists now have an extensive repertoire of treatment modalities available to them. From careful determination of the history, painstaking physical examination, and review of investigation results and lab findings, treatment goals are determined and the appropriate treatment modalities are chosen. With correct sequencing and timing of the treatment a good therapeutic result can be achieved.

SUGGESTED READING

Bethune D. Neurophysiological facilitation of respiration in the unconscious adult patient. Physiother Can 1986; 27(5):241–246.

Cherniack RM, Cherniack L, Naimark A. Respiration in health and disease. Philadelphia: WB Saunders, 1972.

Frownfelter DL. Chest physical therapy and pulmonary rehabilitation. Chicago: Year Book, 1978.

Gross D, King M. High frequency chest wall compression: a new noninvasive method of chest physiotherapy for mucocilliary clearance. Physiother Can 1984; 137–139.

Holody B, Goldberg H. The effect of mechanical vibration physiotherapy on arterial oxygenation in acutely ill patients with atelectasis or pneumonia. Respir Dis 1981; 124:372–375.

Irwin S, Tecklin JS, eds. Cardiopulmonary physical therapy. St. Louis: CV Mosby, 1985:167.

Kigin CM. Chest physiotherapy for the postoperative or traumatic injury patient. Phys Ther 1981; 61(12):1724–1736.

Koloczkowski W. Guidelines to chest assessment. Physiother Can 1985; 22(4):204–205.

Reinisch ES. Functional approach to chest physical therapy. Phys Ther 1978; 58(8):972–975.

Schlenker JD. The pathogenesis of postoperative atelectasis. Arch Surg 1973; 107:846–850.

Sutton PP, Pavia D. Chest physiotherapy: a review. Eur J Respir Dis 1982; 63:188–201.

RESPIRATORY CARE FOR THE SPINAL CORD INJURED PATIENT

PEGGY CLOUGH, B.S., M.S.

Comprehensive, ongoing respiratory care for spinal cord injury (SCI) patients, is a necessary part of a total rehabilitation program. Pulmonary compromise continues to be one of the leading causes of morbidity and mortality for SCI patients both in the acute period following SCI and throughout their lives. Ventilatory compromise is caused by a number of kinesiologic and physiologic factors that are interrelated. These factors result in increased work of breathing coupled with decreased efficiency in clearing bronchial secretions (Fig. 1). How these factors interrelate, in a particular patient with a specific level of injury during the acute post-traumatic period and then chronically, requires a careful respiratory evaluation. Specific treatment interventions can then be utilized to remediate or minimize the effects of the various pulmonary problems.

EVALUATION

The major components of a respiratory evaluation are respiratory pattern, ventilatory status, respiratory rate (RR), forced vital capacity (FVC), tidal volume (TV), maximum inspiratory mouth pressure (PImax), chest wall expansion, breath sounds, cough effort, and sputum production. Each of these parameters is not assessed daily. Evaluation of specific parameters becomes more or less important as the SCI patient progresses through rehabilitation, has acute pulmonary problems, or as the physical therapist uses different treatment modalities. However, respiratory pattern and rate should always be noted.

Respiratory Pattern

Respiratory pattern is evaluated using inspection and palpation. The areas of excursion, symmetry of movement, and the musculature used to accomplish the movement are noted. Immediately after SCI, there is often paradoxical movement of the thorax—on inspiration the chest wall is drawn inward, and during expiration the chest wall moves outward. This para-doxical movement of the thorax is caused by the paralysis of the external intercostal muscles, which normally expand the chest, and by the action of the diaphragm, which creates an increased negative pleural space pressure and sucks the flaccid chest wall inward. Exaggerated outward abdominal wall movement also occurs during inspiration because of the paralysis of the abdominal muscles and unopposed descent of the diaphragm. The cervical accessory muscles of inspiration are usually active in an effort to contribute to the tidal volume. Asymmetry of chest wall excursion is noted by comparing movement of the right and left sides of the thorax during the respiratory cycle. Asymmetry may indicate an incomplete SCI with some sparing, an underlying pulmonary pathology, an asymmetrical neurologic impairment, or a concomitant musculoskeletal injury. For example, a flail left hemithorax would show increased paradoxical movement on the left. Over time, as the SCI patient experiences increased tone in the chest wall musculature and is better able to use the accessory inspiratory musculature, paradoxical excursion is reduced. This abnormal breathing pattern can again become significant during increased ventilatory loading as occurs with a pulmonary infection.

The evaluation of diaphragmatic function is especially critical. Diaphragmatic excursion can be palpated anteriorly using one hand placed midline on the upper abdomen directly below the xiphoid process. The fingers should be spread with the index finger just below the xiphoid process and the little finger at the patient's waist. Using this method, good diaphragmatic excursion would be palpated under the first three fingers. Diaphragmatic excursion can also be determined using mediate or indirect percussion. This method is performed over the posterior thorax with the patient sitting (a position that can be very difficult for an acute SCI patient). The palpation method is preferred because it uses the same hand placement as tactile cueing to enhance diaphragmatic excursion; thus, the therapist is in both an evaluation and a treatment mode.

Diaphragmatic strength and endurance can be assessed by noting the change in diaphragmatic excursion when the patient is instructed to take a tidal volume and then a forced vital capacity. Knowing the change in diaphragmatic excursion between these two ventilatory maneuvers, and what percentage the tidal volume is of the vital capacity gives an indication of how hard the diaphragm is working with each respiratory cycle. The amount of time adequate oxygenation can be maintained before some mechanical ven-

Figure 1 Pulmonary compromise in spinal cord injury

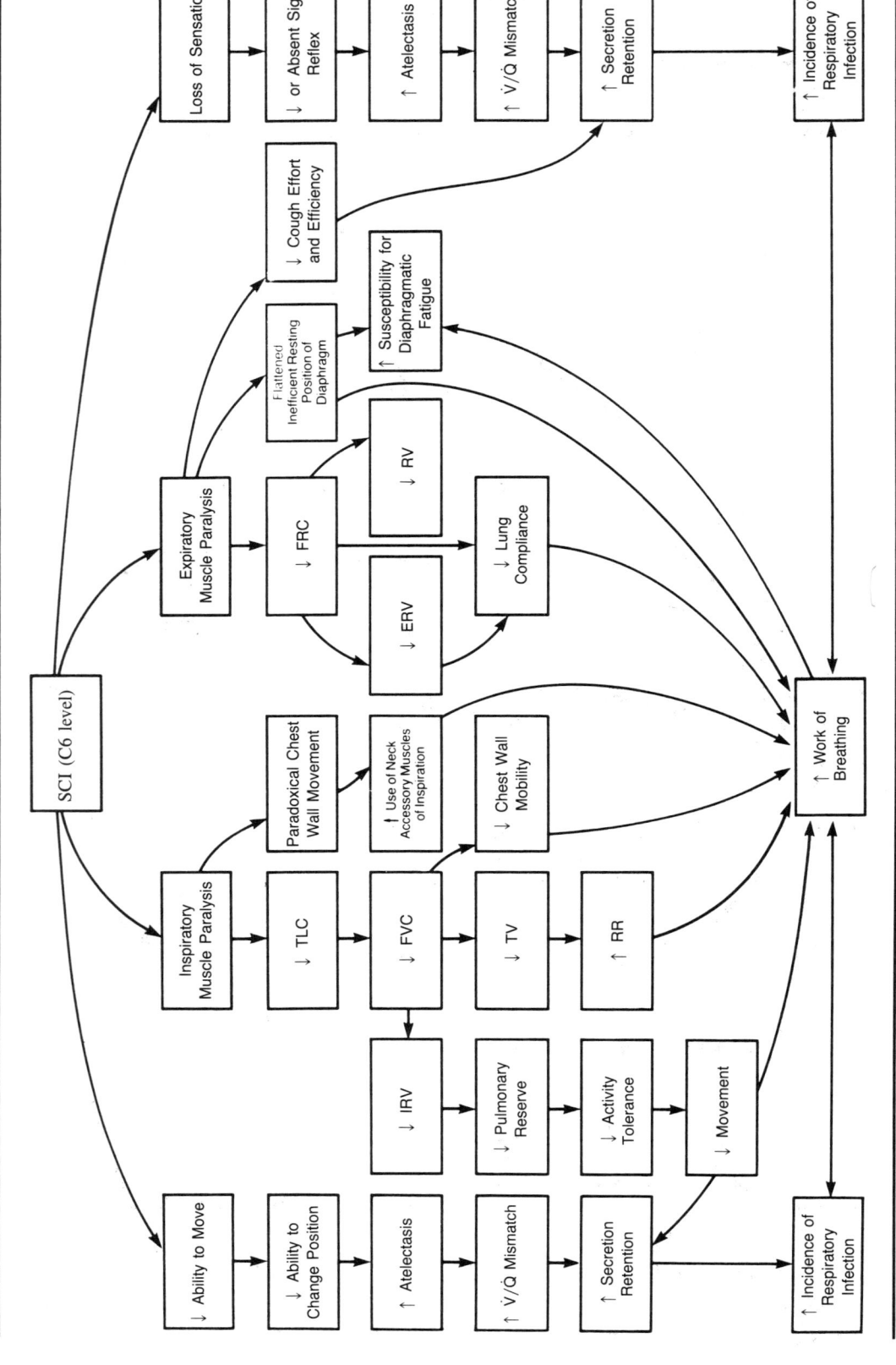

P. Clough 1987

Abbreviations are spinal cord injury (SCI), decreased ($\downarrow$), increased ($\uparrow$), total lung capacity (TLC), forced vital capacity (FVC), inspiratory reserve volume (IRV), tidal volume (TV), respiratory rate (RR), functional residual capacity (FRC), expiratory reserve volume (ERV), residual volume (RV), ventilation ($\dot{V}$), perfusion ($\dot{Q}$).

tilatory assistance is needed gives a crude measure of diaphragmatic endurance. Maximum inspiratory mouth pressure is another indirect measure of endurance, which will be discussed separately.

Ventilatory Status

Ventilatory status is evaluated by inspection and chart review. Three areas are noted; airway, mechanical support, and use of oxygen. The physical therapist can easily see if breathing is through the natural anatomic airway or via an endotracheal or tracheostomy tube. If an endotracheal tube is in place, suctioning is easier, but the patient is only able to approximate a weak cough and is unable to vocalize. With a tracheostomy tube, it is again easy to suction and with the cuff deflated and the tracheostomy tube plugged, the patient can speak and perform an assisted cough. Both these artificial airways allow ventilation to be mechanically supported continuously or intermittently. However, these airways bypass the upper respiratory tract so that the inspired gases are usually not as well humidified. This can cause bronchial irritation and increased secretion production. Assessment of mechanical support of ventilation means noting the type of ventilator and the ventilator settings; particularly, mode, respiratory rate, tidal volume, sigh frequency and volume, inspired O_2 concentration (FiO_2), and weaning status so that the physical therapist can plan an appropriate treatment program. The use of O_2 should always be noted, whether the patient is on or off a ventilator. During treatment, the physical therapist should ensure that nothing impairs O_2 delivery.

Respiratory Rate

Respiratory rate should be counted for 30 seconds and multiplied by two to determine the number of breaths per minute (bpm). In adults, the normal rate is 12 to 18 bpm. Because tidal volume is decreased in SCI patients, respiratory rate is usually increased. Changes in respiratory rate can indicate a change in pulmonary status. The timing of the respiratory cycle can also be evaluated; this evaluation includes both the regularity of the rhythm and the inspiratory to expiratory ratio.

Pulmonary Function Tests

Forced vital capacity, tidal volume, and maximum inspiratory mouth pressure are simple pulmonary function measures that can be performed at the bedside. These tests may be performed by the physical therapist or the respiratory therapist. The information gained should be used in treatment planning by the physical therapist. The FVC, TV, and the ratio

of these volumes gives a measure of ventilatory ability, pulmonary reserve, and the effort the patient can generate. These pulmonary function measures are also used to determine ability to be weaned from a ventilator and ventilatory status during weaning trials. Before a timed or intermittent mandatory ventilation (IMV) weaning protocol is initiated, the patient should have a FVC of 10 to 15 ml per kilogram ideal body weight and an inspiratory mouth pressure of at least -20 cm H_2O.

The PImax is also an indirect measure of diaphragmatic strength and endurance and can be utilized when doing diaphragmatic muscle training. Serial tracking of the length of time spent off the ventilator using diaphragmatic breathing is another measure of diaphragmatic endurance. The ability to maintain a FVC over time using periodic checks is a third indirect measure of diaphragmatic strength and endurance.

With an acute cervical SCI, an acute FVC is approximately 30 percent of normal. During the first 4 months following injury, this value usually doubles. Directly following SCI, all lung volumes are reduced except residual volume (RV), which can be markedly increased during the flaccid stage. Chronic SCI patients show characteristic restrictive impairment with all lung volumes decreased and flow rates essentially normal. Immediately following SCI, PImax usually falls about 50 percent from the normal value of -110 to -150 cm H_2O. During the first 4 months following injury, this value usually improves.

Chest Wall Mobility

Chest wall excursion is evaluated using inspection, palpation, and a chest expansometer. Noting how the chest wall moves during the respiratory cycle is part of the evaluation of the breathing pattern. This general information on chest wall expansion can be gained from inspection and palpation. However, for objective quantifiable information on chest wall expansion, a chest expansometer reading or circumferential measurement using a tape measure must be taken. A chest expansometer is made up of two separate tape measures extending in opposite directions from the same plastic case. Chest expansion measurements are usually taken at the level of the eighth and twelfth thoracic spinous processes.

The entire excursion of the thorax can be measured using a tape measure and taking inspiration and expiration circumferential measurements at both levels. The patient is instructed to take a deep breath in and then to exhale forcefully down to residual volume with measurements taken at full inspiration and at full expiration. Each hemithorax can be measured individually using an expansometer. The expansometer is held against the vertebral column at the appropriate level. The two tape measures are brought around the chest and crossed in front. The midsternal line is marked with a skin pencil. The patient is then instructed to take a deep breath and to blow it all out forcefully, the two readings are taken from each of the tape measures where they cross the pencil mark. With SCI patients experiencing paradoxical breathing, chest excursion is a negative number. Although circumferential measurements and chest expansometer measurements are more accurate with the patient upright, circumferential measurements can be performed with the patient supine, which makes these measurements more practical during the acute phase. However, using an expansometer provides more information because the excursion of each hemithorax is noted and can be compared.

Auscultation

Breath sounds are evaluated daily through auscultation during the acute post injury phase and, whenever changes in other pulmonary parameters (temperature, respiratory rate, pattern, sputum production) warrrant it, during the chronic rehabilitative phase. Because of decreased lung volumes following SCI, breath sounds often sound quiet or distant. Patients are asked to breathe through the mouth using very deep breaths. If the patient is unable to move sufficient gas spontaneously, he or she can be auscultated while on a ventilator. Both the anterior and posterior chest walls should be auscultated so that both the upper and lower lobes can be assessed. The sitting position is ideal for auscultation, but usually immediately following injury auscultation has to be accomplished in the sidelying position. The presence of abnormal and adventitious breath sounds most frequently indicates areas of atelectasis or increased secretions, both of which require active treatment.

Cough Effort and Sputum Production

Cough and sputum production are evaluated by listening to the strength and wetness of the cough effort and by noting the amount, color, and viscosity of secretions. With paralysis of the abdominal musculature the cough is weak and ineffective, and an important body defense mechanism against respiratory infection is lost. If the cough is not efficient in clearing secretions then using and teaching assisted coughing maneuvers is an important part of the treatment program.

TREATMENT

In order to meet the needs of the individual patient, the respiratory treatment program should be based on the following:

1. The level of injury and subsequent neurologic deficits;
2. The time since the acute SCI (acute vs chronic phase);
3. Any underlying or concomitant pulmonary pathology;
4. The physical therapy assessment of current respiratory status;
5. The stability of the fracture or dislocation site;
6. Any other concomitant medical problem; and
7. The ability and willingness of the patient to cooperate with treatment.

Breathing Exercises

Breathing exercises are the foundation of the respiratory treatment program. Knowing the neurologic level and completeness of injury is important in determining the appropriate breathing exercises to be included in the pulmonary program. Patients at the C2 level have only pharyngeal and laryngeal muscles innervated by the intact cranial nerves and so only glossopharyngeal breathing (GPB) exercises are appropriate. These should not be started until the patient is medically stable and are discussed later in the chapter. From C5 to T1 the patient has only the diaphragm and cervical accessory muscles innervated. The external and internal intercostals are innervated from T1 through T12. As the level of injury moves lower, more intercostals become active. The abdominals are innervated from T5 to T12.

Breathing exercises can be initiated with high-level (C6) ventilator-dependent patients in order to facilitate weaning from the ventilator. Exercises to promote diaphragmatic excursion and endurance are best performed during a conventional timed wean at the beginning of the period off the ventilator. If an IMV weaning protocol is used, active diaphragmatic exercises can begin when the IMV setting is at 8 or below. The goal is to make the remaining respiratory musculature, particularly the diaphragm, as efficient as possible and to increase slowly the strength and endurance of the respiratory muscles. Unlike other pulmonary pathologies, the physical therapist working with SCI patients is not only interested in the contraction and descent of the diaphragm, but also its return to its resting position. Because of the paralysis of the abdominal muscles, the diaphragm's resting position is lowered. The diaphragm's flattened resting position compromises the length-tension relationship of the diaphragm's muscle fibers, decreases the possible excursion of the diaphragm, and increases the likelihood of diaphragmatic fatigue. In the upright posture, gravity pulls the diaphragm even lower and increases its inefficiency. Initially, therefore, diaphragmatic breathing should be practised supine. There are three simple ways to assist the diaphragm's ascent during exhalation so that the next contraction can be more efficient: placing the patient approximately 30 degrees head down recruits gravity to move the abdominal contents against the under surface of the diaphragm, moving it upward; using 5 to 10 lbs of sandbag weights over the abdomen has the same result. However, both of these techniques make the diaphragm work against an added resistance during its active contraction. This resistance might be desirable later in rehabilitation, but may be too strenuous when the patient is weaning from the ventilator. Using firm hand pressures over the upper abdomen during exhalation and then releasing the pressure and allowing full excursion of the diaphragm during inhalation is the method of choice during early weaning trials. During IMV weans, "paired" breathing is used. "Paired" breathing means pairing one mandatory ventilator-delivered breath with one or two spontaneous breaths using the diaphragm. The timing of the ventilator and spontaneous breaths is accomplished by careful verbal cueing, pursed lip exhalation to slow the respiratory rate, and assisted full exhalation using firm hand pressures over the lower rib cage and upper abdomen. During conventional weans, the timing of each breathing cycle does not have to be so meticulous; however, the patient should be encouraged to work towards a normal TV and RR. To increase TV and decrease RR, deep slow breathing patterns are stressed. Patients are instructed to breathe in through the nose, if possible, to warm and humidify the inhaled gas. Artificial airways and mouth breathing do not humidify the inhaled gas as efficiently as the nose. Delivery of dry gas to the airways is irritating and can cause increased secretion production and bronchoconstriction both of which increase the work of breathing. Pursed lip exhalation is sometimes used to slow the respiratory rate, increase TV, slow flow rates, and decrease $\dot{V}/\dot{Q}$ mismatching. Inflation-hold is another breathing technique often used with SCI patients. This technique has been shown to be effective in raising the PaO_2 and in decreasing atelectasis. SCI patients with injuries above the T1 level have lost an effective automatic sigh mechanism and the technique of inflation-hold is partially able to remediate this loss. These same patients often hypoventilate and therefore have lowered PaO_2 values, which again can be partially compensated by the inflation-hold technique. This maneuver is easily taught: the patient is instructed to take a deep breath and, at full inspiration, is asked to inhale a little more air. These instructions have the patient effectively holding at total lung capacity (TLC) while trying to pull in just a little more air.

SCI patients (C6 level) also have intact neck musculature that can contribute to increasing the ventilatory efficiency. The neck muscles should be inhibited, using relaxation techniques, if they are actively engaged in trying to lift the thorax with each inspiration. This respiratory pattern is grossly inefficient, raises O_2 consumption, and quickly fatigues the patient. However, developing some consistent tone in these muscles, so that they act as a stabilizing force for the upper thorax, increases the efficiency of the diaphragm by opposing its downward pull on the thorax during contraction. The coordinated muscular activity of the cervical accessory muscles and the diaphragm increases the vertical chest excursion and decreases the work of breathing.

Patients are often very anxious during weaning trials. Therefore, it is necessary that the physical therapist be familiar with the ventilator and airway and the techniques to be used. The therapist's confidence and skill can do a great deal to facilitate patient trust.

As the weaning process progresses, diaphragmatic exercises are continued to increase the excursion of the diaphragm on each contraction until a satisfactory tidal volume can be achieved consistently. Incentive spirometry, using a volume dependent spirometer, is initiated as early as possible. Use of an incentive spirometer encourages the patient to work toward adequate tidal volumes and to practise vital capacity maneuvers because it provides immediate visual feedback. The inspirometer also uses the physiologic principles of an inflation-hold breathing maneuver that acts as a sigh for the patient. Introducing the incentive spirometer is the first step in having the patient assume responsibility for the pulmonary program.

As spontaneous breathing time increases, exercises to increase diaphragmatic endurance and strength can be added. Diaphragmatic endurance and strength can be enhanced in three ways. First, time spent using active diaphragmatic breathing can be increased. This technique is a natural progression of the weaning process and enhances diaphragmatic endurance (though probably doing little for diaphragmatic strength). Using an inspiratory muscle trainer, which provides progressive levels of resistance to inspiration, is the second way to increase diaphragmatic endurance and, to a lesser degree, diaphragmatic strength in SCI patients. Use of an inspiratory muscle trainer is often preferred because the patients can assume responsibility for these exercises after being trained to use the device. Independence in using the inspiratory muscle trainer is important because these exercises must be continued in order for diaphragmatic endurance to be maintained. Loading the upper abdomen with weights is the third method of improving diaphragmatic endurance and strength. Usually, low levels of resistance are employed (1 to 30 lbs). Endurance can be increased over time by having the diaphragm contract and push against this added resistance.

Positioning

Positioning and turning the SCI patient is an important part of the prophylactic treatment regimen not only to maintain skin integrity, but also to maintain adequate aeration of all lung segments. It has been clearly demonstrated that the position of the thorax affects the distribution of both gas and blood flow within the lung. The dependent areas of the lung are best ventilated and perfused. However, the uppermost portion of the lungs have a larger resting volume and are therefore better expanded; at the same time blood flow to this area is decreased. Thus, the area of greatest expansion is not the area that is best ventilated. To understand this paradox, the physical therapist must realize that ventilation is the volume change per unit resting volume. In the upright position, the base of the lung has both a larger volume change with each breath and a smaller resting volume than the apex, thereby making ventilation greater at the base of the lung. Therefore, positioning can be used to increase ventilation or expansion of any lung segment. This is accomplished with a turning or positioning schedule that places the patient supine, sidelying, prone, head down, and head up for different parts of the day. Varied sequential positioning can be accomplished via standard positioning techniques in a conventional hospital bed or via a specialized bed such as the Roto rest bed, the rocking bed, the stryker frame, or the circle electric bed.

Once the patient is out of bed and in the upright position, sitting or standing, an abdominal binder should be fitted. The binder or corset supports the abdominal wall improving the efficiency of the diaphragm by assisting it to return to its normal resting position after each breath. Binders can significantly increase respiratory efficiency, exercise tolerance, voice projection and can also contribute to the stability of the trunk. The corset must be fitted properly extending from the tenth rib to over the iliac crests. The upper buckles should not be as snug as the lower buckles in order to allow for diaphragmatic excursion. Often patients prefer not to use abdominal binders because of the time and effort needed to apply them. However, early in the rehabilitation program, abdominal binders can make a significant difference in performance because the corset increases endurance for the total exercise program. Later, some patients develop sufficient abdominal wall spasticity so that use of the abdominal binder can be discontinued with no change noted in respiratory efficiency or exercise tolerance. Other patients continue to derive benefits from an abdominal binder throughout their lives. If an abdominal binder is to be used, the patient and family need careful instruction in its application and in doing skin checks of the area when it is removed.

Bronchial Hygiene

Postural drainage and percussion are utilized frequently with SCI patients because of their weak cough and impaired ability in clearing secretions. Whenever the physical therapist's evaluation reveals evidence of excess secretions in the lungs or segmental/lobar consolidation, these techniques can prove helpful. Postural drainage is a simple technique that makes use of gravity to pull excess bronchial secretions from the lung periphery, centrally so that the patient can cough them out or the patient can be effectively suctioned. Postural drainage is not done prophylactically. Indeed drainage of excess bronchial secretions cannot be accomplished until there are bronchial secretions for gravity to act upon. The most important factors in achieving good results using postural drainage are (1) a careful examination of the chest so that the correct positions are used and (2) the ability to aerate the segments being drained. If the patient is unable to cooperate with the treatment, the use of a ventilator or manual bagging can be used, but will not yield the same results as the patient's spontaneous deep breathing. If the patient is receiving bronchodilators via respiratory therapy, results are enhanced if postural drainage can follow the respiratory therapy treatment. The amount of time allocated to each of the selected drainage positions depends upon how closely the position approximates the classic drainage position for the segment being drained, the amount and viscosity of secretions, and the patient's tolerance to the treatment. Most SCI patients tolerate postural drainage very well. However, because a significant percentage of SCI patients have also suffered a closed head injury, precautions must be taken. During the acute period directly following the injury, increased intracranial pressure may occur so that head down positions need to be used cautiously and, in some cases, modified.

Percussion and vibration are mechanical techniques applied over the chest wall. These techniques are used to create turbulence in the airflow, which moves in and out with each breath. The turbulent airflow is more likely to move excess bronchial secretions adherent to the bronchial mucosa than is the normal laminar airflow. Because these techniques are used in conjunction with postural drainage, the secretions are moved centrally by gravity to where they can be expectorated. Percussion is performed throughout the respiratory cycle using a cupped hand. The entire rim of the hand must come into firm, but not heavy, contact with the chest wall. Percussion is performed on the chest wall, which overlies the segment being drained. SCI patients usually tolerate percussion well. Caution must be used until the spine is stabilized. Other medical conditions (i.e., fractured ribs, coagulation disorders, osteoporosis, hemoptysis, and uncontrolled seizure disorders) need to be considered before initiating percussion. Vibration is less effective with SCI patients because of the paradoxical movement of the chest wall during the breathing cycle. Vibration is usually performed only during expiration, and the therapist's vibrating hands follow the chest wall. With SCI the chest wall may be moving out instead of in during expiration thus making transmission of the vibration to the underlying lung tissue difficult. Vibration can be used to effectively trigger a cough reflex when applied directly over the carina just following a deep breath or bagging maneuver. Vibrating over the carina is an effective way to assist clearing secretions and is often used just before suctioning the acute SCI patient who has an artificial airway in place.

Assisted Coughing

One of the most common pulmonary techniques taught to the SCI patient is an assisted cough. Patients with injury levels above T12 have weak or no abdominal musculature, making this maneuver necessary. The normal cough is made up of three parts (1) the ability to take a deep breath, (2) the ability to close the respiratory system by contracting the vocal cords, and (3) the ability to build up the pressure in the thorax and push the air out forcefully by using abdominal and internal intercostal muscle contraction. The SCI patient's ability to do the first, as well as the third, part of a normal cough is usually absent or limited. Therefore, breathing exercises, use of the incentive spirometer, and ventilatory muscle training are all part of assisting or enhancing the effectiveness of the cough effort. Quickly delivering a deep breath using a ventilator or a bagging maneuver just prior to the cough effort is another way of enhancing the cough. The larger the volume of air captured within the lungs the faster the expiratory flow rates, due to the lung's natural recoil, and so the more effective the cough.

To compensate for the lack of the abdominal musculature and internal intercostals, a variety of different mechanical techniques can be employed. The two most effective and commonly used abdominal assist techniques are described. Both have advantages and disadvantages and can be modified in a variety of ways to meet specific needs.

The more commonly performed technique positions the patient supine with the head of the bed flat. The therapist's hands are placed flat against the upper abdomen in midline directly below the xiphoid process. The patient is instructed to take a deep breath in and the therapist allows his or her own hands to rest on the upper abdomen as the diaphragm descends and the abdomen protrudes. Then the patient is instructed to cough out two or three times. With each cough effort pressure is applied in and upward. The

therapist uses locked elbows to generate sufficient abdominal pressure. The patient is asked to cough two times in quick succession off a single breath because this type of staged coughing has been shown to be more effective in clearing secretions.—This maneuver is very much like the Heimlich maneuver used with choking victims.—The advantages of this maneuver are that it is easy to perform and teach, it can be done safely even with an unstable spine, and it does increase the efficiency of the cough. The disadvantages are that it decreases the thoracic volume in only the vertical diameter, and it cannot be performed over recent abdominal wounds.

The second way of supplying external support for a cough utilizes the principles of proprioceptive neuromuscular facilitation (PNF). The patient is positioned sidelying with the head of the bed flat. On inspiration, the patient's shoulder is rotated forward and the patient's hip back in order to stretch the upper hemithorax and to facilitate a deep breath. At the end of a deep inspiration the patient is instructed to cough two or three times; simultaneously, the thorax is derotated and the shoulder and hip approximated quickly via two or three manual pushes to facilitate the cough. This decreases the thoracic volume in all three planes of motion and significantly increases the expiratory flow rate, thereby making the cough effort more effective. The advantages of this maneuver are that it facilitates a deep breath by stretching the rib cage on inspiration; it decreases the thoracic volume in all three diameters, vertical, transverse, and anteroposterior; and it can be performed on patients with abdominal wounds. The disadvantages are that it takes more skill and practice to perform and, because of the quick derotation of the thorax, cannot be used with an unstable spine. If a patient can tolerate both assisted coughing maneuvers, the second almost always results in the more productive cough.

Chest Wall Mobilization

Chest wall mobility is decreased in SCI patients with paralysis of chest wall musculature (T9 and above). This decreased mobility of the chest wall makes it harder to expand during inspiration and therefore increases the work of breathing. Mobilization of the chest wall can be accomplished in a number of ways both actively and passively. The patient should be taught at least one active way in which to stretch the chest wall. Active maneuvers include any patient activity that spreads the ribs, including air shift maneuvers and GPB. Two examples of functional activities that were designed for a completely different purpose, but which also serve to increase chest wall mobility are rolling with the arms used as a pendulum and exaggerated side-to-side leans (in a wheelchair) for pressure relief. An air shift maneuver combines a diaphragmatic breath with breath holding. The patient inhales a deep diaphragmatic breath, closes the glottis, and then relaxes the diaphragm. In the supine position with the diaphragm relaxed, gravity compresses the abdominal contents and pushes the diaphragm upwards. This displaces the diaphragmatic breath upward in the lungs and expands the upper thorax. The patient then opens the glottis and exhales. GPB is discussed in the next section.

Passive maneuvers to promote chest wall mobility are positioning, trunk rotation, and pectoral stretching. Sidelying positioning over three to four pillows allows the upper hemithorax a prolonged static stretch, which can be especially helpful if the patient has spasticity in the trunk. Rotation through the trunk as in assisted/resisted rolling or using counter rotation of the shoulder girdle and hip girdle are effective chest mobility exercises. Manual stretching of the pectorals is important to keep the anterior upper chest mobile. Usually a variety of chest wall mobilization techniques should be used for the best results.

Glossopharyngeal Breathing (GPB)

Glossopharyngeal breathing is a specialized breathing technique that can enhance ventilation when there is paralysis of the respiratory muscles. It uses a series of mechanical actions of the lips, tongue, soft palate, pharyngeal and laryngeal muscles to trap and force air into the lungs. This technique is most commonly associated with polio patients but can be useful with quadriplegic patients. When this technique is mastered, the quadriplegic patient gains the following:

1. The ability to sigh, which helps maintain lung compliance and decrease atelectasis;
2. The ability to stretch the chest wall periodically so the work of breathing is not increased;
3. Increased ability to cough and to clear secretions due to the increased volume of air in the chest, which decreases the risk of respiratory infection;

4. Limited ability to maintain adequate ventilation independently in ventilator-dependent patients (which can be critical in a power or equipment failure);
5. Increased speaking volume; and
6. Increased exercise tolerance before dyspnea, which increases the ability to participate in physical and social activities.

Although the benefits can be great, certain requirements must be met before GPB is even attempted. The patient must have voluntary control over the soft palate, tongue, lips, pharyngeal and laryngeal muscles; have the fifth, seventh, ninth, tenth, eleventh, and twelfth cranial nerves intact; be medically stable with no chronic pulmonary disease or acute pulmonary infection; (if a tracheostomy tube has been placed) have a fenestrated, cuffed tracheostomy tube that can be tightly plugged; be able to tolerate being disconnected from the ventilator for 30 seconds or more; be able to follow directions; and be highly motivated to learn the technique.

If the above requirements are met and GPB would be beneficial, then a specific evaluation is undertaken to determine the patient's ability to use the mouth and throat musculature for positive pressure breathing. The steps of the GPB stroke are explained in Table 1. These steps are repeated for each stroke, and usually 10 to 14 strokes make up a GPB breath. After several strokes, there will be feeling of fullness in the chest, the mouth is then opened, and the patient passively exhales.

Learning GPB requires patience and commitment from both the therapist and the patient. Patients have been known to learn the technique in a single session, but the average amount of time needed to learn and perfect GPB is 2 to 3 months. Treatment is begun in a comfortable supine position with the head, neck, and shoulders supported. If the patient is ventilator dependent, the first phase of treatment is to wean the patient from the ventilator. The patient must be able to stay relaxed while off the ventilator 30 to 60 seconds. It may take several sessions to build up endurance, confidence, and trust so that this can be accomplished. Next the patient practises breath control,

TABLE 1   Steps in the GPB Stroke

Step 1	Open the mouth and depress the back of the tongue to the floor of the mouth as in a sucking motion. The pharyngeal space is increased, the floor of the mouth and larynx are depressed, and the glottis remains closed.
Step 2	Close the lips and raise the soft palate to trap the air in the mouth and pharynx. The larynx remains closed.
Step 3	Push the tongue up and backward toward the soft palate in a rolling motion while making a squeezing motion in the throat and opening the larynx. This pushes the air from the mouth and pharynx through the open glottis and into the lungs.
Step 4	Hold the air in the lungs as you would hold your breath with your mouth open. This closes the glottis so the air pumped into the lung cannot escape.

holding his breath with an open mouth. Any movement, which is needed for the GPB stroke, that the physical therapist assesses as weak, can be strengthened by having the patient make certain sounds or mimic mouth and laryngeal movements performed by the therapist. When this has been accomplished, the patient is taught the GPB stroke. This is usually taught by mimicry with the therapist performing the stroke and then the patient. GPB stroking can also be taught step by step but this is slower and can be confusing.

During this treatment phase close observation and feedback by the therapist is essential. Once the patient can demonstrate GPB stroking, the technique has been mastered. However, it is still important for the patient to practise so that rhythm can be established and endurance can be increased.

To make the GPB teaching sessions as successful as possible, try to schedule them early in the day for short periods of time so that the patient is alert and can concentrate. Treatments should not follow meals or strenuous activity. Patients who are totally ventilator dependent can usually add 500 percent to their FVC using GPB. Patients who use GPB to lengthen the time they are independent from the ventilator can usually add 300 percent to their FVC, whereas those who use GPB only for cough and chest wall stretching can usually add 100 percent to their FVC.

Certain precautions need to be taken when teaching GPB or when having patients practise this breathing technique independently. Patients using GPB do raise their intrapleural pressure thus producing a Valsalva effect. Venous blood return is diminished and therefore cardiac output is decreased. This can cause a discernible drop in arterial and pulse pressures. These effects can put undue stress on a patient who is in heart failure and can also cause autonomic dysreflexia by increasing arterial hypertension for short periods following the Valsalva effect. To minimize these effects the total volume of the GPB strokes for a single breath should be limited to one liter. Higher volumes should be used only occasionally for chest stretching and coughing. As the patient becomes adept at GPB, he may report some light-headedness or dizziness when practising the technique to build endurance, this is due to hyperventilation and can be controlled by resting or by decreasing the GPB volumes.

Discourage Smoking

Smoking is a serious health hazard for everyone. It is linked with lung cancer, emphysema, chronic bronchitis, stroke, heart disease, increased respiratory infections, and low birth weights. These effects of smoking take some time to manifest themselves; nevertheless they are just as pronounced in the SCI population as in the normal population. However, the immediate effects of smoking, which can be tolerated

fairly well in a healthy individual, can significantly compromise the respiratory function of a SCI patient, who is already prone to increased respiratory infection, whose work of breathing is increased, and whose pulmonary reserves are decreased.

With a single inhalation of cigarette smoke, airway resistance is increased 200 to 300 percent, thereby increasing the work of breathing. Cigarette smoke damages the cilia so their rhythmic beat becomes discontinuous, thus decreasing the efficiency of this lung clearance mechanism. SCI patients have decreased cough efficiency so impairment of the cilia increases the likelihood of repeated respiratory infections. Cigarette smoke is irritating to the bronchial mucosa, which results in mucus gland hypertrophy and increased mucus production. In SCI patients, clearing secretions is difficult and having more secretions to clear only compounds the problem. Smoking also causes a decrease in the FVC (which is already significantly decreased due to paralysis of the chest wall musculature); and impairs inspired gas distribution causing ventilation/perfusion disturbances that further contribute to hypoventilation hypoxia problems. Because of these concerns all members of the rehabilitation team should actively discourage cigarette smoking; it should not be allowed in any of the treatment areas or common patient areas because of its harmful effects to the smoker and, via second-hand smoke, to others in the area.

Patient and Family Education

The patient and family are involved in the pulmonary portion of the treatment program throughout rehabilitation. All SCI patients and their caregivers are taught the signs and symptoms of pulmonary distress. This includes monitoring fluid intake, temperature, dyspnea, increased respiratory rate or effort, cough and sputum production.

By discharge, the patient should be able to demonstrate all the breathing maneuvers he has been using. This might include diaphragmatic breathing, use of an inspirometer, pursed lip exhalation, use of an inspiratory muscle trainer, weighted diaphragmatic resistive exercises, GPB, or if innervated, strengthening exercises for the intercostals and abdominals. If the patient uses an abdominal binder, the caregiver must be able to apply it correctly. Any SCI patients with a cervical injury and their caregivers should be taught postural drainage and percussion, whether it was used during their rehabilitation or not (i.e., when to utilize the technique and how to perform it). For SCI patients with thoracic or lumbar injuries this bronchial hygiene technique is taught if it was used during rehabilitation or if there is a positive pulmonary history.

Assisted coughing is taught to all patients lacking

abdominal strength. Upon discharge the patient should be able to demonstrate and use at least one active chest wall mobilization technique. In addition, the caregiver should be able to demonstrate one passive chest wall mobilization technique. The importance of vigilance in assessing the pulmonary status and consistency in carrying out the pulmonary portion of the home program should be stressed and written instructions should be provided.

SUGGESTED READING

Alvarez SE, Peterson M, Lunsford BR. Respiratory treatment of the adult patient with spinal cord injury. Phys Ther 1981; 61:1737–1745.

Axen K, Pineda H, Shunfenthal I, et al. Diaphragmatic function following cervical cord injury: neurally mediated improvement. Arch Phys Med Rehabil 1985; 66:219–222.

Belman MJ, Sieck GC. The ventilatory muscles: fatigue, endurance and training. Chest 1982; 82:761–766.

Clough P, Lindenauer D, Hayes M, et al. Guidelines for routine respiratory care of patients with spinal cord injury. Phys Ther 1986; 66:1395–1402.

DeTroyer A, Heilborn A. Respiratory mechanics in quadriplegia: the respiratory function of the intercostal muscles. Am Rev Respir Dis 1980; 122:591–600.

Fugl-Meyer AR, Grimby G. Respiration in tetraplegia and in hemiplegia: a review. Int Rehabil Med 1984; 6:186–190.

Gross D, Ladd HW, Riley EJ, et al. The effect of training on strength and endurance of the diaphragm in quadriplegia. Am J Med 1980; 68:27–35.

Hornstein S, Ledsome JR. Ventilatory muscle training in acute quadriplegia. Physiother Can 1986; 38:145–149.

Montero JC, Feldman DJ, Montero D. Effects of glossopharyngeal breathing on respiratory function after cervical cord transection. Arch Phys Med Rehabil 1967; 48:650–653.

Sobush D, Dunning M III, McDonald K. Exercise prescription components for respiratory muscle training: past, present, and future. Respir Care 1985; 30:34–42.

VENTILATORY MUSCLE TRAINING

BRENDA M. LOVERIDGE, B.P.T., M.Sc., Ph.D.
SHAYNA HORNSTEIN, B.Sc., P.T.

Ventilatory muscle endurance training (VMT) is being incorporated into rehabilitation programs for cervical cord injured individuals and, although a clear understanding of the effects is still being defined through research, sufficient evidence exists to support the application of VMT with this population. Loss of function of intercostal and abdominal muscles accounts for part of the reduction in vital capacity observed in quadriplegics. Many quadriplegics tend to have a decreased tidal volume and an increased frequency of breathing compared to normal individuals. However, many patients are able to maintain normal blood gases following the acute postinjury period. Microatelectasis is present in the basal segments of the lung in many high level quadriplegics and is thought to persist indefinitely.

Weak skeletal muscles tire more readily than muscles of normal strength, and it has been suggested that respiratory muscle weakness and subsequent fatigue may contribute to the general fatigue, dyspnea, exercise intolerance, and possibly the respiratory complications observed in quadriplegics. Respiratory complications are of particular concern in high cervical cord injured patients as such complications are still a frequent cause of acute respiratory failure and death. It is not unreasonable to assume that respiratory muscle weakness may be a factor contributing to this failure. Whereas a direct connection between respiratory muscle fatigue and respiratory failure has not been proven in quadriplegics, any improvement in respiratory muscle function through training may minimize the effects of fatigue and perhaps provide such patients with more reserve than they would otherwise have had in the face of respiratory infections.

It has been demonstrated that the strength and endurance of the ventilatory muscles in quadriplegics can be improved with training. However, little objective evidence exists in the literature to demonstrate the effects these improvements have on ventilation or exercise performance. Subjective improvements have been reported following training such as being able to sit for longer periods of time before becoming fatigued, having "more energy" and less shortness of breath in all activities, experiencing improved sleep, and feeling that their breathing is "easier." Recently, in a study with chronic stable C6 and C7 quadriplegics with complete motor loss, we observed a trend towards an increased resting tidal volume, decreased frequency of breathing and altered inspiratory timing mechanism following increases in strength and endurance of the respiratory muscles. It appears that some quadriplegics tend to spend a longer time during inspiration (Ti) relative to total time (Ttot) during each breathing cycle. It has been shown in normal subjects that a prolonged Ti/Ttot predisposes the ventilatory muscles to fatigue. It has been postulated that this occurs because the inspiratory muscles are contracted for a longer period of time than they have to relax during each breathing cycle, thereby resulting in insufficient time for relaxation and recovery of the diaphragm. The presence of a prolonged Ti/Ttot in quadriplegics suggests that these individuals may be predisposed to fatigue as demonstrated in normal subjects. The fact that the Ti/Ttot decreased towards normal following endurance training, coupled with the changes in tidal volume and frequency, suggest that such training may induce positive effects on resting ventilation in quadriplegics. The subjective improvements reported by this group may indeed reflect an objective change in breathing pattern. However, more studies in larger populations are needed to confirm these findings. Though inconclusive, current evidence suggests significant improvements in ventilation and in performance of activities of daily living in quadriplegics following ventilatory muscle endurance training.

It has been demonstrated that upper limb endurance training can improve ventilatory muscle performance in populations other than quadriplegics; however, there is no data to support this hypothesis for quadriplegics. It must also be kept in mind that many quadriplegics have limited intact upper limb musculature; therefore, even if upper limb training may produce improvement in the ventilatory muscles, the effect may be smaller in quadriplegics than has been found in other groups.

PATIENT ASSESSMENT

Cardiorespiratory History

1. Ensure that the patient is medically stable before initiating testing and training and that this treatment is approved by the patient's physician. Do not institute testing in patients with known coronary ar-

tery disease, or in patients over the age of 35 without a resting electrocardiogram (ECG). If the patient is receiving supplemental oxygen, yet is otherwise medically stable, oxygen must be incorporated into the inspiratory side of the testing and training valve using additional tubing. Ventilatory muscle endurance testing and training appears to be a relatively safe technique, and no untoward signs and symptoms are usually observed.

2. Include preinjury cardiac and respiratory history.

3. Assess lesion level, complete or incomplete motor and sensory loss.

4. Note level of functional activity. (Distance wheeled in 3 minutes can be used as a measure of function). Quantify activities of daily living that result in shortness of breath (SOB) (e.g., SOB while eating, talking, wheeling). Measure length of time spent sitting before undue fatigue is felt.

5. Measure forced vital capacity (FVC), forced expiratory volume (FEV) 1.0, and inspiratory capacity (IC).

Inspiratory Muscle Strength Testing

Maximum inspiratory mouth pressure (MIP) is the clinical index used to assess ventilatory muscle strength. While MIP is greatest in individuals when measured at residual volume (RV), part of the pressure recorded reflects elastic recoil of lungs. Also, it is difficult to assess whether an individual is at RV each time you repeat the measurement. MIP is best measured at functional residual capacity (FRC) where the pressure generated better reflects the action of the inspiratory muscles alone. The correlation between vital capacity and MIP is a weak one. A relatively normal vital capacity may be found in some quadriplegics despite a marked decrease in ventilatory muscle strength and endurance. For this reason, it is important to measure ventilatory muscle strength and endurance independently, and not to rely on vital capacity as the sole indicator of respiratory muscle weakness.

To measure MIP, the patient wears nose clips and breathes in and out of a mouthpiece connected to a pressure manometer with a Y connecter open to room air. At the end of a normal breath, the room air con-

nector is blocked and the patient is instructed to pull in as hard as possible, thereby generating a negative pressure. Ideally, there should be a small air leak in the system, during the generation of inspiratory pressure, to prevent patients from sucking in their cheeks and producing an artificially higher pressure as a result of this maneuver than is reflected by the strength of the inspiratory muscles. As this is an effort-dependent measurement, it must be repeated until three measurements within 5 percent of each other are recorded. MIP is the average of these three best efforts.

It is important to record the position in which the measurement was made and to retest the patient in the same position to document improvements in MIP. Quadriplegics can usually generate higher pressures in the supine position, particularly in the earlier phases post injury. In sitting, the diaphragm cannot function as effectively as a result of the loss of intercostal and abdominal muscles. In supine, these effects are not as detrimental since the abdominal contents can still exert a positive effect on diaphragm action. For example, a patient 2 to 3 months post injury may generate a pressure of -60 cm H_2O in supine, but only be able to generate a pressure of -40 cm H_2O in the sitting posture.

The range of inspiratory pressures found in quadriplegics is quite variable, but generally individuals with higher cervical cord injuries generate less inspiratory pressure than those with lower cervical cord injuries due to direct weakness of the diaphragm (Table 1). However, even in quadriplegics with lesions at the same level, quite large differences in pressures can be observed.

It is clear that some quadriplegics demonstrate considerable muscle weakness even 1 year post injury, whereas others appear to maintain a relatively normal MIP. There are no data following patients prospectively post injury to ascertain if there are any factors in common between patients with low or higher pressures. The highest inspiratory pressures were observed in competitive wheelchair trained athletes.

Inspiratory Muscle Endurance Testing

There are almost as many different approaches to measuring ventilatory muscle endurance as there

TABLE 1 Maximum Inspiratory Mouth Pressures (at FRC) Recorded in Patients with Complete Motor Loss Following Traumatic Cervical Cord Injury

Time Post Injury	Position	Range of Pressures ($-cm\ H_2O$)
2 to 4 weeks	supine	20 to 40
<1 year	sitting	20 to 90
>1 year	sitting	40 to 110
Normal males	sitting	110 ± 31

are research articles on the subject. Ventilatory muscle endurance is a measure of the resistance against which the patient can breathe for a given period of time. It is important that the technique be safe, clinically easy to administer, and provide an index of endurance that can plot patient improvement. Without an index to measure improvement, compliance to training regimes is a much more difficult task.

In keeping with these points the following is a suggested format for testing endurance with quadriplegics:

1. To ensure comfort and improve compliance, pad the nose clip and select a mouthpiece that is comfortable for the individual.

2. Monitor responses during the test, i.e., ECG and subjective symptoms. Heart rate should not increase more than 20 beats above resting, no arrhythmias should develop. There should be no undue fatigue, dizziness, or lightheadedness (which may suggest CO_2 retention). Any of these findings suggest that this resistor is too difficult for the patient.

3. Record MIP.

4. Prior to resistor selection, spend the first two sessions having the patient breathe through the device with a negligible resistance to allow time for familiarization with the technique and adjustment to breathing through a mouthpiece.

5. Select a resistor that requires the generation of a pressure equal to approximately 50 percent MIP or one that is challenging for 5 to 10 minutes. For example, if a patient can only generate ± 20 cm H_2O, a resistor with a 5 mm diameter may be all that the patient can tolerate for the first few days of training.

6. Have the patient wear noseclips and breathe through the resistor for 5 minutes followed by a 10 minute rest.

7. In the absence of any untoward signs and symptoms, repeat the test having the patient breathe against an increasingly difficult resistor for 5 minutes interspersed with 10 minute rests, up to a resistance no greater than 80 percent MIP. In patients early post injury, two or three sessions may be required to determine endurance accurately.

8. Record the highest resistance the patient can breathe against comfortably for 5 minutes without any untoward signs or symptoms. This provides a baseline measurement of endurance and also identifies the resistor to use for the initial training sessions.

ENDURANCE TRAINING

The intensity, frequency, and duration of training required to produce significant improvements in inspiratory muscle strength and endurance is unclear. Improvement has been observed in both frequent low intensity, and infrequent, high intensity protocols with

stable chronic quadriplegics. It is important that the individual does not progress too quickly as inspiratory muscle fatigue may be induced. The adverse consequences of chronic fatigue in quadriplegics are not clear and must be avoided. Consequently, the safest training regime at the present time is one that uses an interval training format. It is also the format with which the greatest degree of compliance is achieved. Breathing against a resistance is often viewed as boring, and during longer exercise protocols (15 minutes of continuous exercise) quadriplegics complain of increased saliva formation, which necessitates frequent swallowing, aching of the jaw, from holding the mouthpiece in place; and individuals with chronic sinus drainage complain of a feeling of gagging, caused by secretions that drain better during these maneuvers than normally. In contrast, 5-minute exercise sessions interspersed with short rests are better tolerated. Interval-training formats have proven successful in other skeletal muscle training regimes and seem particularly suited to training the ventilatory muscles, as they both minimize fatigue and other negative side effects experienced when these exercises are performed.

The training resistor should be the highest resistor that the individual can breathe against comfortably for 5 minutes during the testing procedure. Underestimate rather than overestimate the training program in the early stages. Instruct the subjects to breathe at their own rate and depth. It has been suggested that a fixed breathing pattern may result in more effective training, but to date the data are not sufficient enough to provide specific guidelines. Watch for the same signs and symptoms as stated in the testing format and decrease the training resistor if any of these signs appear. Training should be discontinued or the resistance decreased if the patient is suffering from any acute infections.

Suggested Guidelines for Endurance Training

Zero to 3 Months Post Injury

Begin with 5 to 10 minutes of exercise a minimum of twice daily, including a 2-minute rest after each 5-minute interval. Retest MIP and endurance every 2 to 3 weeks to establish a new training resistance and to plot improvement. Progress to 15 minutes of exercise twice daily when two 10-minute sessions have been well tolerated for at least 2 weeks. Maintain an interval training protocol with 5 minutes of exercise followed by 2 minutes of rest. In some patients, an increased resistance requires a decrease in exercise time for the first few sessions.

Do not allow progression until breathing is comfortably tolerated at each stage. Do not increase the resistor, the exercise time, nor the position of training simultaneously.

Three to 6 Months Post Injury

Ensure that once there is progression from training in a supine position to training in a sitting position there is a retest to establish a new training resistance. MIP is less for most patients initially in the sitting position and a lower training resistance is frequently required. Continue with two 10-minute sessions daily until this is well tolerated in the sitting position. Then progress to 15-minute exercise sessions continuing with an interval training rotation of 3 to 5 minutes of exercise followed by 2 minutes of rest. Decrease the training frequency to 5 times per week when the patient has progressed to 15-minute exercise sessions.

Maintenance Program

Prior to discharge, reassess the individual in accordance with the guidelines listed earlier. Instruct the patient in a maintenance program and where possible, have them attend for follow-up assessments at 3-monthly intervals for the first year post injury. The frequency and duration for maintenance programs has yet to be determined; however, 15 minutes once daily, 3 to 4 days per week is in accordance with other skeletal muscle training regimes and is a reasonable starting point for a maintenance program. The follow-up assessments provide the opportunity to ensure that the gains achieved during the initial training program are being maintained. If losses in ventilatory muscle strength and endurance are occurring, the patient will become aware of increased difficulty with the training resistor.

SUGGESTED READING

Gross D, Ladd HW, Riley EJ, Macklem PT, Grassino A. The effect of training on strength and endurance of the diaphragm in quadriplegia. Am J Med 1980; 68:27–35.

Hornstein S, Ledsome JR. Ventilatory muscle training in acute quadriplegia. Physiother Can 1986; 38(3):145–149.

Ledsome JR, Sharp JM. Pulmonary function in acute cervical spinal cord injury. Am Rev Resp Dis 1981; 124:41–44.

Loveridge B, Badour M, Dubo H, Younes M. Ventilatory muscle endurance training in quadriplegia: effects on breathing pattern. Am Rev Resp Dis 1986; 135(Suppl 5):A193.

McKinley AC, Auchincloss JH Jr, Gilbert R, Nicholas JJ. Pulmonary function, ventilatory control and respiratory complications in quadriplegic subjects. Am Rev Resp Dis 1969; 100:526–532.

INSPIRATORY MUSCLE TRAINING: AN ADJUNCT TO WEANING

LORETTA L. LANGIS, B.Sc., P.T.
CATHERINE ANDERSON, B.Sc., B.H.Sc. (PT)

Patients in intensive care provide physical therapists with many challenges. Since precursors to intensive care admissions can range from trauma, organ system failure, and sepsis to neurologic compromise and organ transplantation, the complexity of problems and the length of stay can vary greatly. Mechanical ventilation is frequently required and may need to be maintained for prolonged periods of time while the underlying pathology is the focus of management.

When the need for mechanical ventilation appears no longer necessary, it has been our experience that approximately 3 to 5 percent of intensive care patients do not wean from the ventilator by popular conventional methods. It is believed that in these patients the respiratory muscles have become weakened and/or fatigued and cannot tolerate the sustained repetitive task of breathing. The cause of this weakness or fatigue can be one or a combination of the following factors: prolonged increased work of breathing, inadequate nutrition, catabolic nutritive states, and disuse atrophy secondary to the ventilation itself. It would follow that some form of program specifically designed to increase the strength and endurance of the respiratory muscles would be of benefit.

Although a paucity of literature exists with specific reference to training of the inspiratory muscles of ventilatory-dependent patients, the similarity in composition between respiratory muscles and skeletal muscles makes the application of sound skeletal muscle training principles to respiratory muscles both feasible and pragmatic. In the training program, which is outlined in this chapter, we have striven to combine current knowledge of respiratory muscle physiology with exercise physiology to gain a maximal training effect. The results that would be expected, and which have been obtained, are increased strength and endurance of inspiratory muscles with eventual weaning from ventilatory dependence.

CRITERIA FOR SELECTION OF PATIENTS

Criteria for patient selection include the following:

1. The patient must demonstrate an inability to wean from mechanical ventilation by popular conventional* means.
2. The patient must be reasonably free from sepsis (i.e., white blood cell count within normal limits, negative blood cultures, normal temperature and carbon dioxide production—V_{CO_2}).
3. The patient must be hemodynamically stable.
4. Nutritional level must be adequate to meet metabolic demands.
5. The patient should be free from acute pulmonary infection.
6. Electrolytes should be within normal ranges (specifically, inorganic phosphate, magnesium and calcium).

DESCRIPTION OF TECHNIQUE

Apparatus

Figure 1 illustrates the apparatus used for training. The trainer consists of pediatric endotracheal tube connectors (varying in size from 3.5–7.0 mm) and 2 plastic ventilator connectors 15 and 22 mm. The ventilator with training and monitoring equipment consists of a manometer (for measuring tidal volumes) in line close to trach connector; a trainer—connected in the inspiratory limb of the ventilator close to the "Y"; a one way flow valve—connected in the expiratory limb of the ventilator close to the "Y"; (the ventilator used for clinical trials is the Monaghan: trainer may be adapted for use with other ventilator types).

Baseline Measurements

These measurements include the following:

1. Respiratory rate
2. Tidal volume
3. Minute volume
4. Peak negative inspiratory pressure (PNIP)
5. Pattern of breathing
6. Dyspnea
7. Heart rate
8. Blood pressure
9. Electromyography of diaphragm (optional).

---

* Although different institutions have preferred methods of weaning patients, most will try various means, (such as the intermittent mandatory ventilation route or trial-by-fire), before determining a patient is ventilatory dependent.

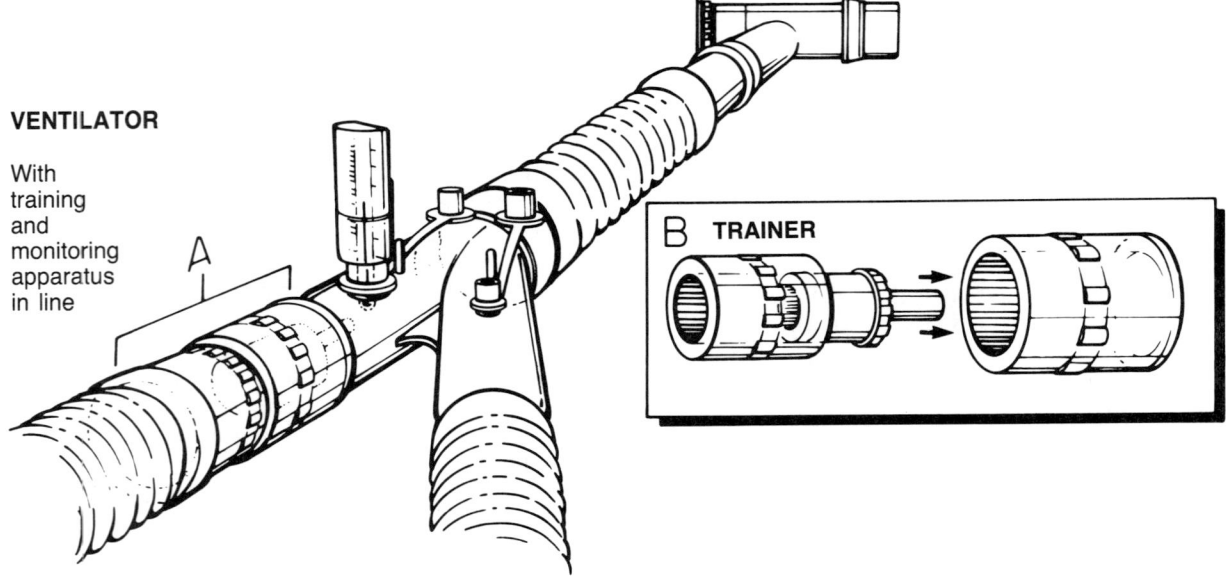

Figure 1 Apparatus used for inspiratory muscle training: *A*, Ventilator with training and monitoring apparatus in line; *B*, Trainer.

Training Technique

Prior to initiating training the patient should have 24 to 48 hours of full respiratory rest.

Night rest is essential to the training program. The patient must be placed on intermittent mandatory ventilation (IMV) during the evening (2200 to 0600 hours) such that virtually no spontaneous respirations occur.

During the day, the patient should be placed on intermittent mandatory ventilation such that the spontaneous respirations are 30 breaths per minute (bpm) or less.

The training session should begin by collection and analysis of the baseline measurements (listed previously). Throughout the training session careful monitoring of these parameters is essential as respiratory muscle fatigue should be avoided.

The resistor, one-way flow valve, the manometer should be placed in the ventilator circuit, as outlined in the Apparatus section (see Fig. IA), and the patient placed on continuous positive airway pressure (CPAP) (if previously on positive end expiratory pressure [PEEP] while being ventilated). Training continues for up to 15 minutes or until one of the criteria for stopping treatment has been met.

Criteria for Stopping Treatment

Criteria for stopping treatment include observation of the following:

1. persistent or extreme shortness of breath;
2. paradoxical breathing pattern or abdominal bounce;
3. respiratory rate greater than forty bpm in conjunction with other clinical findings (such as dyspnea and increased blood pressure);
4. blood pressure above acceptable limits for the individual patient; or
5. fifteen minute time interval up.

Progression of Training and Weaning

When the patient is able to train for 15 minutes twice a day for 1 to 2 days without the criteria for stopping (except time interval) having been met, the resistor size in the trainer should be changed.

The lumen of the resistor can be decreased 0.5 to 1.0 mm as tolerance indicates (i.e., resistor changed from a 6.0 mm to a 5.0 mm endotracheal tube connector).

As strength and endurance increases, the IMV required to maintain a daily respiratory rate less than 30 bpm should decrease.

When the patient has progressed to the stage of being able to maintain respiratory rate during the day at less than thirty on CPAP or T-piece then the evening rest periods can be gradually shortened. When breathing has been spontaneous for 48 hours without any difficulties, the patient is ready to be placed on oxygen mask or tracheostomy mask.

MECHANISM OF ACTION AND ANTICIPATED RESULTS

As with any exercise program designed to increase the strength and endurance of a group of muscles, this inspiratory muscle training program requires that the inspiratory muscles contract against a load (i.e., the inspiratory resistor) for a number of repetitions (i.e., breaths). As with skeletal muscles, the breathing muscles become adapted over time to cope better with the increased work added to the system. On a cellular basis, this adaptation may include the following muscle changes: increased capillary density, increased size and number of muscle cell mitochondria, increased mitochondrial enzymes, increased concentration of glycogen, and increased proportion of fatigue-resistant fiber type. On a larger, more clinical scale this adaptation may include: increased peak negative inspiratory force, increased tidal volumes and vital capacity, increased endurance, and decreased cardiovascular requirement for the same breathing effort.

The end result of the program is an individual whose inspiratory muscles have been maximized such that they are able to sustain respiration without the assistance of mechanical ventilation, and as such patients are able to cope with natural increases in work, such as are caused by chest infection, without undue fatigue.

Case Study (Example)

Mrs. M. a 78-year-old female was admitted to hospital for investigation of an abdominal mass. After major debulking surgery to remove the tumor, Mrs. M. was admitted to intensive care for management of respiratory distress. Past medical history includes inactive tuberculosis, which left the right upper and left lower lobes of her lungs scarred and nonfunctional, and congestive heart failure with frequent bouts of pulmonary edema.

After 4 weeks of intensive care management (complicated by sepsis), it became apparent that Mrs. M. was ventilatory dependent and was not going to wean by conventional means. Respiratory muscle training was initiated.

Treatment Regimen

DAY 1
IMV6 during the day—respiratory rate 30 bpm
IMV14 overnight (2000 to 0600 hours)—no spontaneous respirations

Training—6.0 mm resistor
4 minutes × 2
Reasons for stopping
1. Shortness of breath

2. Increased blood pressure
3. Increased respiratory rate

PNIP—8 cm H_2O

DAY 10
IMV5 during the day—respiratory rate 28 to 30 bpm
IMV12 overnight—no spontaneous respirations

Training—6.0 mm resistor
15 minutes × 2
Reason for stopping
1. Time interval

PNIP—12 cm H_2O

DAY 11
IMV5 during the day—respiratory rate as on day 10
IMV12 overnight—respiratory rate as on day 10

Training—5.0 mm resistor
6 minutes × 2
Reasons for stopping
1. As on day 1

PNIP—14 cm H_2O

DAY 15
IMV4 during the day—respiratory rate 24 to 28 bpm
IMV10 overnight—no spontaneous respirations
Training—5.0 mm resistor
15 minutes × 2
Reason for stopping
1. Time interval

PNIP—18 cm H_2O

DAY 16
IMV4 during the day—respiratory rate as on day 15
IMV10 overnight—respiratory rate as on day 15

Training—4.5 mm resistor
5 minutes × 2
Reasons for stopping
1. As on day 1

PNIP—18 cm H_2O

DAY 20
IMV2 during the day—respiratory rate 24 to 18 bpm
IMV8 during the evening—occasional spontaneous respiration

Training—4.5 mm resistor
15 minutes × 2
Reason for stopping
1. Time interval

PNIP—-22 cm H_2O

DAY 22
CPAP5 during the day—respiratory rate 24 to 28 bpm
IMV6 during the evening

Training—4.5 mm resistor

15 minutes × 2
Reason for stopping
1. Time interval

PNIP——−28 cm H_2O

DAY 26
CPAP5 during the day and evening respiratory rate
24 to 28 bpm

No training

PNIP——−30 cm H_2O

DAY 28
Mrs. M. weaned from ventilator put on tracheostomy mask
—respiratory rate 22 to 26 bpm

PNIP——−32 cm H_2O

SUGGESTED READING

Braun N. Respiratory muscle dysfunction. Heart Lung 1984; 13(4): 327–332.

Gross D, et al. The effect of training on strength and endurance of the diaphragm in quadriplegics. Am J Med 1980; 68:27–35.

Keens TG, Chen V. Cellular adaptations of the ventilatory muscles to chronic increases in respiratory load. J Appl Physiol 1978; 44:905–908.

Kim MJ. Respiratory muscle training: implications for patient care. Heart Lung 1984; 13(4):333–339.

Leith DE, Bradley M. Ventilatory muscle strength and endurance training. J Appl Physiol 1973; 41:508–516.

Macklem PT. Respiratory muscles: the vital pump. Chest 1980; 78: 753–758.

IMPORTANCE OF MOBILITY IN CHEST CARE

DEBRA R. SEBURN, B.S.R.

Chest care is incomplete without mobility whether the patient is immediately postoperative, confined to bed, in an intensive care unit or in a long-term care setting. In some cases, taking the person for a walk may be the most effective chest treatment that a therapist has to offer.

In this chapter, "mobility" refers to any physical activity included in the treatment regimen, based on an assessment of the patient's ability and desire to optimize it. Mobility may simply involve active and/or passive range of motion exercises, routine position changes, circulatory bed exercises or transfers. It refers to ambulation and thus involves any of the aids that may be required to accomplish ambulation.

The goal of this chapter is to share an approach to mobility based on observations of its effectiveness; an approach that may be unique to therapists The physiologic basis for mobility in chest care is not to be discussed in detail.

WHY GET PEOPLE MOVING?

The historical impetus to move patients was to prevent or minimize the complications of bed rest. These complications include atelectasis of dependent lobes, deep vein thrombosis, pulmonary emboli, skin ulcers, joint stiffness, contractures, and muscle weakness. Today, given our understanding of the effects of immobilization on all the body systems, positioning and mobility are essential components in chest physical therapy.

Posture has been shown repeatedly to influence pulmonary volume and regional ventilation-perfusion ratios. Also since respiratory excursion is linked to the movement of the ribs and diaphragm, any position that restricts such movement may restrict the capacity of the thorax. Some of the changes that occur in the respiratory system when a normal individual moves from sitting to supine lying include decreased vital capacity, functional residual capacity, residual volume, and FEV_1 closure of the small airways in dependent regions and changes in the pulmonary blood flow distribution. A patient requiring treatment for respiratory disease or postoperative complications may show reduced pulmonary function from airway disease, infection, fear of deep breathing and coughing, or pain. It is clear that a further reduction, attributable to posture or immobility, is not only unnecessary but also potentially harmful.

The sitting position is mechanically favorable for inspiration with less restricted descent of the diaphragm, for expiration, for recruiting the accessory breathing muscles in the shoulder girdles and cervical region, and for generating a more effective cough. Pulmonary function studies confirm that sitting erect (or seated leaning forward for chronic airways limited patients) is the position of choice over supine, prone or the frequently observed half-slumped lying posture. Therefore, patients who are at risk because of low pulmonary capacity should be seated upright as early as possible.

The same principle is extended to patients confined to bed, since routine changes in position affect the ventilation-perfusion ratio to different parts of the lungs and help to decrease any regional defects and the potential for atelectasis. Although regular position changes are required, based on the lung pathology, the therapist may suggest that more time be spent in one position. For example, oxygenation is improved in adults with unilateral pulmonary disease if the patient is placed in sidelying with the normal lung dependent.

Further work has shown conclusively that exercise improves ventilatory muscle function, and increases chest expansion and tidal volume. Activity facilitates secretion removal; it is common for a patient to have a more productive cough following a walk or a change of bed position. At rest, inspiration time equals approximately one half expiration time; these times tend to equalize during exercise. The latter serves to confirm the need for mobility.

Psychological Benefits

The psychological benefits of increased mobility deserve special attention. It is well known, although not understood, that exercise makes a person feel good about themselves and makes them better able to cope with their present situation. Activity promotes relaxation and the potential for increased pain tolerance. With increased activity, both the patient and staff have a sense of accomplishment. The patient receives positive feedback from staff, other patients, and visitors, and is therefore likely perceived as "doing well." It has been noted that on inquiry about a patient's progress the caregiver frequently reports the degree of mobility first. For example "Mr. P. is feeling better today. He sat in the chair twice." Activity is used as an understandable measure of wellness.

The ultimate goal of mobility in chest care is to assist patients to maintain and/or regain maximum performance as soon as they are able. In addition, routine early mobilization may decrease the need for long-term chest treatment.

TIMING

The timing of any treatment, whether it requires active or passive participation, influences the success of the treatment and the cooperation of the patient. The following are elements of timing to consider in mobilizing patients:

1. It is ideal to plan with the patient what the activity will be and when he would like to do it.
2. Consider the time of day when the individual has the most energy and what other things are anticipated during the day. The goal is to provide a balance between rest and activity while progressively increasing activity. For example, walking just after a bath or a meal is not optimal for the debilitated patient.
3. Communication and coordination with other staff is essential to avoid conflicts with other procedures and to ensure that help is available if it is required.
4. Consider the schedule of pain medication to ensure adequate pain control. This is most applicable to intensive care and postoperative patients.
5. Aim to be consistent with the treatment time.
6. Plan the treatment time to derive more psychological benefits and to promote "normalcy." For example, you may plan for someone to be sitting for meals and for visitors.
7. It may be useful to note your intended appointment time on a nursing cardex, in the progress notes, and for long term patients, at the bedside.

MOBILITY ASSESSMENT

The depth and details of the assessment for mobility depend upon history, length of illness, and premorbid ability. It is practical to take a functional approach to mobility unless the therapist anticipates focusing on a specified pathology. The latter requires a more detailed assessment of the specific function or joint. Observation is an important part of the assessment.

Subjective

Review of the chart and discussion with the patient, his family, or nurse is completed to determine level of consciousness and orientation, ability to communicate, premorbid exercise tolerance, and current level of mobility including use of aids. It is useful to know what activity has been done already that day to assess its effect on his tolerance.

Objective

Cardiopulmonary. Pulse, blood pressure, and temperature may be noted on a bedside chart. Blood gas analysis helps to assess the extent of lung pathology, expected exercise tolerance, and need for supplementary oxygen.

Musculoskeletal. To assess range of motion, ask the patient to lift his arms over his head and reach the back of his neck, to flex and extend his knees, hips, and ankles, and to rotate his trunk left and right. This may be done supine (except trunk rotation) or sitting, although sitting allows observation of balance and coordination. Look for stiff, painful, or swollen joints, joint contractures, and soft tissue limitation.

Strength. Assessment can be easily combined with range of motion; assess trunk strength, quadriceps, and gastrocs (in standing). Strength in shoulder depressors, biceps, and triceps is most important when crutches or a walker will be used. Grip strength may be assessed grossly by having the patient squeeze the therapist's hand.

Balance. Assess static and dynamic balance in sitting and standing positions.

This assessment promotes a functional approach to mobility and upon completion the therapist has determined any contraindications to activity, the degree of assistance required (including aids), and current exercise tolerance.

APPROACH: THE ESSENTIAL ELEMENT

The most success may be expected when the treatment is planned to emphasize ability. This planning requires realistic goals and is ideal if the patient can be included in the goal setting. It is important to provide simple, objective measures of progress for the patient and the therapist, such as time sitting, distance walked, pre- and post-activity pulse, and change in respiratory rate.

The energy costs of daily activities to weak and debilitated patients are easily underestimated by healthy individuals. The therapist has a important role not only in encouraging activity but also in regulating it. A chart of the energy costs (in METS) of simple activities of daily living can be a useful and objective teaching tool for both patient, family, and other staff.

Observation is an essential component of treatment; patients who are particularly weak or uncomfortable often develop their own method of moving. Therapists should be open to this and must examine the goals of treatment before recommending change. Safety must always be the first consideration.

TIPS FOR MOBILITY

1. SAFETY FIRST: (a) seek adequate help for the safety of the therapist and the patient; (b) be sure that brakes are applied to bed, wheelchair or commode. When the bed brakes are inadequate, it is best to recruit someone to stabilize it (a towel wrapped around the wheel also provides additional security); (c) plan and clear the intended pathway as much as possible; (d) demonstrate to patients any pieces of furniture, such as overbed tables, which are on castors and do not provide support safely; (e) remove as much equipment from the patient as possible for the walk or transfer—disconnect and unplug feeding lines, nasogastric tubes, and cardiac monitoring. Many patients can be disconnected briefly from a ventilator to facilitate transfer from the bed to the chair if they have an adequate spontaneous respiration rate (usually on an IMV or CPAP circuit with low PEEP); (f) it is useful to be competent in operating any mechanical lifts that are available to you. They may be great energy savers and provide safety in the transfer of heavy, dependent patients who may otherwise be confined to bed; (g) communicate to the nursing staff the tolerance, level of assistance and the aids that a patient requires to mobilize safely.

2. Plan sufficient time to allow the person to do as much as possible alone and encourage them to do so. Advising patients to take their time seems to relieve stress and to improve performance without significantly lengthening the treatment time.

3. Allow the patients enough time to sit at the edge of the bed to orient themselves and regain balance before proceeding to more difficult tasks. Those who are elderly or have been bedridden for longer

periods are more prone to the effects of postural hypotension and thus require more time.

4. "Limb-loading" may be useful for patients who are confused, elderly, or markedly weak. It is suggested that a sustained downward pressure applied at the knees prior to transfer or standing may stimulate a stronger response to weight bearing.

5. Transfers from sitting to standing are facilitated by assisting the patient to move to the edge of the bed or chair and to lean forward to move the center of gravity over the feet before trying to stand upright.

6. Patients with advanced chronic lung disease who are recovering from an acute exacerbation or from surgery may require oxygen in the initial stages of mobility. It is more important that they go for a walk with the oxygen support than remain sedentary without it. This is an example in which the oxygen enables the patient to increase his exercise tolerance without becoming dependent on it.

Mobility is an integral part of chest physical therapy and maximal patient activity requires few supplies. The most important "equipment" is the therapist's approach and focus on the patient's ability. The timing and planning of treatment with ongoing assessment are key factors in its effectiveness. Although skill in assessing ability and prognosis for improvement may become almost instinctive, it is important to retain objective measurements to communicate to the patient, other staff, and colleagues.

SUGGESTED READING

Crosbie WJ, Myles S. An investigation in the effect of postural modification on some aspects of normal pulmonary function. Physiother 1985; 71(7):311–314.

Dean E. Effect of body position on pulmonary function. Phys Ther 1985; 65(5):613–618.

Gillespie DJ, Rehder K. Body position and ventilation—perfusion relationships in unilateral pulmonary disease. Chest 1987; 91(1):75–79.

Grosmaire EK. Use of patient positioning to improve PaO$_2$: a review. Heart Lung 1983; 12:650–653.

PREOPERATIVE AND POSTOPERATIVE CHEST CARE

LINDA M. COUSINS, B.Sc. (PT)
HELEN A. JOHNSON, B.Sc. (PT)

It is well known that respiratory complications can occur following surgery, and "post-op chest physical therapy" is frequently among the routine postoperative orders. In many centers "pre-op" chest physical therapy is also requested. This chapter reviews aspects of pre- and postoperative chest care which we have found effective in our setting.

After surgery, especially that of a thoracic, spinal or high abdominal nature a well documented cycle develops. Incisional pain and fear of moving cause splinting, or inhibition of the depth of breathing. This and other factors can quickly lead to atelectasis, and may progress to or be accompanied by secretion retention and pneumonia. History of smoking, postural or skeletal abnormalities, recurrent lung infections, chronic lung disease, and immobility place patients at increased risk. These respiratory complications can seriously hinder recovery and can even be life threatening, especially in the very young or the elderly. They can also be easily minimized or prevented by preoperative teaching and early postoperative follow-up.

Preoperative contact has proven beneficial in many ways. The patient gains insight into what to expect in the postoperative course and many questions and fears can be answered. The patient becomes familiar with the therapist, thereby enhancing memory and compliance. Similarly the therapist becomes familiar with the patient, thereby improving efficiency and problem-solving postoperatively. The preoperative visit is ideally made the day before surgery. It consists of a brief explanation of the type of incision, various tubes and lines which may be present, pain medications, and the time course of mobilization out of bed. The effects of anesthesia, pain, and immobility on breathing are reviewed to help the patient understand the concept of prevention of complications. Deep breathing techniques are taught and the patient is introduced to incentive spirometry where appropriate. Brief mention may be made of other physical therapy techniques that may be utilized to facilitate depth of breathing and mobilization of secretions. Methods to support the incision during coughing and moving about are demonstrated. The importance of frequent position changes (including alternate sidelying and sitting) is stressed and the patient is encouraged to move all limbs actively through range of motion as appropriate. Finally, a basic chest assessment is performed to screen for presence of preoperative pathology and other risk factors.

Postoperative chest care should begin as soon as possible. There is considerable evidence for atelectasis beginning as early as 1 to 2 hours and peaking at 12 to 24 hours after surgery. Early assessment may detect developing pathology and alert both patient and nursing staff. Gentle manual techniques such as manual pressures, squeezing, and posterior lifts are particularly effective and may be sufficient to improve the breathing pattern in the initial postoperative period. Adequate pain control is of primary importance to allow the patient to cooperate. The main emphasis is on increased depth of breathing, for example by using deep inspirations with 3-second breath hold and on regular change of position in bed. The patients are instructed to use the incentive spirometer for 10 breaths at the appropriate setting every hour that they are awake.

If significant pathology is diagnosed further treatment measures are initiated. These often include manual techniques of a more vigorous nature such as shaking, rib springing, clapping, and percussion. Mechanical vibration, assisted coughing, and suctioning are used as required. According to the nature of the procedure, the patient is assisted in mobilization out of bed by nursing or physical therapy staff as soon as appropriate. Most general surgery patients require follow-up for 2 or 3 days unless serious difficulties are encountered. Cardiac and thoracic surgery patients typically experience a somewhat slower rate of recovery with more complicating factors and require more intensive involvement.

CARDIOVASCULAR SURGERY

Patients undergoing surgery for coronary artery bypass, valve replacement or repair, Wolfe-Parkinson-White (WPW) correction, or other cardiac procedure via median sternotomy have a greater risk of developing respiratory complications and require more physical therapy intervention.

In a retrospective audit of 50 patients in our institution (excluding the WPW procedure) greater than 90 percent were found to have developed some degree of left lower lobe atelectasis postoperatively. Other common complications include pneumonia, pleural effusions and pulmonary edema. In addition, in the immediate postoperative period in the intensive care unit (ICU), and occasionally beyond, hypo- or hypertension and cardiac arrhythmias can be of major concern. These particular factors affect the type and amount of physical therapy treatment that can be carried out. Later problems are often in the area of mobility, with decreased range of motion of the shoulders or knees attributable to painful sternotomy or leg incisions, and limited endurance attributable to cardiac instability or deconditioning.

Preoperatively, the usual teaching is given with regard to prevention of complications, deep breathing and coughing, and the use of the incentive spirometer. Time is also spent presenting the tubes, lines, and monitors, in addition to the general ICU atmosphere and routines, with which the patient is faced upon regaining consciousness. Routine physical therapy follow-up is described including prophylactic use of the mechanical vibrator and manual treatment techniques to the left lower lobe. The provision of this extensive amount of information seems to help alleviate anxiety and to improve cooperation and compliance in the majority of patients in the early postoperative period. Routine bed mobility, foot and ankle exercises, in addition to active or active-assisted hip and knee flexion and unilateral shoulder flexion are taught for use in the immediate postoperative period. The progression of mobility from dangling at the bedside on the first postoperative day, up in a chair on the second, and ambulation from the third day onward is described. Brief mention is also made of the mobility class and of forthcoming preparation for exercise to be done on discharge. Although much of this additional material is also covered by nursing in preoperative teaching, we find the repetition helpful, especially in areas such as use of analgesics, importance of frequent position change, and early mobilization.

The preoperative assessment looks at both chest status and mobility, and should include a subjective evaluation of endurance. It may also be necessary to include more specific evaluation of strength, gait, or neurologic findings.

The patient is not usually seen on the day of surgery unless initial postoperative chest x-ray film shows a significant area of collapse, in which case treatment with the mechanical vibrator and manual techniques, such as squeezing, shaking, and bouncing, may be used.

On the first postoperative day the patient is usually seen following extubation. An assessment is carried out and routine deep breathing, coughing, and use of the incentive spirometer are reviewed. Circulatory and range of motion exercises are carried out as taught preoperatively. Treatment is applied to the left lower lobe and any other areas indicated by assessment findings. The mechanical vibrator is used for 15 to 20 minutes followed by techniques such as manual pressures, squeezing, shaking, and bouncing.

The patient is assisted with supported coughing if secretions are present.

At this point postoperatively, it is important to be aware of signs of pulmonary edema, which can severely compromise respiratory status, that is not amenable to physical therapy treatment, and usually requires medical treatment with diuretics such as furosemide. One interesting and often misconstrued finding on assessment is that of widespread fine wheezes on auscultation. In the presence of a positive fluid balance in a postcardiac surgery patient wheezes are often a result of pulmonary edema and therefore, do not respond to salbutamol inhalations. Patients following mitral valve replacement more often have difficulties with pulmonary edema because of their preoperative elevations in pulmonary vascular pressures.

Cardiac arrhythmias, attributable to myocardial irritability or ischemia, may preclude treatment in the immediate postoperative period or may limit turning if they are position induced. Marked hypotension or hemodynamic instability may also preclude treatment at this time. Hypertension does not contraindicate treatment, but caution must be exercised in the effort expended in carrying out exercises and in changing position. Usually, assisting with range of motion and turning and decreasing the number of repetitions of each exercise from 10 to five is sufficient to prevent excessive elevations in blood pressure.

A similar treatment regime is followed while in ICU and upon transfer to the floor on the second or third postoperative day. As explained preoperatively, assistance is also provided with increasing mobility level. During this period, nursing staff in the ICU and sometimes on the ward are asked to assist with chest care by using the mechanical vibrator on specified areas once or twice in the evening. This is in addition to routine follow-up consisting of encouragement of deep breathing, coughing, and hourly use of the incentive spirometer.

Once on the ward, physical therapy chest care is continued as long as necessary. In this period, problems with fluid balance must continue to be monitored for. In particular, patients tend to develop left pleural effusions, which may not require physical therapy treatment, but if large enough may require thoracentesis to resolve.

Problems with limited mobility become more apparent in this period due in particular to decreased cardiac condition or to a painful leg incision. The main role of physical therapy is to maintain range of motion of the hip and knee and to encourage progressive ambulation as tolerated. All patients attend a mobility class, which consists of active upper and lower extremity and trunk exercises and education regarding activity level and exercise at home.

Patients undergoing surgery for WPW syndrome or other aberrant pathways are usually young and frequently male. It is interesting to note that we encounter difficulties (i.e., poor pain tolerance, reluctance to carry out deep breathing and coughing and reluctance to increase mobility) more frequently with these patients than with the older population of coronary artery or valvular disease patients.

THORACIC SURGERY

In cardiac or pulmonary surgery via a thoracotomy incision there is a particular set of unique problems and requirements. Patients tend to be more stable in the immediate postoperative period, and in our center are rarely admitted to the ICU postoperatively. However, they do have a greater risk of developing significant atelectasis and/or respiratory infections and pneumonia. This is primarily due to the painfulness of the incision and the patient's resulting reluctance to deep breathe and cough. Many of these patients also have chronic airways limitation as a result of the heavy smoking often associated with the lung cancer necessitating the surgery. These patients also have more resulting postural and general mobility problems than do many other surgical patients.

With these patients, preoperative teaching is of an intermediate level between that done with the general surgery and that done with the aforementioned cardiovascular surgery. Emphasis is placed on the effects of pain on breathing and the importance of regular deep breathing and coughing. The chest tube is mentioned and explained. Exercises to maintain and improve shoulder range of motion are taught and further exercises for trunk mobility and posture are mentioned.

Postoperatively, these patients are routinely admitted to a respiratory observation unit (ROU), where close monitoring by nursing is provided, with cardiac and various respiratory monitors available. If admitted to the ROU early enough in the day, the patient is seen on the day of surgery. An assessment is carried out and, although the patient is often drowsy, deep breathing, coughing, and use of the incentive spirometer are initiated. Gentle manual techniques such as manual pressures, bouncing, squeezing, and posterior lifts may be used to improve the depth of breathing and to facilitate secretion mobilization. If assessment findings suggest that atelectasis or secretion retention have already begun to develop, more extensive treatment may be provided. This may include the use of the mechanical vibrator and other techniques as previously described. Again, nursing may be asked to carry out treatment using the mechanical vibrator and to insure regular use of the incentive spi-

rometer as well as deep breathing and coughing. During this period and the first few postoperative days adequate pain relief is particularly important; patients may require the provision of demand analgesia or an epidural catheter. As part of the management of these patients, pain and its control are monitored closely.

Treatment is often required twice daily in the initial postoperative period and may be continued for up to 2 weeks or more. This again consists of mechanical vibration and manual techniques, such as squeezing, shaking, bouncing, rotations, and side stretches. Foot and ankle exercises and auto-assisted or active shoulder range on the operative side are reviewed on the first postoperative day and continued thereafter. Mobility is progressed at a similar rate as after cardiovascular surgery, but may progress more slowly because of pain and the necessity of having some chest tubes connected to wall suction for some time postoperatively. In the first postoperative week—usually once the chest tube has been removed—trunk rotation and side flexion exercises are begun in addition to posture education. Postural problems are frequent with these patients, with a tendency to side flexion toward the operative side and to elevation of the contralateral shoulder. More specific exercises may be required for some patients to deal with these problems.

The basic principles of pre- and postoperative care vary little with different patient populations. Preoperative assessment and teaching provide a useful baseline for the therapist and promote patient understanding and compliance postoperatively. Postoperative care consists of instruction in and monitoring of deep breathing, supported coughing and hourly use of the incentive spirometer where indicated. Further treatment is provided depending on assessment findings. Specific problems are encountered with cardiovascular and thoracic surgery patients, some of which alter physical therapy treatment provided, and some of which necessitate it. Many provide an interesting challenge to the physical therapist, and all make up a significant portion of the patient population cared for by the cardiopulmonary physical therapist.

SUGGESTED READING

Bethune D. Neurophysiological facilitation of respiration in the unconscious adult patient. Physiother Can 1975; Oct:241–245.

Guymer AJ. Handling the patient with speech and swallowing problems. Physiother Can 1986; 72:276–280.

Netter FH. Controlling disorders of respiration. In: CIBA collection of medical illustrations. Vol 7: the respiratory system. Summit, NJ: CIBA, 1979:75.

Smith A. Neurology and neurosurgery. In: Frownfelter D. Chest physical therapy and pulmonary rehabilitation. Chicago: Year Book, 1979:265.

BREATHING PATTERNS IN CHRONIC OBSTRUCTIVE PULMONARY DISEASE

BRENDA M. LOVERIDGE, B.P.T., M.Sc., Ph.D.

Chronic obstructive pulmonary disease (COPD) is progressively disabling, and there appears to be a fairly consistent change in breathing pattern as the disease becomes more severe. Patients appear to alter their breathing patterns to meet their ventilatory needs in response to ever increasing pulmonary derangements, probably based on alterations in lung and chest wall mechanics, which are relatively irreversible. These changes appear to produce a resetting of the central neural mechanisms controlling ventilation.

In order to assist patients in optimizing the function that remains, it is important to understand clearly how breathing differs in patients with COPD as compared to normal subjects, and to understand why these changes may have occurred. With this understanding a more realistic approach to respiratory rehabilitation can be developed. This chapter develops such a framework.

BREATHING PATTERN IN COPD

During the last 3 years we have examined breathing patterns in 22 patients with COPD with varying degrees of mechanical impairment, and blood gas alterations, and compared this data to that observed in an age matched normal control population. Our observations on breathing patterns are supported by many other reports in the literature. The findings from our studies are used to exemplify the changes that occur in COPD patients. We studied 4 groups; group 1 (6 patients) had FEV 1.0 25 to 50 percent predicted (moderate), group 2 (8 patients) had FEV 1.0 less than 25 percent predicted (severe). Both groups 1 and 2 had PaO_2 more than 55 mm Hg and were not hypercapnic. Group 3 (8 patients) had FEV 1.0 less than 25 percent predicted and were hypoxemic and hypercapnic at rest and receiving supplemental home oxygen (chronic respiratory failure); group 4 (8 patients) were an age- and sex-matched normal control population.

Breathing patterns were assessed in these patients using inductance coils around the ribcage and abdomen. The coils were summed and calibrated against a known volume source to convert the signal to a volume measurement. This technique was validated in our laboratory and has been successfully employed in a wide variety of patient populations. It allows breathing to be monitored at rest without the patient having to breathe on a mouthpiece; this in itself causes changes in breathing. A computer assisted program allowed the collection of 30 to 45 minutes of breathing with each subject providing as representative a sample of resting breathing as possible.

Changes in resting breathing were apparent in patients with moderate obstruction as compared to normal controls. These COPD patients had a significantly increased frequency of breathing (f) with a rate of 20 breaths per minute, as compared to 16 per minute in normals, but maintained a normal tidal volume (Vt) and, therefore, had an increased minute ventilation (Ve). COPD subjects also significantly shortened the length of time spent during inspiration (Ti), and therefore, had to increase significantly their mean inspiratory flow rate to maintain Vt (Fig. 1). There are two options for increasing Vt: one is to lengthen inspiratory time and maintain the same mean inspiratory flow; the other is to increase mean inspiratory flow and maintain an unchanged inspiratory time. Combinations of the two could also obviously produce the same net increase in Vt. As the level of mechanical impairment becomes more limiting (group 2), mean frequency of breathing increases further to 23 breaths per minute, and Vt drops approximately 110 ml as a result of further shortening of inspiratory time. The small increase in frequency was offset by the small decrease in Vt so that Ve remained unchanged.

Patients in group 3 who had similar mechanical impairment to patients in the severe group 2, but who also had hypoxemia and hypercapnia, showed a markedly different breathing pattern. Patients in group 3 no longer maintained Ve. These patients had a significantly decreased mean inspiratory flow, which, when coupled with a shortened inspiratory time (as found in all COPD patients), prevented them from maintaining Vt. Although mean frequency increased slightly (24 per minute), it was not sufficient to balance the significant drop in Vt, and therefore, minute ventilation fell. Whereas it cannot be proven that the blood gas alterations are secondary to the breathing pattern changes in this group, it is an acceptable hypothesis. A decreased Vt and increased frequency implies a greater deadspace ventilation (higher Vd/Vt) and, therefore, a lower alveolar ventilation. This rapid

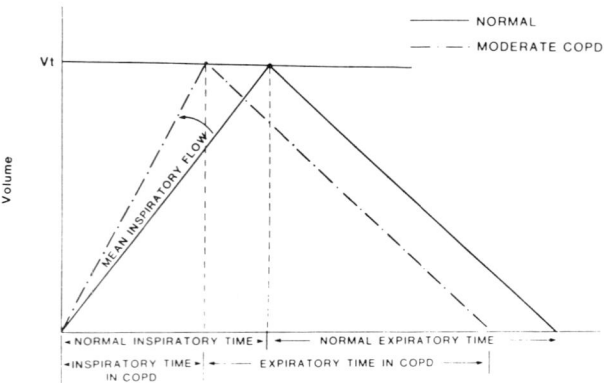

Figure 1 Mean respiratory cycle for normal subjects (——) and COPD patients with moderate disease (—·—·). As inspiratory time shortens in COPD, mean inspiratory flow (slope) must increase to maintain tidal volume (Vt).

shallow breathing pattern has long been associated with CO_2 retention in COPD patients. The drop in Ve observed and the subsequent alveolar hypoventilation may lead to the hypoxemia and hypercapnia observed in these patients. A summary of the mean spirogram for all groups is illustrated in Figure 2. The trend towards a more restrictive breathing pattern with progression of the disease becomes quite apparent.

We also found that breathing becomes less variable in COPD. That is, in COPD patients Vt, Ve, and inspiratory timing vary less from breath to breath than they do in normal subjects. Their breathing pattern is more fixed and monotonous in nature. The decreased variability was observed in patients in group 1 with only moderate disease, and remained unchanged in patients with more severe disease in spite of worsening mechanics. Patients with moderate COPD also

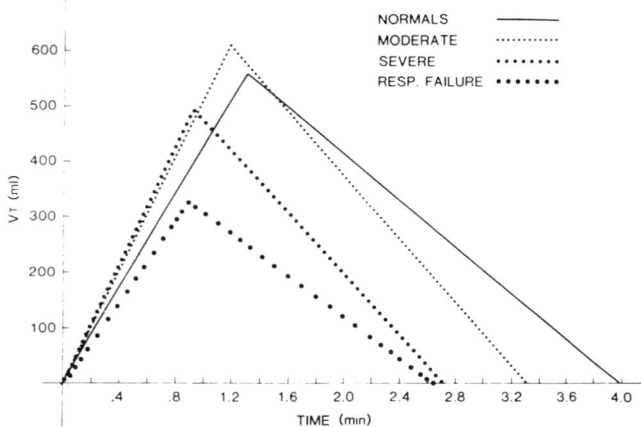

Figure 2 Comparison of the mean spirogram for the moderate, severe, and respiratory failure COPD subjects with a mean spirogram of an age-matched normal control group.

do not sigh (take big breaths) as frequently as do normal subjects, and patients with severe obstructive disease rarely sigh at all. Perhaps taking big breaths is too costly in terms of energy expenditure. However, the decreased variability in breathing in COPD could not be explained purely on the basis of a difference in the number of big breaths between COPD patients and normals, for when sighs were removed from the analysis, the decreased variability remained. The results suggest a more fixed output from the respiratory control centers in COPD. In the face of prolonged loading of the respiratory system, as seen in COPD patients who take many years to develop significant disease, it appears that the respiratory centers adapt and optimize breathing to meet this demand. However, as in all situations, such adaptations are not without cost. The COPD patient's breathing becomes more fixed, big breaths are not regularly taken, and there is more susceptibility to airway closure, especially in the face of added insults such as acute infections.

There obviously are strategies open to COPD patients to improve their ventilation. They need only increase frequency, or increase Vt, or a combination of both to improve minute ventilation. Consider frequency first. Patients with only moderate impairment already have a mean frequency of 20 per minute, and this increases progressively with disease severity. Increasing frequency adds greatly to the oxygen cost of ventilation. The respiratory muscles use much more oxygen as frequency increases, so that further increases in frequency could prove too costly. What about Vt? Again patients with moderate disease significantly shorten inspiratory time, which alone would cause a drop in Vt. To compensate, patients markedly increase mean inspiratory flow, and thereby maintain Vt. Mean inspiratory flow can be viewed as representative both of the drive to breathe and of the inspiratory effort; given abnormal lungs in COPD the ventilatory muscles have to work considerably harder than in normal just to maintain a normal Vt. It is unlikely that patients can increase mean inspiratory flow much more, as it is often double that of a normal individual during resting breathing. Why then, do patients shorten inspiratory time so early in their disease? Simply lengthening inspiratory time would allow an increase in Vt. It has been suggested that a prolonged inspiratory time relative to the total time spent in one complete respiratory cycle (one inspiration and expiration) can produce inspiratory muscle fatigue, and that perhaps the body adapts in ways that spare the ventilatory muscles from a fatigue situation. Although unproven, the hypothesis claims that fatigue would occur with a longer inspiratory time because the ventilatory muscles would be contracting for a relatively long period of time and have less time to recover during the following shortened expiration. Regardless of the reason, the ratio of inspiratory time to total cycle time is the same in all COPD patients as in normal subjects. It does not change even with severe disease or in chronic respiratory failure. It is tempting to suggest that the respiratory system finds this fixed ratio optimal, for as yet undefined reasons, and does not increase tidal volume by lengthening inspiratory time at the expense of expiratory time.

Although statistically insignificant, Vt begins to fall in patients with severe disease without respiratory failure. Whether this represents an early phase in the development of chronic respiratory failure is speculative, but plausible. Compared to patients with equally severe disease but without respiratory failure, patients in chronic respiratory failure have a decreased drive to breathe (mean inspiratory flow drops) and Vt falls precipitiously, as inspiratory time remains shortened. Whether the decreased mean inspiratory flow of chronic respiratory failure represents the development of ventilatory muscle fatigue, central neural fatigue, or other changes in central control is unclear. What is clear is that with reduced inspiratory flow and tidal volume, ventilatory demands can no longer be met, and blood gas derangements become apparent.

Further supporting evidence that COPD patients select their own optimal breathing pattern comes from studies examining the effects of added expiratory loads on dynamic compression or collapse of airways in patients with COPD. One of the conclusions from these studies was that making patients alter their breathing worsens the dynamic compression of major airways. It appears that patients who experience flow limitation and dynamic compression on expiration (a common finding in patients with severe airflow obstruction), breathe in such a manner as to minimize the effects of dynamic compression of their airways as much as possible.

PATIENT MANAGEMENT

Given that patients may have selected the breathing pattern that is optimal for their condition and that altering the pattern could worsen dynamic compression of airways, produce inspiratory muscle fatigue, or adversely effect ventilation in other ways, is it logical for physical therapists to try to alter resting breathing in these patients? In the past, it was generally viewed that patients should be encouraged to adopt a "normal" pattern of breathing (as this was considered to be optimal) and discouraged from using accessory muscles of breathing because of the high oxygen costs associated with such maneuvers. Such theories should no longer be viewed as the foundation on which to build therapeutic regimens for breathing exercises in this patient population. These patients do not have a normal respiratory system, and the mechanical impairment is not reversible. The changes have

occurred over many years and, at least in part, represent alterations in central control mechanisms. Therefore, trying to change a COPD patient's breathing to match that of a subject with normal mechanics does not make much sense. That is probably at least part of the reason why studies trying to show that such patients can alter their breathing pattern at rest and maintain these alterations outside of the controlled experimental situation have failed.

Where does this leave breathing exercises in the management of patients with COPD in the relatively stable stages of their disease process? What techniques should be employed?

First, we should stop teaching "diaphragmatic" or "unilateral" breathing exercises or any other breathing exercise that aims to alter resting breathing pattern in stable COPD patients. It is a waste of their time and ours. Such exercises have never been shown to be of any benefit, and may have encouraged a pattern that in fact was detrimental. The patient's choice of resting breathing pattern is probably the best. However, that does not preclude teaching how to cope with episodes of dyspnea through the use of relaxation techniques, the lean forward position, and pursed lip breathing, which helps to slow down rate of breathing. Most patients recover from dyspnea more quickly using one or more of these procedures. Teaching the patient how to cope with the limitations of the disease is an important objective.

Efforts should concentrate on improving general exercise tolerance, including both upper limb and lower limb exercises as much as is possible within the limits of the disease. This ensures that the patient can function at his maximum and provides some reserve, however limited, to assist in dealing with the next acute episode of the disease. Even if the only measurable index of improvement following an increase in exercise tolerance is a lessening of dyspnea, or a general feeling of well being, these should be considered worthwhile. Whether such general reconditioning exercise has a positive effect on the ventilatory muscles has yet to be proven. Ventilatory muscle endurance training may have a role to play in some patients with COPD either through specific inspiratory muscle training, or limb endurance training or a combination of both. However, the research with ventilatory muscle training in COPD patients is not yet sufficiently complete to warrant routine widespread application of such measures. Much is yet unknown regarding which COPD patients, if any, develop inspiratory muscle fatigue. Furthermore, in patients who may demonstrate inspiratory muscle weakness and lack of endurance, it might be that these muscles should be rested, as opposed to exercised. For the present, these techniques should be tested in controlled clinical studies, where their true value can be determined, and not be part of routine care for the COPD patient.

SUGGESTED READING

Loveridge B, West P, Anthonisen NR, Kryger MH. Breathing patterns in patients with chronic obstructive pulmonary disease. Am Rev Respir Dis 1984; 130:730–733.

Loveridge B, West P, Kryger MH, Anthonisen NR. Alterations in breathing patterns with progression of chronic obstructive pulmonary disease. Am Rev Respir Dis 1986; 134:930–934.

Parrot S, Saunier C, Gautier H, Milic-Emili J, Saboul G. Breathing pattern hypercapnia in patients with obstructive pulmonary disease. Am Rev Respir Dis 1980; 121:985–991.

Sorli J, Grassino A, Lorange G, Milic-Emili J. Control of breathing in patients with chronic obstructive lung disease. Clin Sci Molec Med 1978; 54:295–304.

EXERCISE IN CARDIAC REHABILITATION

DIANA HOLMES HOPKINS-ROSSEEL, B.Sc.
(PT)

Cardiac rehabilitation is a comprehensive program designed to restore and maintain the coronary patient's function at an optimum level—physically, psychologically, and socially. This process begins early in the hospital stay and continues beyond the stage of convalescence. Only relatively recently has the concept of secondary prevention been acknowledged. Now, known risk factors for the development of ischemic heart disease can be evaluated and minimized through lifestyle changes (Table 1).

Cardiovascular (CV), or aerobic, exercise is an integral component of the cardiac rehabilitation program. The specific goal of the CV exercise component is identical to that of the cardiac rehabilitation program in general—to improve quality of life. The benefits of the exercise component are both proven and speculative. It is known that early ambulation decreases the adverse effects of bed rest or deconditioning (Table 2). Postcoronary exercise also effectively increases cardiac efficiency by decreasing heart rate and myocardial oxygen consumption at a given workload. The heart muscle is then more resistant to ischemia or excess catecholamines (stress hormones). Other objective benefits include higher peak exercise capacity, more efficient performance of muscular work at submaximal workloads, and improved carbohydrate metabolism. In addition, blood lipid levels (particularly triglycerides) may be reduced, and high-density lipoproteins (HDL) may increase. Systolic blood pressure may be lowered, and skeletal muscles become stronger and more oxygen efficient.

On a more subjective level, a postcoronary CV exercise regimen increases the patient's self confidence and sense of well-being. Exercise may promote relaxation by relieving tension and thus becomes a healthy way to manage stress. Further, exercise (postmyocardial infarction and postcardiac surgery) can be a healthy alternative for unhealthy behaviors such as eating or smoking. In addition, it definitely helps with weight control by burning calories. In psychological terms, group exercise provides support and offers an opportunity to socialize, whereas individual exercise provides an opportunity for solitude and reflection.

A typical cardiac rehabilitation program includes four phases of exercise: the acute, inpatient phase; the convalescent phase; the conditioning phase; and the maintenance phase.

At all levels, sessions should include a warmup, aerobic exercise, and cooldown as follows:

1. *Warmup*: Calisthenics and low-level exercise should be selected to *gradually* increase the workload of the heart and to prepare the muscles for exercise (should include both stretching and gravity-resisted strengthening exercises).
2. *Exercise*: An ideal exercise uses the large muscle groups in a rhythmic fashion, for a sustained period of time, at a prescribed heart rate (e.g., walking, bicycling, rowing, crosscountry skiing, swimming).
3. *Cooldown*: Select low-level exercise and relaxation breathing exercises to gradually decrease the workload of the heart.

EXERCISE PHASES IN CARDIAC REHABILITATION

Phase I: The Acute Phase

This phase may begin as early as day three postmyocardial infarction (MI) or coronary artery bypass surgery and continues throughout the hospital stay. The acute phase is characterized by three very low-level exercise sessions per day. Patients progress at their own individual rate through a predetermined step program. A sample program is provided in Table 3. Patients need not complete the entire step program prior to discharge.

Phase II: The Convalescent Phase

Significant tissue healing occurs during the convalescent phase; there remains a risk of further tissue damage should the patient be allowed to exercise without close monitoring. Therefore, patients perform one session per week under the direct supervision of a member of the cardiac rehabilitation team to ensure safe performance and progression of the prescribed exercise routine. This session is done in a group setting to allow for interaction and tends to be the best forum for patients to voice their fears and complaints surrounding their disease. The duration of this phase is usually 6 to 12 weeks. It is often preceded by a modified exercise tolerance test (METT) to determine a safe level of exercise prior to discharge, in addition to providing the patient with a heart rate (HR) guide-

TABLE 1   Risk Factors for Developing Coronary Artery Disease

Uncontrollable factors
  Advanced age
  Male gender
  Postmenopausal state
  Heredity

Controllable factors
  Cigarette smoking
  Hypertension
  Hyperlipidemia (elevated blood lipid levels)
  Obesity
  Diabetes
  Sedentary lifestyle
  Stress level/personality type

line. These exercises are prescribed to help prevent deconditioning and muscle weakness.

Exercise Prescription for Phase II

Type: Select a leisurely walk or stationary bicycling without resistance (Table 4).
Frequency: Complete once daily (one session per week to be directly supervised and monitored by a member of the cardiac rehabilitation team).
Duration: Gradual increase in aerobic exercise from 5 minutes to 30 minutes.

Target Heart Rate*: 70 percent of HR attained during METT or 15 bpm below ischemic level (or symptomatic level).

Phase III: The Conditioning Phase

This is a 12-week period of supervised conditioning exercise designed to help the patient acquire the training benefits described earlier. The patient requires a standard exercise tolerance test (ETT) before participating in this phase of the exercise program.

Exercise Prescription For Phase III

Type: Select walking, jogging, stationary bicycling with increasing resistance, stationary rowing.
Frequency: Do three to five times per week (all sessions under direct supervision with cardiac monitoring).
Duration: Session should last 20 to 30 minutes.
Target Heart Rate: Goal is 70 to 85 percent of the maximum HR attained during the ETT.

---

* HR recommendation post-MI—less than 100 bpm
  HR recommendation postcardiac surgery—less than 120 bpm
  HR recommendation for patients receiving beta-blockade medications—15 bpm above resting HR.

TABLE 2   The Adverse Effects of Bedrest or Deconditioning

Thrombophlebitis	Atelectasis
Orthostatic hypotension	Negative nitrogen and protein
Reflex tachycardia	balance
Decreased lung volume and	Decreased skeletal muscle mass,
vital capacity	strength and flexibility
Decreased physical work	
capacity	

TABLE 3   Phase I Step Program

STEP 1		Active or active-assisted range of motion (ROM) exercises to bilateral (*B*), upper extremities (*UE*), and lower extremities (*LE*) in bed.
STEP 2		Active ROM exercise of (*B*)*LE* in sitting.
STEP 3	*Warmup*	Active ROM exercises of (*B*)*LE* in sitting (~ 1 min).
	Exercise	Ambulate 25 to 50 feet.
	Cooldown	Intermittent deep breathing exercises in sitting (5 min).
STEP 4	*Warm-up*	Active ROM exercises (*B*)*LE* in standing (~ 1 min).
	Exercise	Ambulate 1 min.
	Cooldown	Deep breathing in sitting (5 min).
STEP 5	*Warmup*	Active ROM exercises of (*B*)*UE* and *LE* standing (2 min).
	Exercise	Ambulate or cycle without resistance for 2 min.
	Cooldown	Deep breathing in sitting (5 min).
STEP 6	*Warmup*	Active ROM exercises (*B*)*UE* and *LE* standing (~ 2 min).
	Exercise	Ambulate/cycle for 3 min.
	Cooldown	Deep breathing in sitting (5 min).
STEP 7	*Warmup*	Active ROM exercises (*B*)*UE* and *LE* standing (~ 2 min).
	Exercise	Ambulate/cycle for 4 min.
	Cooldown	Deep breathing in sitting (5 min).
STEP 8	*Warmup*	Active ROM exercises (*B*)*UE* and *LE* standing (~ 2 min).
	Exercise	Ambulate/cycle for 5 min.
	Cooldown	Deep breathing in sitting (5 min).

TABLE 4   Phase II Exercise Program

Warmup Exercises
  Standing with arms abducted to 90°. Rotate arms forwards and
    backwards—10 repetitions (reps) in each direction.
  Slight knee bends standing—10 reps
  Trunk side-flexion standing—10 reps each direction
  Marching on the spot—20 steps
  Trunk rotation—10 reps to each side
  Leg lifts forward (hip flex)—10 reps each leg
  Shoulder girdle protraction or retraction—10 reps each direction
  Leg lifts to the side (hip abduction)—10 reps each leg

Walking Program
  Week
  1   5 min—leisurely pace
  2   10 min—leisurely pace
  3   15 min—leisurely pace
  4   20 min—leisurely pace
  5   25 min—leisurely pace
  6   30 min—leisurely pace
  7   30 min—leisurely pace
  8   30 min—slightly increased pace

  Stationary bicycling without resistance can be substituted

Cooldown Activities
  Walk at a slow, ambling pace or stand in one place shifting body weight
    from one leg to the other for 1 to 2 min.
  Sitting in a relaxed position perform 4 sets of 3 diaphragmatic deep breaths
    with 1 min rest in between each set as follows:
      in nose, out through nose
      in nose, out through mouth
      in mouth, out through nose
      in mouth, out through mouth

Often a second ETT is performed at the end of 12 weeks to determine the exercise capacity attained.

Phase IV: The Maintenance Phase

This is often the most difficult phase in that full responsibility must be taken by the patient for the exercise program. It becomes increasingly difficult for a high level of motivation to be maintained. The patient is encouraged to continue his exercising at the level achieved during the conditioning phase of the program, three to four times per week for the rest of his life. At this point, further options for the aerobic component of the exercise program can be discussed and implemented; return for outpatient monitoring is necessary only if complications arise.

It is important that we mention the parameters used to monitor cardiac status. During all inpatient sessions and outpatient visits, heart rate, blood pressure, and cardiac rhythm (usually via a two-lead telemetry monitor) are recorded prior to exercise, at intervals during exercise (not to exceed 5 minutes), and 3 to 5 minutes post exercise. When exercising is done without supervision, pulse is monitored by the patient prior to exercising, once while exercising, and post cooldown. These findings are coupled with the patient's symptoms (Table 5) to determine exercise tolerance and personal safety.

Candidates for the exercise component of a cardiac rehabilitation program include patients in the following categories: postmyocardial infarction; post coronary artery bypass surgery; postvalvular surgery

TABLE 5   Symptoms Indicating Possible Ischemia

Angina
Shortness of breath or difficulty breathing
Dizziness or nausea
Irregular heart beats (palpitations)
Diaphoresis
Extreme fatigue

NB   If one or more of these symptoms occurs with activity patient should *stop and rest* (take nitroglycerin for angina if prescribed) and report the symptoms to the doctor and the cardiac rehabilitation team.

as well as those with stable angina. These candidates must have written physician authorization, stable vital signs, and total absence of certain preclusive symptoms—namely, continued ischemia, left ventricular failure, serious circulatory impairment, uncontrolled hypertension, serious arrhythmias, conduction defects, or significant dysfunction of other organ systems.

PRECAUTIONS PRIOR TO INITIATING EXERCISE

1. Record vital signs, cardiac rhythm, and symptoms.
2. Avoid exercise for 1 to 2 hours after a meal.
3. Avoid breath holding.
4. Avoid isometric exercises.
5. Avoid exercise during extremely hot or cold weather.
6. Ensure appropriate clothing is worn.
7. Avoid uneven terrain during phases I and II.
8. Avoid smoking for at least 1 hour prior to exercise (smoking should be discontinued altogether).
9. Ensure that any exercises undertaken can accommodate any preexisting disabilities or medical conditions.

CONTRAINDICATIONS TO INITIATING EXERCISE

1. Severe or acute heart failure.
2. Recurrent malignant arrhythmias (atrial or ventricular).
3. Unstable ST segment; angina at rest.
4. Second or third degree heart block.
5. Persistent hypotension (less than 90 mm Hg).
6. Uncontrolled hypertension.
7. Severe aortic stenosis.
8. Acute systemic illness or fever.
9. Acute pericarditis or myocarditis.
10. Recent embolism.
11. Thrombophlebitis.
12. Dissecting aneurysm.
13. Symptomatic ventricular aneurysm.
14. Orthopaedic problems prohibiting exercise.

CONTRAINDICATIONS TO CONTINUING EXERCISE

1. (a) Unusual heart rate increase—greater than 20 bpm above resting HR in Phase I.
   (b) Drop of systolic BP greater than 15 mm Hg; systolic greater than 180, diastolic greater than 100.
2. Excessive BP rise.

3. Failure of monitoring equipment.
4. Lightheadedness, confusion, ataxia, pallor, cyanosis, dyspnea, nausea, fatigue, new regurgitation murmur, pulmonary rales.
5. Onset of angina with exercise.
6. Onset of dysrhythmias; supraventricular tachycardia (SVT), ventricular tachycardia (VT), frequent premature ventricular contractions (PVCs), couplets, multifocal PVCs; second or third degree heart block; inappropriate bradycardia.
7. ST segment displacement.
8. Severe leg claudication.

Modifications of the exercise protocol will likely be indicated for patients who are initially complicated and continue to demonstrate the following:

1. Large infarction clinically, although stable after 2 or 3 days.
2. Resting tachycardia (100) or inappropriate heart rate increased with activities of daily living (ADL).
3. BP failing to rise or dropping with ADL.
4. ECG revealing greater than 6 PVCs per minute with ADL.
5. Angina or undue fatigue with ADL.

Exercise is not an isolated component of the cardiac rehabilitation program. Safely performed and properly monitored exercise can positively affect psychological, social and physiological status. Patients often demonstrate increased confidence and a greater improvement in mood. Promotion of an early return to work or to a premorbid lifestyle helps the patient socially. Exercise has physiological benefits that help to decrease many of the risk factors for coronary artery disease both directly and indirectly.

Exercise has not been proven to improve the prognosis of patients with coronary artery disease; however, as a single means of intervention in a comprehensive cardiac rehabilitation program, it is vital in contributing to the patient's quality of life.

SUGGESTED READING

Alpert JS. The heart attack handbook. Boston: Little, Brown, 1985.

American College of Sports Medicine. Guidelines for graded exercise testing and exercise prescription. 3rd. ed. Philadelphia: Lea & Febiger, 1980.

American Heart Association. The exercise standards book. Dallas: American Heart Association 70–041–A, 1979.

Irwin S, Tecklin JS, eds. Cardiopulmonary physical therapy. St. Louis: CV Mosby, 1985:3–166.

Shephard RJ. Prognostic valve of exercise testing for ischemic heart disease. Br J Sports Med 1982; 15(4): 220–229.

Sokolow M, McIlroy MM. Clinical cardiology. Los Altos, CA: Lange Medical Publications, 1981.

Wenger NK. Rehabilitation of the coronary patient status 1986. Prog Cardiovasc Dis 1986; 29(3):181–204.

MUSCULOSKELETAL PHYSICAL THERAPY

MASSAGE: CURRENT APPLICATION

HANS W. BLASER, R.P.T., M.C.P.A.

The clinical success of massage and soft-tissue manipulation has often eluded scientific explanation. The inability to provide scientific verification for these treatment procedures has unfortunately resulted in professional scepticism, which undermines the credibility of this form of therapy. Although the use of and benefits from sophisticated high-tech equipment has continued to grow, massage and soft-tissue manipulation should not be ignored as a very valuable form of treatment.

Throughout my professional career, I have had a strong interest in the development and use of massage therapy. Manual assessment and therapy in the clinical setting have demonstrated both versatility and effectiveness as a means of care for chronic soft-tissue dysfunction resulting from trauma, stress, or disease. The holistic principle, on which massage therapy is founded, focuses on the use of different massage techniques to resolve physical pathology and restore harmony within the physiologic system. When such therapeutic techniques are used in combination with other physical therapy modalities, such as remedial gymnastics, relaxation techniques, heat or cold, and mobilization and manipulation, the results can be quite dramatic. Therefore, professionals should not hesitate to use this form of therapy when indicated.

INDICATIONS FOR MASSAGE THERAPY

The vast majority of patients seen in a general physical therapy practice are those with conditions which have progressively deteriorated over a period of several months or years. A large percentage of the difficulties experienced by patients are the results of myofascial disorders. These conditions are particularly well suited for massage therapy techniques because

of the manner in which these physiologic disturbances develop.

The patient is often unaware of the insidious build up of symptoms and pain patterns, which can lead to a physiologic "crisis." Emotional, psychological, and physical stresses in the workplace, at home, and in the everyday social environment can become significant contributing factors. Stress and tension factors are also found to hinder the healing processes after physical trauma and in existing medical conditions. Since minor traumatic incidences, such as joint and muscle strains, are often "forgotten" a pattern of "trigger points" can develop thereby resulting in periodic painful spasms. Such a situation often leads to a patient's habitual and subsconscious contracting of muscles (guarding), even during sleep. Eventually this response pattern leads to musculoskeletal dysfunction and/or circulatory disturbances. It is under these circumstances that *remedial massage techniques* provide a positive therapeutic modality. The choice of the appropriate massage technique is diverse and includes such "regular procedures" as effleurage, pétrissage, friction, kneading, vibration, and percussion. Although the mechanical, physiologic, psychological, and reflex effects of these therapeutic procedures are well known and accepted, a brief summary of these techniques follows.

Effleurage. A superficial or deep stroking movement, effleurage is usually used to assist venous and lymphatic return in the extremities. It is also used to explore and evaluate areas of tenderness and soft-tissue irregularities or to passively stretch specific muscle groups. Effleurage has mostly a relaxing effect.

Pétrissage. With its wringing, squeezing, kneading, and skinrolling manipulations pétrissage intends to free inter-tissue adhesions and to increase circulation. Besides the mechanical effect, it has a strong stimulating and reflex effect especially with skinrolling.

Friction. Friction or deep compression is done to manipulate and separate deep tissue adhesions. This is accomplished by movements across fibers, such as in tendon or ligamentous structures; longitudinal or circular movements intend to release muscle spasms and to soften tissue nodules and indurations.

Tapotement. Tapotement or striking movement, such as hacking, cupping, slapping, pincement, or beating, has a very stimulating effect and can either be superficial or deep. The finer movements are used in selected neurologic conditions, the heavier ones in specific muscle conditioning programs. However, this form of treatment is now almost totally replaced by equipment providing measurable input and results.

Vibration. Vibration or shaking does loosen up soft tissue and enhances circulation. It can be soothing or stimulating according to intensity and speed. It is usually used on overfatigued muscles, flatulence, or specific joint lesions. Mechanical vibrators with preset cadence are used in neurologic disorders, such as strokes, for stimulating purposes.

The modalities of choice in the care of complex problems of acute and chronic pain and dysfunction are as follows:

1. Myofascial triggerpoint therapy to release dormant or acutely painful muscle nodules (ischemic compression) and
2. Connective tissue massage, to intrinsically affect the body's basic functions.

Both modes are used independently or in combination according to findings.

As an extension to the above, the following treatment options provide viable therapeutic results

1. Psychophysiologic methods of relaxation
2. Remedial gymnastics; rhythmic movement therapy to enhance balanced and harmonious muscle interaction, usually in an oblique or rotational pattern
3. Therapeutic touch, to influence the patient's energy fields for healing purposes and pain control
4. Foot reflexology (zone therapy) to effect responses in tissue or organs within the same zone.

These methods are diverse and go beyond the scope of this chapter and will therefore not be addressed here. During the 30 years of my professional career I have had the opportunity to use each of the techniques mentioned previously. The decision to incorporate particular therapeutic techniques was the result in part of curiosity, but also represented a predetermined choice of therapy for a given physiologic condition. In some instances, "desperation" and frustration, because of lack of results with other modalities, encouraged consideration of alternative methods of care. All the massage techniques employed provided satisfactory results when chosen with care and executed with proper skill.

For some therapists, massage may appear too simplistic or too strenuous a mode of therapy. For others the development and the use of this artful skill

seems too time consuming. However, the application of this therapeutic technique should certainly not be considered in this manner, especially if one considers its effectiveness in the treatment of specific conditions.

CRITERIA FOR CHOOSING A SPECIFIC TECHNIQUE(S)

Literally all conditions presenting myofascial pain and dysfunction warrant examination by touch and palpation and manual examination of the joint complexes involved. In the case of joint dysfunction as a primary concern, the assessment definitely would include the examination of all the muscles serving this joint to determine the existence of muscle shortening and/or trigger points. Myofascial trigger points are hyperirritable spots or areas in a muscle or its fascia. When such findings exist this indicates possible nutritional deficiencies to the area resulting from such things as overloading, fatigue, chilling, psychological stress or postural and skeletal abnormalities.

Examination for Trigger Points

A thorough history taking is essential, including work and leisure time activities in order to evaluate musculoskeletal restrictions associated with varied pain patterns. The patient is usually in a properly supported and relaxed prone position with the arms at his sides. *A visual evaluation* of the back's appearance focuses on skin depressions, or elevations, puffiness or drawn in bands, indications of uneven muscle tone, spasms or nodules. The patient's head position should be actively changed from left to right to neutral to eliminate guarding or preferred positioning. The spinal curves are observed and deviations from a "norm" noted such as irregular spinous processes or "flattened" areas as frequently found on T2, 3, 4 levels. The interrelationship of the C, T, and L-curves are a strong indicator of primary, secondary, or tertiary stress levels. This "picture" is subsequently confirmed (or corrected) by palpating the skin for taut bands, adhesions, edema, or tenderness. (This procedure also provides indications of possible connective tissue irregularities with consequences to the function or dysfunction of organs or systems). The muscles are searched for trigger points with the middle three fingers of each hand to maintain even contact and to facilitate the "feel" of the area of search. This assures best the proper evaluation of the trigger points. A strong interrelationship between C, T, and L-spine does exist in that, for example, a right thoracic trigger point (or spasm) contributes to associate trigger points on the left C-spine and left sacroiliac (SI) joint and/or crest. An *acute trigger point* is always tender, and painful on compression. Its presence prevents full lengthening of the muscle and may give rise to autonomic phenomena, such as vasoconstriction, gooseflesh, hypersecretion, and referred pain. A *latent trigger point* may be quiet and will only be painful by palpation. A *secondary* myofascial trigger point may be found in synergistic or antagonistic muscles due to overload. *Satellite* trigger points may exist in a muscle within the same zone of reference. Myofascial trigger points should be distinguished from periosteal and nonmuscular trigger points.

Trigger Point Therapy. Trigger point therapy is the key in the elimination of the conditions mentioned above. *Acute situations* have to be approached with caution so as not to cause adverse reactions and increased pain. For effective *pain relief* either of the following procedures are helpful.

1. Ice application for 15 minutes through wet towelling directly to the trigger points.
2. Moist heat for twenty minutes just proximal to the area.
3. Ultrasound for 8 minutes at 0.5 to 0.8 watts/cm^2 applied closely around the trigger points in overlapping circular fashion.
4. Transcutaneous electrical nerve stimulation (TENS) to acupuncture points serving the same zone.

Massage in *subacute and dormant* trigger points with minimal referred pain is the single most effective mode of care for their elimination. *The treatment* starts with light effleurage given in an accommodating circular fashion followed with uninterrupted touch with finger-pétrissage, working systematically on all muscles in the proximity of the trigger points. After this preparation of the surrounding tissue (3 to 4 minutes) the trigger point is firmly pressed upon (15 to 20 pounds), usually with one thumb guided by the index and thumb of the other hand to prevent "rolling off." The pressure, or very small circular deep friction, is maintained for between 5 to 12 seconds with gradual release and a gentle superficial finishing stroke. One should feel the tension melting away from under the fingers. A single subacute trigger point can usually be inactivated in one treatment. To prevent possible soreness and to increase the benefits of therapy a hot-pack may be applied *after* the treatment. Follow-up exercises should be thoroughly discussed including posture at work, as well as during leisure time activities.

In cases of multiple trigger points such as presented in habitual poor posture with asymmetrical muscle pull (stress) in the paraspinal complex, the procedures are essentially the same. Such conditions would necessitate a series of trigger point treatments usually starting with the upper thoracic spine, extending to both shoulders and following the spine in both directions. The patient should be taught ischemic compression techniques, body awareness and good posture, as well as activity modification, stretch and strengthening exercises. In longstanding (chronic) cases, movement therapy is used to restore harmonious function; friction massage is often used to improve intertissue mobility; deep kneading is added to aid in the absorption of metabolites, and skinrolling is used to stimulate the subcutaneous tissues' circulation and to restore its resilance.

Connective Tissue Massage. This type of massage is a segment related reflex therapy. The connective tissue layers (or fascia) are situated between skin and muscles and envelop all organs, viscera, and so forth. The fascia contain both sensory and motor nerve fibers controlling blood supply, water conservation, and sensitivity to pain. This tissue is of major physiologic importance in the balance of water and salt contents within the body, as well as for acid-base equalization and therefore electric and osmotic stabilization. Deep-seated pain and pathologic conditions associated with visceral diseases, or diseases associated with pathology of circulation, manifest their existence with visual and palpable changes in the skin of the same spinal nerve segment. This increased tension between epidermis and dermis leads to thickenings, band-like depressions, and atrophy or hypertrophy of muscles. Those visual and palpable changes form a guide for diagnosis and corrective treatment. By means of pulling strokes with the tip of one finger, a stretching and separating of the skin from the underlying tissue is achieved. In a strict predetermined pattern, the appropriate nerve endings are stimulated for a normalizing response.

Connective tissue massage is a modality with great potential and power to heal. In selected conditions, by restoring the negative repair functions, circulatory disorders leading to possible organ damage or tissue necrosis can be prevented. Connective tissue massage is often a vital link in the chain of physiotherapeutic procedures; however, considerable skill and discipline are required to use this technique effectively. Conditions responding well to connective tissue massage are circulatory disturbances, such as intermittent claudications, Reynaud's disease, Sudeck's atrophy, subacute thrombophlebitis, scleroderma; brachial neuralgia, myalgia, periarthritis, epicondylitis, and scars also respond well. Extraordinary results have been achieved in orthopaedic conditions, such as chronic or recurrent SI dysfunction, frozen shoulder, and slow healing fractures with extensive soft-tissue involvement.

As indicated in this chapter, massage techniques are effectively used either singly or in combination with other physical therapy modalities. They positively influence pathology, stress, tension, mood, and of course, the symptoms of pain. Despite the many beneficial effects associated with this mode of care there appears to be a reluctance by professionals to use and discuss these procedures and their results. The lack of means to scientifically explain the success of massage modalities continues to be a major obstacle. However, the practitioners utilizing those treatment techniques fully appreciate and enjoy their broader scope of practice, which also enhances the patient's understanding for effective whole body care.

SUGGESTED READING

Dicke E, Schliack H, Wolff A. A manual of reflexive therapy of the connective tissue. Scarsdale, NY: Sidney S Simon, 1978.

Tappan FM. Healing massage techniques. Reston, Va: Reston Publishing, 1980.

Travell JG, Simons DG. Myofascial pain and dysfunction. Baltimore, MD: Williams & Wilkins, 1983.

ORTHOPAEDIC MANUAL THERAPY: CYRIAX APPROACH

DAVID J. MAGEE, B.A., Dip. P.T., B.P.T., M.Sc., Ph.D.

The Cyriax approach was developed and published by James Cyriax, a British orthopaedic physician. This comprehensive regimen of assessment of orthopaedic conditions offered the concept of examination by selective tension. Cyriax divided all soft tissues into two basic types: (1) contractile tissue, which consists of muscles, tendons, and their attachments; and (2) inert or noncontractile tissue.

Contractile tissue is tested by placing the joint, over which the muscles moved in the resting position, so that the stress on the inert tissues, when the muscles contract, is at a minimum. The patient is then asked to perform a strong isometric contraction. If the contraction is strong and pain free, it indicates there is no problem with the muscle or muscles being tested. If the contraction is strong (relative) and painful, it indicates an injury to the muscle being tested (first or second degree strain?), to the tendon (tendinitis?), or to the bony attachment. If the contraction is weak and painful, it indicates a rather severe injury around the joint such as a fracture. The weakness demonstrated is primarily caused by reflex inhibition. The fourth and final result when testing contractile tissue is a weak and painless contraction. This result could indicate a rupture of the muscle being tested (third degree strain) or dysfunction of the nerve supplying the muscle.

Whereas contractile tissue is tested by gauging strength and pain, inert tissue is tested by measuring range of motion and pain. Thus, the inert tissues are selectively stretched by moving the joint passively and actively through as full a range as possible. Concurrently, the examiner notes the amount of range obtained in each direction, the amount of pain caused by the movement and, finally, what the movement felt like at the end of the range of motion. This last determinant is referred to as end feel and was determined by applying gentle overpressure at the end of the movement.

Cyriax described three normal end feels. The first is called bone to bone, and is described as a hard unyielding sensation, which is painless. An example of this type of end feel is found at the end of normal elbow extension. The second normal end feel is called soft tissue approximation. This end feel is felt as a yielding compression that stops further movement. An example of this end feel is felt at the end of knee flexion. The third normal end feel is tissue stretch, which is by far the most common type in the body. With this type of end feel, there is a resisting arrest of movement with slight give (i.e., it possesses some resistance). Examples of this type of end feel are lateral rotation of the shoulder or extension of the fingers.

In addition to the normal end feels, there are a number of abnormal end feels described by Cyriax. The first one is muscle spasm, which is invoked by movement resulting in a sudden dramatic arrest of that movement and is often accompanied by pain. The end feel is sudden and hard and, as Cyriax says, exhibits the feeling of a "vibrant twang." In other words, the muscle reflexly stops the movement because of pain. The second type of abnormal end feel is a capsular end feel, which has a very similar feeling to normal tissue stretch end feel, but the range of movement is obviously reduced. As the capsule is usually thickened due to pathology, there is not quite as much give as in a normal tissue stretch end feel, in fact, it is more akin to stretching a leather belt. In this particular case, the capsule of the joint is postulated to be affected. The third end feel is called an empty end feel and is detected when considerable pain is produced by movement. Additional movement is obviously impossible because of pain, although there appears to be no real mechanical resistance to the movement. Typical examples of conditions causing this particular type of end feel are neoplasms and acute subacromial bursitis. Springy block is the name given to the fourth abnormal end feel. With this end feel, there is a rebound effect, which occurs at the extreme of the range of motion. Cyriax feels this end feel is indicative of an internal derangement, such as a torn meniscus in a knee. According to Cyriax, the final type of abnormal end feel is what is called a bone to bone end feel. This end feel is similar to the normal bone to bone end feel, but the bone to bone sensation occurs before the normal end of range of movement occurs.

Like contractile tissue, the testing of inert tissues may result in one of four findings or patterns. The first pattern is one that indicates there is no problem with the inert tissues being tested. In this case, the range of motion is full, there is no pain, and the end feel is normal for that joint. The second possible pattern of restriction is one of pain with limitation of movement in some directions and an abnormal end feel. Examples of this type of pattern are seen with a first or second degree ligament sprain or a local adhesion. If, on testing inert tissue, movement is limited but pain free with an abnormal end feel, it is an example of the third inert pattern and usually indicates symptomless osteoarthritis. The final pattern of restriction is one of pain and limitation of range of motion in every direction (it does not have to be the same amount of limitation in every direction) and an abnormal end feel. This finding indicates that the entire joint is affected and that a capsular pattern is also evident. Cyriax felt—and it has been shown—that if the capsule is affected each joint has its own specific pattern of restriction. Capsular pattern is defined as a pattern of proportional limitation of different movements in the joint. An example of the capsular patterns are shown in Table 1.

ASSESSMENT

Cyriax developed a concept of assessment in a logical set pattern to determine which tissues are at fault. He began with the history followed by observation, examination, palpation, and treatment.

History

The history included as complete a medical history as possible, including a history of the present illness in addition to past problems, and revolved around the patient's interpretation of the problem and the amount of pain and discomfort he is experiencing.

Observation

The second part of the examination is the "looking" phase and is called observation. In this phase the examiner strictly "watches" the patient and notes posture, movement, general and detailed posture, manner, attitude and willingness to cooperate.

TABLE 1   Common Capsular Patterns of Joints

Joint(s)	Restriction*
Temporomandibular	Limitation of mouth opening
Occipitoatlanto	Extension, side flexion equally limited
Cervical spine	Side flexion and rotation equally limited, extension
Glenohumeral	Lateral rotation, abduction, medial rotation
Sternoclavicular	Pain at extreme of range of movement
Acromioclavicular	Pain at extreme of range of movement
Humeroulnar	Flexion, extension
Radiohumeral	Flexion, extension supination, pronation
Promimal radioulnar	Supination, pronation
Distal radioulnar	Full range of movement, pain at extremes of rotation
Wrist	Flexion and extension equally limited
Trapeziometacarpal	Abduction, extension
Metacarpophalangeal and interphalangeal	Flexion, extension
Thoracic spine	Side flexion and rotation equally limited, extension
Lumbar spine	Side flexion and rotation equally limited, extension
Sacroiliac, symphysis pubis, and sacrococcygeal	Pain when joints are stressed
Hip†	Flexion, abduction, medial rotation (but in some cases medial rotation is most limited)
Knee	Flexion, extension
Tibiofibular	Pain when joint stressed
Talocrural	Plantar flexion, dorsiflexion
Talocalcaneal (subtalar)	Limitation of varus range of movement
Midtarsal	Dorsiflexion, plantar flexion, adduction, and medial rotation
First metatarsophalangeal	Extension, flexion
Second to fifth metatarsophalangeal	Variable
Interphalangeal	Flexion, extension

* Movements are listed in order of restriction.
† For the hip, flexion, abduction, and medial rotation are always the movements most limited in a capsular pattern; however, the order of restriction may vary.
From Magee D. Orthopedic physical assessment. Philadelphia: WB Saunders, 1987.

Examination

The third part of the assessment is the examination. Active movements are done first to demonstrate the patient's willingness to do the movement, the joint range possible, and the muscle power necessary to do the movement. The passive movements are then performed by the examiner to test the inert structures around each of the involved joints. When doing the active and passive movements, the examiner should note where in the range of motion the pain occurs, the ability of the patient to do the movement and whether trick movements are performed. The passive movements are followed by resisted isometric movements to test contractile tissue. Following these tests, reflexes, cutaneous sensory distribution (dermatomes), myotomes, and sclerotomes may be tested if faults in these structures are suspected.

Palpation

The final part of the assessment is palpation, which is carried out in a systematic fashion to ensure all necessary structures are examined.

TREATMENT

Cyriax felt the goal of treatment was to restore normal pain-free range of motion. He felt that most soft tissue conditions could be treated by injection, transverse frictions, traction, and/or manipulation. The first, injection, is beyond the scope of this chapter; the last, manipulation, is advocated by Cyriax only in select cases where the end feel is correct to carry out the manipulation and all contraindications to manipulation are absent. For example, Cyriax felt the intervertebral disc could be reduced by manipulation. He felt that reduction by manipulation was possible when one or more active movements was painful or limited and when dural signs such as straight leg raising and coughing causing increased pain were present. However, any cord signs would be absent, so there would be no spastic gait or positive Babinski sign. As examples, contractile tissue signs would also be absent or minimal and there would be minimal root signs such as affected dermatomes, myotomes, sclerotomes or reflex changes. Combined with the manipulation was very strong traction—both used to reduce the intervertebral disc.

Cyriax also advocated the use of traction in select cases such as early nuclear protrusions, stability, for reduction, or as a prophylactic measure. He felt traction is more worthwhile in the lumbar spine, especially for pulpy disc protrusions, and in these cases, he advocated the use of very strong traction (80 to 100 kg).

Cyriax's main forte, as far as treatment by physical therapists is concerned, is in the use of transverse frictions for treating soft tissue injuries. Provided they are done as advocated by Cyriax, transverse frictions can be a very useful addition to the therapist's repertoire of treatment techniques. Cyriax offers eight criteria for proper transverse frictions. The frictions must be applied to the right spot and at right angles to the fibers of the affected tissue. The therapist's fingers and the patient's skin must move as one while the friction is given with sufficient sweep. The transverse frictions must be given deep enough and for a long enough time to have an effect on the tissues that need treatment. Pressure augments, but does not replace, the frictions, which must be given for 10 to 15 minutes to be effective. The patient must be placed in a comfortable position to ensure relaxation during the treatment. If a muscle is to be frictioned, it must be relaxed so that the frictions can be applied to the appropriate area of the muscle However, if treatment is to a tendon, the tendon should be kept taut so that the frictions can "smooth off" the gliding surface between the tendon and the sheath.

TREATMENT TECHNIQUES

Transverse Frictions to the Supraspinatus Tendon

For all transverse friction techniques, it is essential that the patient and therapist be properly positioned for the treatment to be effective. For this technique, the patient flexes the elbow of the arm to be treated to 90 degrees and places the forearm behind the back, with the elbow "tucked in" to the side, to bring the supraspinatus tendon anterior, where it is easily treated. The patient is then put in a half lying position so that the arm is fixed in adduction and medial rotation (Fig. 1). In this position, the supraspinatus tendon may be palpated and treated as it passes forward over the head of the humerus to the greater tuberosity.

The therapist then positions him/herself in order to use the hand on the same side as the arm being treated (i.e., the right hand is used if the right supraspinatus tendon is to be treated).

Face the patient's shoulder and place the tip of the index finger over the tendon with the distal interphalangeal joint flexed. The index finger is reinforced with the middle finger, while the thumb provides a counter pressure. The most tender aspect of the tendon is found (not the bone, which may also be tender) and transverse frictions are applied in a side motion by flexing and extending the wrist with the thumb as the fulcrum. The sweep should be about 2 cm. The frictions must be applied for about 15 minutes at least twice a week. Relief is usually obtained in 4 to 6 weeks.

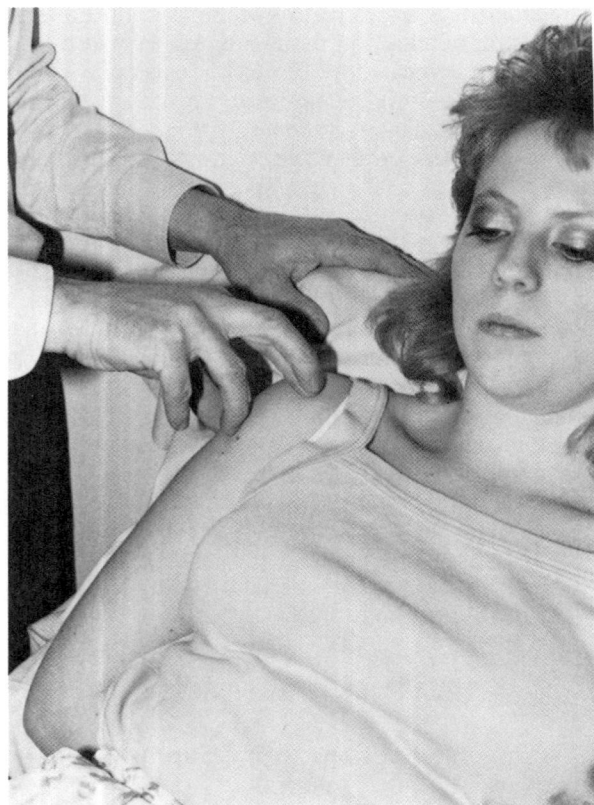

Figure 1 Transverse frictions to the supraspinatus tendon.

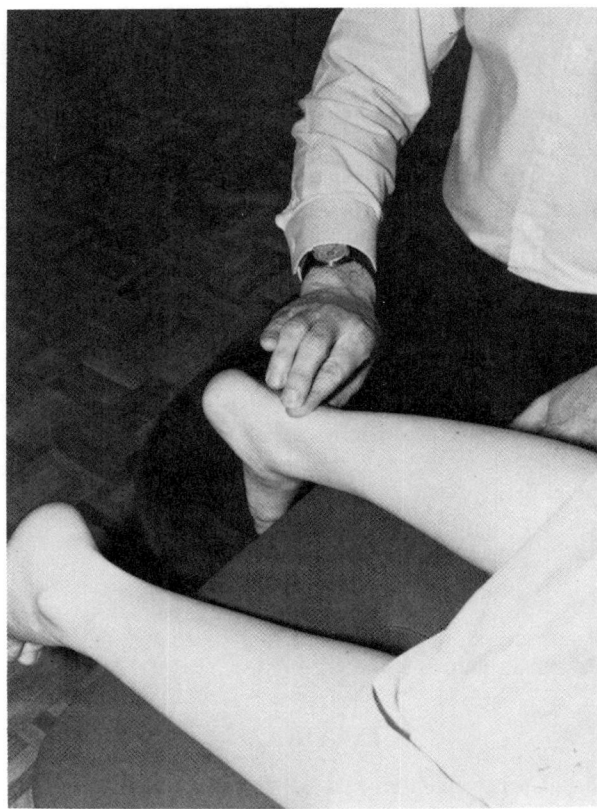

Figure 2 Transverse frictions to the posterior aspect of the Achilles tendon.

Transverse Frictions to the Achilles Tendon

There are four techniques for applying transverse frictions depending on whether the lesion is on the posterior, side, or anterior aspect of the tendon. The therapist must take the time to ensure that he is treating the proper aspect of the tendon. For all four techniques, the patient lies prone.

If the lesion lies in the posterior aspect, the tendon is put "on stretch" by the therapist using his leg to push the foot (which is over the edge of the treatment table) into dorsiflexion. Using the index finger, reinforced by the middle finger, transverse frictions are applied in a side to side motion (Fig. 2) by flexing and extending the elbow. The sweep should be about 2 cm.

If the lesion is adjacent to its insertion into the bone, the patient moves up the treatment table so that the foot is held in full plantar flexion. This position relaxes the tendon so the therapist can indent the tendon and have access to the fibers inserting into the calcaneus. Using both hands, the therapist places both thumbs on the plantar surface and both index fingers (one over the other for reinforcement) over the lesion (Fig. 3) forming a circle. The index fingers are pushed

down hard onto the calcaneus and the fingers are drawn to and fro across the area by moving the forearms.

If the lesion is on one or both sides of the tendon, the tendon is again put on stretch (the therapist's leg holds the ankle in dorsiflexion over the edge of the treatment table). The sides of the tendon are then grasped by the thumb and fingers (Fig. 4). Transverse

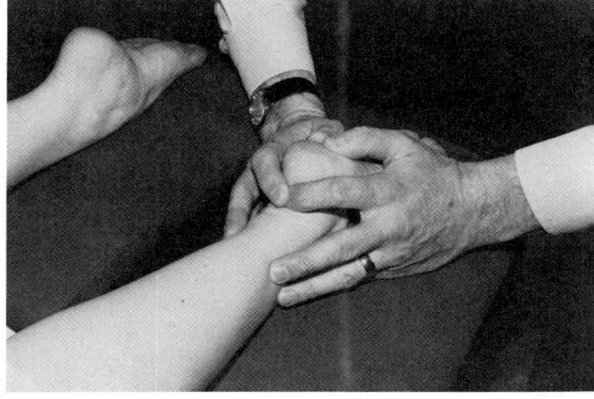

Figure 3 Transverse frictions to the posterior aspect of the Achilles tendon at the bone-tendon interface.

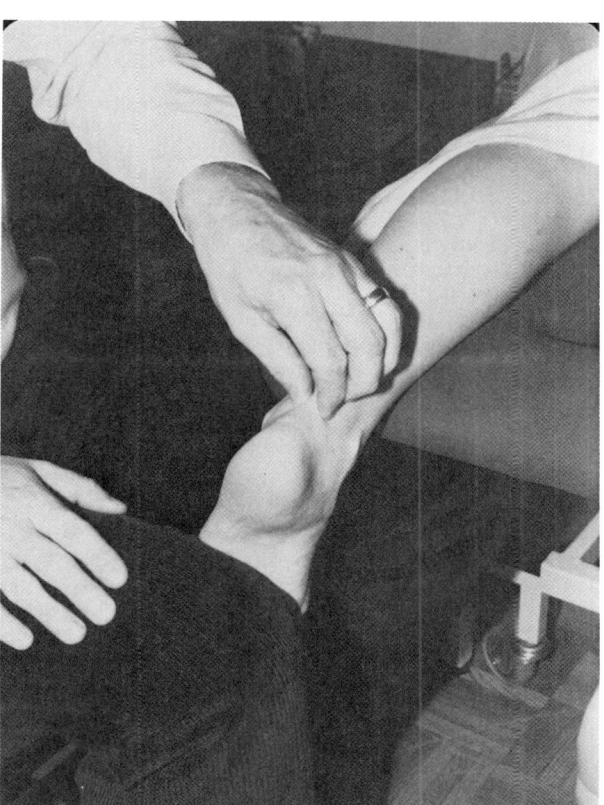

Figure 4 Transverse frictions to the side(s) of the Achilles tendon.

frictions are imparted by sliding the digits forward and backward over the affected area of the tendon while the thumb acts as a pivot point. Either side of the tendon may be done with proper positioning.

To apply transverse frictions to the anterior as-

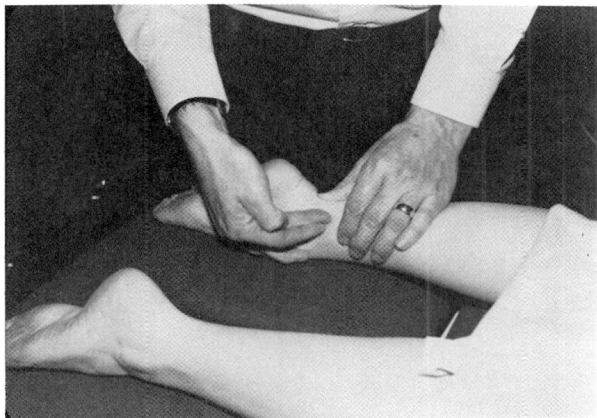

Figure 5 Transverse frictions to the anterior aspect of the Achilles tendon.

pect of the Achilles tendon, the foot is fully plantar flexed and lying on the treatment table. The relaxed tendon is then pushed laterally as far as possible with the thumb of one hand. The anterior aspect of the tendon and the lesion are then palpated with the ring or middle finger of the other hand (Fig. 5). The transverse frictions are applied by supinating and pronating the forearm while the fingers, hand, and arm are held in a straight line.

Traction to the Cervical Spine

Cyriax advocated the use of very strong traction forces to cause a separation of the vertebrae in the cervical spine. He advocated these strong pulls because he felt that spinal problems are primarily the result of pathology to the intervertebral disc. Cyriax felt that the application of strong traction forces results in the reduction of a herniated disc. Because of the strong forces applied by the therapist using his body weight, it is necessary that the patient be well stabilized. The patient's head is held in the standard fashion (one hand around occiput and one hand around chin). The therapist's body is positioned so that the feet act as a pivot point held against the legs of the

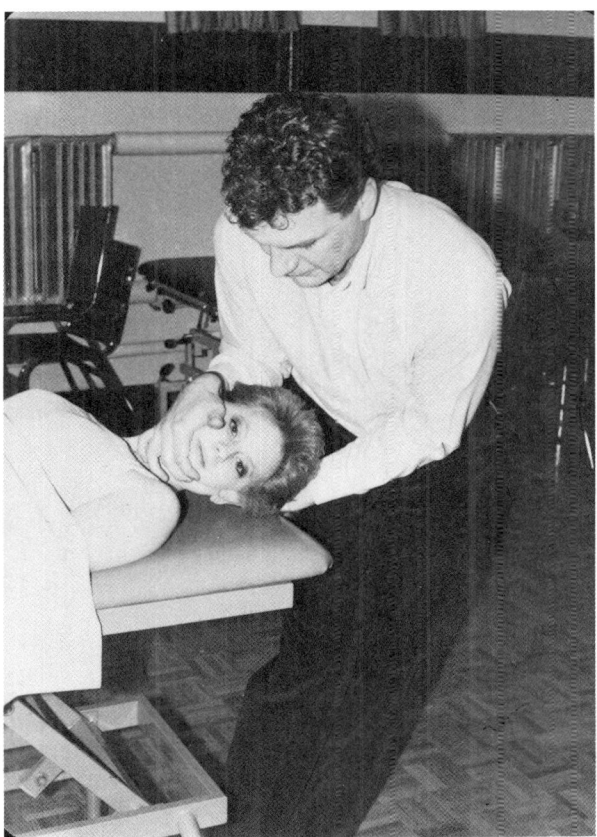

Figure 6 Traction and rotation of the cervical spine.

treatment table. If rotation is also to be applied, the feet face in the direction of the rotation (Fig. 6). If side flexion is to be applied, the feet face in the opposite direction.

Sometimes, Cyriax suggests it would be appropriate for an assistant to fix the treatment couch or the legs or shoulders of the patient to provide a stable base against which the therapist can pull.

The above techniques are given as examples of Cyriax's approach to treatment. Many other examples are illustrated in his books. If these techniques, in addition to Cyriax's assessment techniques are carried out properly, a more definitive diagnosis can be obtained and proper treatment can be implemented.

SUGGESTED READING

Cyriax J. Examination of the spinal column. Physiother 1970; 56: 2–6.

Cyriax J. Manipulation—by laymen or physiotherapists. Physiother Can 1971; 23:236–238.

Cyriax J. Textbook of orthopedic medicine. Volume 1—Diagnosis of soft tissue lesions. London: Bailliere Tendall, 1982.

Cyriax J. Textbook of orthopedic medicine. Volume 2—Treatment by manipulation, massage and injection. London: Bailliere Tendall, 1980.

Cyriax J. The knee. Physiother 1971; 57:203–206.

Cyriax J. The pros and cons of manipulation. Lancet 1964; March: 571–573.

Magee D. Orthopedic physical assessment. Philadelphia: WB Saunders, 1987.

ORTHOPAEDIC MANUAL THERAPY: KALTENBORN APPROACH

DAVID J. MAGEE, B.A., Dip. P.T., B.P.T., M.Sc., Ph.D.

Developed by Freddy Kaltenborn, a physical therapist and chiropractor from Norway, the Kaltenborn approach incorporates the Cyriax method of examination, but also looks at specific accessory movements of traction, compression, and gliding in the joint.

ASSESSMENT

Kaltenborn advocates the sequence of case history, present status, preliminary diagnosis, treatment, and final diagnosis. The case history involves a history of the present problem in addition to past history and related personal and family history. The present status involves assessment and examination. Based on the assessment, Kaltenborn recommends an initial treatment and, when the patient returns, a final diagnosis can be made based on the reaction to the initial treatment.

In his assessment scheme, Kaltenborn advocates the Five-Five assessment scheme of Dr. Herbert Frisch, an orthopaedic surgeon, as well as those of James Cyriax. The Frisch scheme involves five areas—inspection, function, palpation, neurologic tests, and special additional tests. Each of these areas is subdivided into five topics of examination.

During *inspection,* look at posture, body shape, functional movements the patient may or may not be able to perform, the skin, and any aids that may be needed to perform activities of daily living. The second area is function, which involves active, passive, and resisted movements as well as traction and gliding or translatoric (joint play) movement. Functional testing is followed by *palpation.* Palpation involves careful assessment of the following structures by feel: the skin and subcutaneous tissues; muscles and tendons; tendon sheaths and bursae; the joints and surrounding tissue (capsule, ligaments); and, if possible, the nerves and blood vessels. The fourth part of the assessment involves *neurologic tests* in which the examiner tests the nerve trunks, key muscles (myotomes) and reflexes, sensibility (dermatomes and peripheral nerve distribution), motor function and coordination. Finally, Kaltenborn uses any special additional tests that help to further delineate the problem and confirm the diagnosis. These tests include radiography, specific laboratory tests, electrodiagnosis (electroencephalography, electromyography), punctures such as biopsy or aspiration, and finally tests for referred pain.

TREATMENT CONCEPTS

In terms of his treatment, Kaltenborn advocates those ideas of MacConaill which involve ovoid and sellar joints. With the ovoid joint, one joint surface is concave, whereas the other is convex. With sellar joints, each joint surface is both concave and convex (for example, saddle joints). MacConaill broke ovoid and sellar joints down further into modified and unmodified joints. The unmodified ovoids are triaxial ball and socket joints such as the glenohumeral and hip joints. The modified ovoids are the biaxial ellipsoid type joints such as the second, third, fourth, and fifth metacarpophalangeal joints. The unmodified sellar joints were the biaxial saddle joints such as the first metacarpophalangeal joints. The modified sellar joints were uniaxial hinge joints such as the interphalangeal joints.

Kaltenborn took MacConaill's ideas and developed them into joint play treatment techniques. These techniques involved the application of the concave-convex rule. If the fixed joint surface is concave and the mobilized surface is convex, mobilization is carried out in the opposite direction to the direction of restriction. If the fixed joint surface is convex and the mobilized joint surface is concave, mobilization is carried out in the same direction as the direction of restriction. Figure 1 illustrates this concept. Mobilization in these cases is done at the anatomic or pathologic limit of the range of motion.

The techniques used may be direct, indirect, or a combination of both. Direct mobilization implies that the two bones of a specific joint are moved through direct contact with each other. Indirect mobilization implies that other anatomical structures are used for leverage in distracting the surfaces of the two bones. The third technique, a combination of direct and indirect techniques involves localized movement with one hand while applying traction to the joint indirectly with the other hand.

In addition to these concepts, Kaltenborn looks at the close packed (status rigidus) and loose packed (status perlaxus) positions of the joint. In the close packed position of the joint, the surfaces are as con-

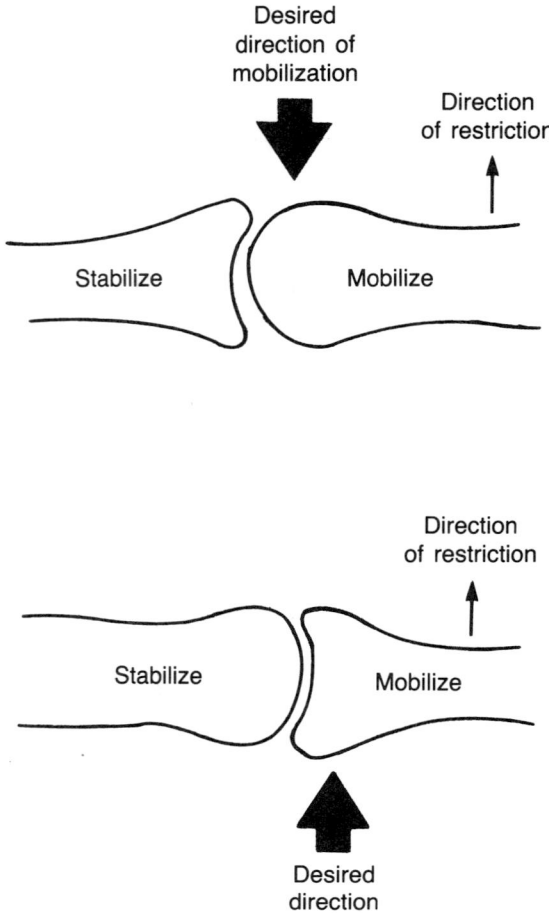

Figure 1 Concave-convex mobilization rule.

(From Kaltenborn FM. Mobilization of the extremity joints. Oslo: Olaf Norlis Bokhandel, 1980: 28).

TABLE 1   Close Packed Positions of Joints

Joint(s)	Position
Facet (spine)	Extension
Temporomandibular	Clenched teeth
Glenohumeral	Abduction and lateral rotation
Acromioclavicular	Arm abducted to 30 degrees
Sternoclavicular	Maximum shoulder elevation
Ulnohumeral (elbow)	Extension
Radiohumeral	Elbow flexed 90 degrees, forearm supinated 5 degrees
Proximal radioulnar	5 degrees supination
Distal radioulnar	5 degrees supination
Radiocarpal (wrist)	Extension with radial deviation
Metacarpophalangeal (fingers)	Full flexion
Metacarpophalangeal (thumb)	Full opposition
Interphalangeal	Full extension
Hip	Full extension and medial rotation*
Knee	Full extension and lateral rotation of tibia
Talocrural (ankle)	Maximum dorsiflexion
Subtalar	Supination
Midtarsal	Supination
Tarsometatarsal	Supination
Metatarsophalangeal	Full extension
Interphalangeal	Full extension

* Some authors (e.g., Kaltenborn) include abduction.

(From Magee DJ. Orthopedic physical assessment. Philadelphia: WB Saunders, 1987: 15).

gruent as possible (there is maximum contact between the two joint surfaces), and the ligaments and capsule are maximally taut. The bones cannot be separated by traction. Testing and treating cannot be performed in this position. In the loose packed position of the joint, the joint surfaces are not congruent, the ligaments are loose, the position of maximum looseness is referred to as the resting position, and is a position that any joint assumes when it is full of fluid as a result of injury. This resting position is optimal for obtaining distraction and movement during tests and joint play treatment procedures. Tables 1 and 2 show the common close packed and loose packed position of various joints.

TREATMENT TECHNIQUES

Kaltenborn felt the traction should be applied in three stages. The first stage, called piccolo, is a trac-tion technique with only sufficient traction to neutralize pressure within the joint without separating the joint surfaces. This type of technique is used for pain relief. With the second traction technique only sufficient traction is applied to "take up the slack" and to tighten the soft tissues surrounding the joint. A third traction technique, which applies even greater pressure, is a distraction technique that stretches the soft tissues about the joint.

Kaltenborn felt that different movements were possible (during mobilization). The first is translatoric or gliding movement. In this case, the bone is moved in a direction that is parallel to the treatment plane; it must not be confused with rolling. With rolling, different new points of one joint surface come in contact with a new point on the opposite joint surface, and the two points on each joint surface are equidistant; whereas with gliding, the same point on one joint surface comes in contact with new points on the other joint surface.

The second movement possible during mobilization is angular or rolling movement. In this case, the bone being moved follows the contour of the fixed bone surface. The third movement is traction, in which one bone is moved in a direction at right angles to

TABLE 2 Resting (Loose Packed) Positions of Joints

Joint(s)	Position
Facet (spine)	Midway between flexion and extension
Temporomandibular	Mouth slightly open (freeway space)
Glenohumeral	55 degrees abduction, 30 degrees horizontal adduction
Acromioclavicular	Arm resting by side in normal physiologic position
Sternoclavicular	Arm resting by side in normal physiologic position
Ulnohumeral (elbow)	70 degrees flexion, 10 degrees supination
Radiohumeral	Full extension and full supination
Proximal radioulnar	70 degrees flexion, 35 degrees supination
Distal radioulnar	10 degrees supination
Radiocarpal (wrist)	Neutral with slight ulnar deviation
Carpometacarpal	Midway between abduction-adduction and flexion-extension
Metacarpophalangeal	Slight flexion
Interphalangeal	Slight flexion
Hip	30 degrees flexion, 30 degrees abduction and slight lateral rotation
Knee	25 degrees flexion
Talocrural (ankle)	10 degrees plantar flexion, midway between maximum inversion and eversion
Subtalar	Midway between extremes of range of movement
Midtarsal	Midway between extremes of range of movement
Tarsometatarsal	Midway between extremes of range of movement
Metatarsophalangeal	Neutral
Interphalangeal	Slight flexion

(From Magee DJ. Orthopedic physical assessment. Philadelphia: WB Saunders, 1987: 14).

the treatment plane. When joint mobilizations are performed, the bone is moved at right angles to the treatment plane. This plane is defined as passing through the joint and lying at a right angle to a line running from the axis of rotation to the middle of the contacting articular surface.

Once the mobility or joint play has been restored to the joint, it is essential that properly taught exercises be performed to maintain the newly acquired range of motion. Although the patient is unable to perform joint play movements actively, the active full range movements done during exercise will maintain the joint play.

PATHOLOGIC CONCEPTS

Kaltenborn felt that disc degeneration went through six stages. In the first stage, the disc has distinctive borders between the annulus fibrosus and the nucleus pulposus. There are no fissures at this stage. In the second stage, called chondrosis incipiens, radial fissures appear in the annulus with no dislocation of the annulus fibrosus. In effect, this stage represents a normal older disc. The third stage is intradiscal dislocation or protrusion within the disc. The annulus ruptures and the nucleus pulposus herniates into the annulus so that the herniation is contained within the disc.

In stage four, there is a latent prolapse. The nucleus pulposus causes outward deformity of the annulus during certain movements, thereby resulting in a soft intermittent protrusion. Stage five is a definite prolapse, with irreversible protrusion of the nuclear contents through a fissure in the annulus. The final stage, or stage six, is regression with nerve root compression and nuclear material absorption.

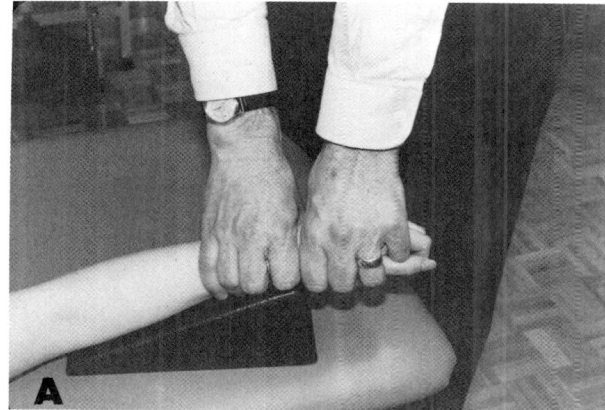

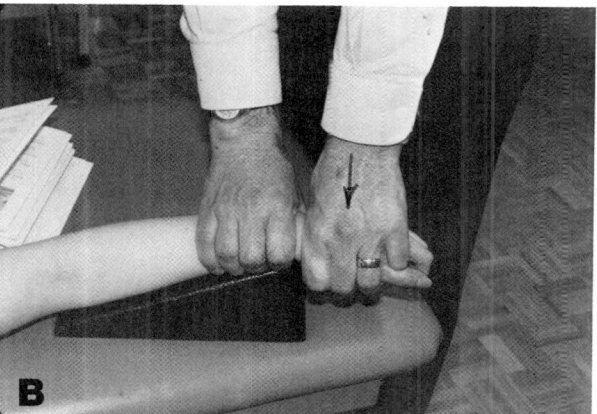

Figure 2 Mobilization of the radiocarpal joint for restricted extension. *A*, starting position; *B*, anterior excursion at radiocarpal joint.

Related to the disc is facet joint pathology. Kaltenborn felt that the facet joint pathology was attributable to pinching of the interarticular meniscus, fat pad, or joint capsule. This pinching results in muscle spasm, which locks a joint. The locking may also be caused by a loose or free body within the joint, such as cartilage or bone. This finding is similar to the condition called osteochondritis dissecans. In addition, facet joint pathology may be caused by subluxation or locking of the facet joint.

TREATMENT TECHNIQUES

Treatment of Radiocarpal Joint for a Restricted Extension

The patient is seated with the anterior aspect of the arm on a wedge so that the radius rests on the wedge—and the proximial row of carpal bones does not—and the hand hangs over the edge of the wedge. The therapist stands facing the ulnar side of the hand with right hand holding and stabilizing the patient's forearm on the wedge. The therapist's left hand holds around the carpal bones on the posterior aspect sta-

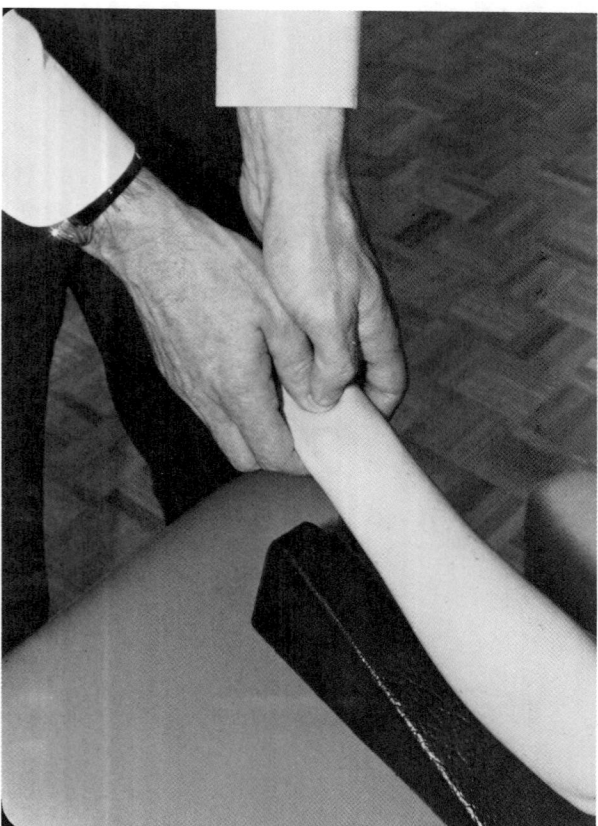

Figure 3 Mobilization of capitate on lunate for hypomobility.

bilizing these bones. The mobilization technique (gliding or traction) is applied in an anterior direction and the carpals are moved anteriorly in relation to the radius (Fig. 2). The amount of anterior pressure applied with the right hand depends on whether pain is the predominant symptom (less "push") or whether hypomobility is the primary symptom (stretch tissues).

Treatment of Hypomobility Between Lunate and Capitate

The patient, with his or her hand forward, sits facing the therapist. The therapist places the little, ring, and middle fingers of both hands around the thenar and hypothenar eminences (Fig. 3) and applies slight traction between the two to separate the carpal bones slightly. The index fingers are placed over each other over the lunate on the anterior surface fixating the lunate. The thumbs are then placed over each other and then over the capitate on the posterior surface. The capitate is then mobilized anteriorly by pushing anteriorly with the thumbs.

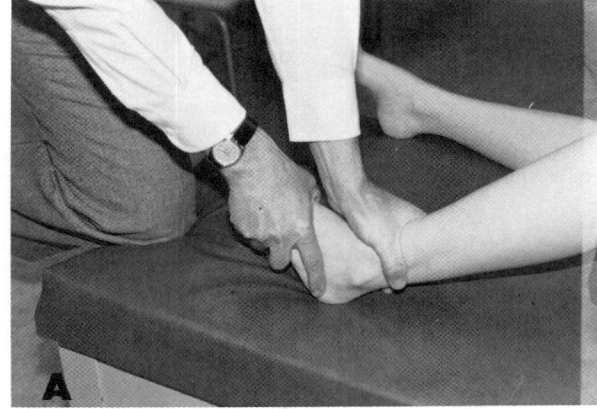

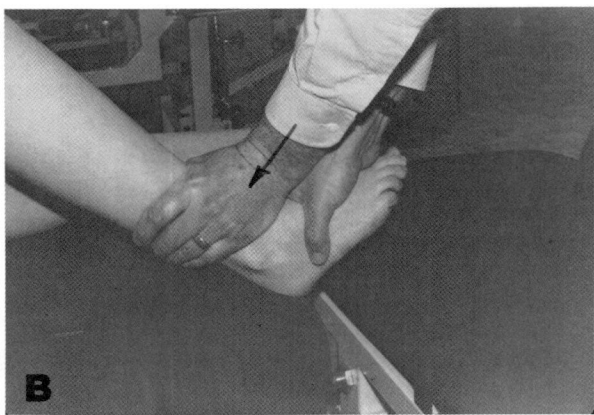

Figure 4 *A*, Mobilization of tibia and fibula on the talus for restricted plantar flexion; *B*, arrow shows direction of pressure.

Treatment for Restricted Plantar Flexion

The patient lies supine on the table with the knee flexed to about 80 degrees; the heel is on the treatment table and the ankle is slightly plantar flexed. The therapist stands facing the leg. The right hand stabilizes and holds the patient's foot around the metatarsal bones, thereby preventing movement of the foot. The left hand encircles and holds the distal aspect of the tibia and fibula with the hypothenar eminence just proximal to the ankle joint. The therapist locks his elbow and leans forward pushing the tibia and fibula back on the talus (Fig. 4).

These techniques are given as examples of Kaltenborn's techniques and how they might be applied. Other examples are described in his book (see Suggested Reading). The techniques are very exacting and require a firm understanding of anatomy including the shape of the bones and biomechanics.

SUGGESTED READING

Kaltenborn FM. Mobilization of the extremity joints Oslo: Olaf Norlis Bokhandel, 1980.
Magee DJ. Orthopedic physical assessment. Philadelphia: WB Saunders, 1987:1.

ORTHOPAEDIC MANUAL THERAPY: MAITLAND APPROACH

DAVID J. MAGEE, B.A., Dip. P.T., B.P.T., M.Sc., Ph.D.

The treatment techniques of Australian physical therapist Geoffrey Maitland are widely used by the physical therapy community.

ASSESSMENT

Maitland's assessment method is meticulous because it provides a guideline to treatment. The patient is assessed after each treatment technique to see if the technique has altered the signs and symptoms in terms of pain, stiffness, and spasm. Any changes give an indication of how vigorous or gentle further assessment and treatment needs to be.

The first part of Maitland's assessment is the **subjective evaluation.** During this evaluation, the therapist notes on a body chart (Fig. 1), the specific area of pain and its quality and any other abnormal sensations, such as paresthesia or anesthesia. In addition, detailed examination of the pain is undertaken by seeking such information as the effect of functional activities on pain and stiffness in terms of severity and length of time symptoms last. As with any assessment, a detailed past and present history is also taken.

The second part of the assessment is an **objective evaluation.** In this part of the assessment, Maitland feels it is necessary to include not only the joints and muscles in the painful area, but also the structures that may refer pain to the area. He feels that there are five groups of patients if the criteria is based on pain and stiffness. First of all, those patients in whom pain is the main problem. In other words, the limitation of movement is caused by pain. It must be understood that the limited movement may be active or passive physiologic movement, accessory (joint play) movement, or any combination of these movements. The second group are those in whom pain and stiffness occur together. In the third group, stiffness is the main problem, and in the fourth group pain is intermittent and/or momentary, but full range of motion is exhibited. Finally, the last group consist of those patients with internal derangement.

Maitland feels that pain and its relation to limited range of motion play a role in determining the grade of mobilization that is to be given. For example, if pain occurs at the end of the range of motion, that is, pain is the dominant symptom, it would indicate there is an active lesion or an extra articular lesion. In this instance, Maitland's grade I, or possibly grade II mobilization, would be performed. If pain and resistance at the end of the range of movement occurred at the same time, this feeling would indicate a capsular problem. In this case, stretching would be carried out with caution with Maitland's grades III and IV being performed. If the end of the range of motion, in other words resistance, is reached before the pain is felt, then stretching may be carried out and grades III and IV mobilizations may be performed with little difficulty.

During the various movement tests, the examiner looks for at least one comparable sign. Maitland defines a comparable sign as a motion or combination of motions that reproduces the pain or the stiffness.

Maitland also put forth the idea of quadrant positions to be used during the objective evaluation. Quadrant positions combine movements that maximally stretch the joint. They are especially evident in ball and socket type of joints, such as the shoulder and hip. For example, in the shoulder start with the arm fully abducted and beside the ear. The arm is then moved laterally away from the head with the arm laterally rotated. At the same time, the scapula is stabilized to prevent it from shrugging. As the arm is moved laterally, a point is reached where the arm comes forward. The position of maximum forward movement is approximately 30 degrees from the sagittal plane. Past this position, the arm rotates immediately. This position is called the quadrant position of the shoulder.

In his assessments, Maitland also advocates the idea of movement diagrams, which measure pain in terms of its intensity in relation to the range of motion. In this way, the examiner is able to tell if pain stopped before the end of range of motion, or whether it reached maximum by the end of range of motion. In addition, the examiner can note whether the pain at rest increased with movement, and whether spasms stopped the movement before the end of range of motion. Resistance from inert tissues could also stop movement before the end of the range.

For example, Figure 2 may be used as an illustration of his movement diagram concept. Maitland states, "a movement diagram is compiled by drawing graphs for the behavior of pain, physical resistance,

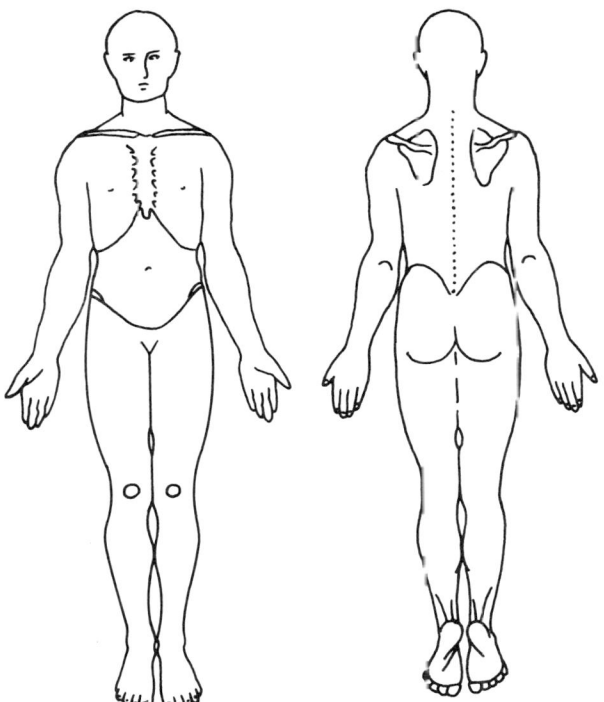

Figure 1 Body chart.

intensity. L indicates the limit of range available (pathologic range of motion), whereas P_2 indicates the intensity of pain at the end of the available range of motion. R_2, standing in this case for physical resistance (no muscle spasm), indicates the reason for the range only going to L. Thus, P_1, L, and R_2 are all in a straight vertical line. The line joining P_1 and P_2 gives an indication of how the pain alters as the joint is moved through the range of motion. In this case, the pain gradually increases up to a little more than half maximum intensity. If pain was the factor that limited the range of motion, it would be located at the same point as R_2. R_1 indicates where resistance begins to be felt, whereas the line joining R_1 and R_2 indicates the resistance increase. S_1 and S_2 indicate where reflex muscle spasm begins and ends during the available range of motion. The slope of the line joining S_1 to S_2 indicates how easily the spasm is provoked. If sloped toward A on the base line, it is easily provoked; if sloped toward B, it is harder to provoke. The strength or amount of spasm is shown by the height of the spasm line.

As Maitland states, "the diagram is compiled showing the behavior of all elements for that particular movement." The therapist can then interpret the relationship of the different factors and base the treatment technique and grade on these factors.

and muscle spasm, depicting the position in the range at which each is felt and the intensity of each." Intensity or quality is indicated by the vertical line (AC) and the horizontal line (AB) represents the normal, nonpathologic, range of motion of that joint in one direction. In the figure, pain (P_1) begins at about one-third of the normal range of motion and increases in

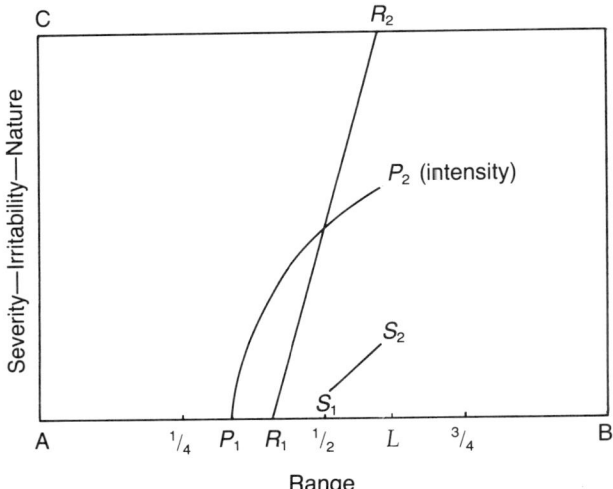

Figure 2 Movement diagram.

TREATMENT

Maitland felt that treatment should be based on signs and symptoms, especially pain and stiffness. He felt that if in the history, there is a great deal of joint irritability; pain on most or all movements; severe pain of particular postures; much limb pain; or postural spasm protecting the joint area, then gentle treatment should be applied. If during testing, active and passive physiologic movement, or accessory movement, the pain is sufficient to produce a facial distortion; if pain and/or parasthesia increase some seconds after the test movement has been completed; if spasm is elicited; or if much pain increases after normal examination, it is again an indication for gentle treatment.

If, in the history, there is moderate pain that becomes static for some time and is generally unvaried in intensity; no pain on joint movement; or pain that soon settles with little limb pain and no exacerbation of any particular posture and no postural spasm, it is an indication for more vigorous treatment. If during testing, the joint irritability is obviously minimal, with no muscle guarding on movement, or there is limitation of movements, more by tissue tension or compression than pain, then again, more vigorous treatment can be applied.

Grades of Mobilization

Maitland advocates the use of four grades when performing mobilizing techniques and these four grades may be fitted into either the physiologic range of movement or the accessory range of movement. Thus, the amount of movement occurring in a small amplitude movement varies. For example, if the small amplitude movement occurs in the physiologic range of shoulder abduction, it might move through 20 or 30 degrees. If it occurs in the accessory movement of lateral distraction, it may involve only a one-quarter inch or less. Generally, mobilization using Maitland's techniques are quite gentle and always within the control of the patient—that is, by contracting his muscles, the patient can stop the therapist from performing the graded mobilization technique. Because Maitland's techniques deal (primarily) with the joints, he advocates this gentle treatment as most effective. Thus, the techniques are more gentle than those advocated by Cyriax, for example. Cyriax feels most spinal problems come from the disc; Maitland feels they come from the facet joints and surrounding tissues.

Maitland's grade I (Fig. 3) is a small amplitude or oscillation of movement, which occurs at the beginning of the range of motion and which is carried out when the joints are reactive or acute and painful.

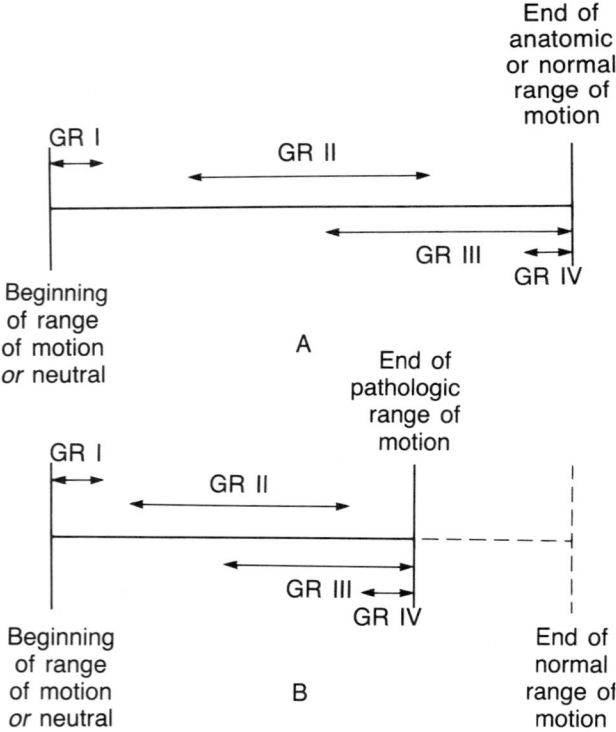

Figure 3 Maitland's grades of mobilization: *A*, normal (anatomic) range of motion; *B*, pathologic range of motion.

Each chosen mobilization technique is carried out two to three times per treatment, with each time having an oscillation duration of 10 seconds with a 15- to 30-second rest period in between. Grade II mobilizations are large amplitude movements, which occur in the middle of the range of motion. Each chosen mobilization technique is carried out approximately three times per treatment with an oscillation duration of 20 to 30 seconds with a rest period of 30 seconds in between. Grade III mobilizations are large amplitude movements at the end of the range of motion. Each chosen mobilization technique is carried out four to five times per treatment with an oscillation duration of 30 to 60 seconds and a rest period of 30 to 60 seconds in between. Grade IV is a small amplitude movement at the end of the range of motion. Each chosen mobilization technique is carried out four to five times per treatment with an oscillation duration of 30 to 60 seconds and a rest period of 30 to 60 seconds.

It should be noted that with each successive grade, the joint will have demonstrated less reactive signs prior to treatment. For example, a joint would be less acute for a grade IV mobilization to be performed, than for a grade I mobilization. For all four grades, Maitland advocates that the oscillations occur at the rate of 2 to 3 per second.

Small amplitude movements are especially effective when the joint condition is irritable or acute as they cause less flareup. Small amplitude movements are used if pain starts early in the range of motion, and if pain intensity increases rapidly. Large amplitude movements are more effective in mobilizing as long as they do not increase pain.

When performing Maitland's mobilizing techniques, the movement should be carried out in the range of motion just prior to where the pain begins. As the range of pain-free movement increases, mobilization can be carried further into the range of motion. A stage may be reached when it is necessary to carry the movement to pain to reach the resistance (usually when the pain is found to begin at the last quarter of the range). This method is necessary when progress is slowed down and a change of technique has not affected progress. When resistance can be felt, the choice is between a large amplitude or small amplitude movement of grade III or IV. Stronger movements tend to produce more local soreness, and large amplitude movements produce less soreness, but may not increase the range of motion as quickly. When a patient has pain in an arc of movement or a catching pain, large amplitude mobilization should be used. With severe pain, gentle small amplitude movement should be used. When there is very little pain, but movement is restricted, grade IV is the only movement that is useful. Grade III mobilizations relieve any local soreness produced by grade IV. If mobilizations produce

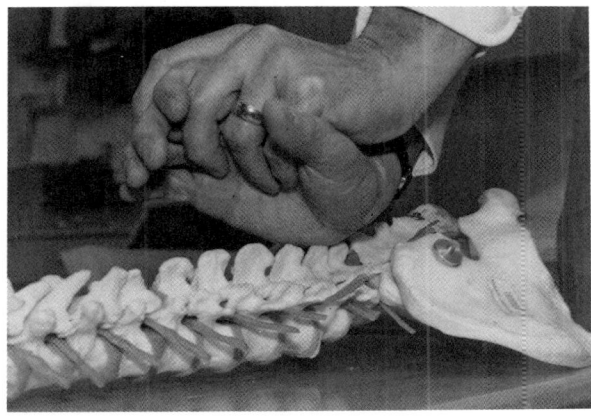

Figure 4 Hand position for applying Maitland's grades III and IV to the lumbar spine.

a quick muscle contraction or muscle spasm, a slower technique with less depth is used. If pain is used as a guide to the depth, spasm is avoided because the pain usually starts earlier in the range than the spasm.

The amount of treatment given in the first day should be considered separately from subsequent treatment sessions; this is because the examination in itself may cause pain. Also, the first stretching of a joint appears to cause more reaction. At the end of the first treatment, the patient should be given a warning that temporary increase in symptoms may follow. The number of mobilizations performed depends on the reaction to previous sessions. Daily treatment or treatment every second day should be instituted to begin with. A stage may be reached when it is difficult to know whether to stop or to carry on. If this occurs, the treatment should be stopped and the patient reassessed in 7 to 14 days to see if there has been any change. The situation may improve without any treatment. The objective is to use the gentlest techniques, which produce the desired results, and to modify the

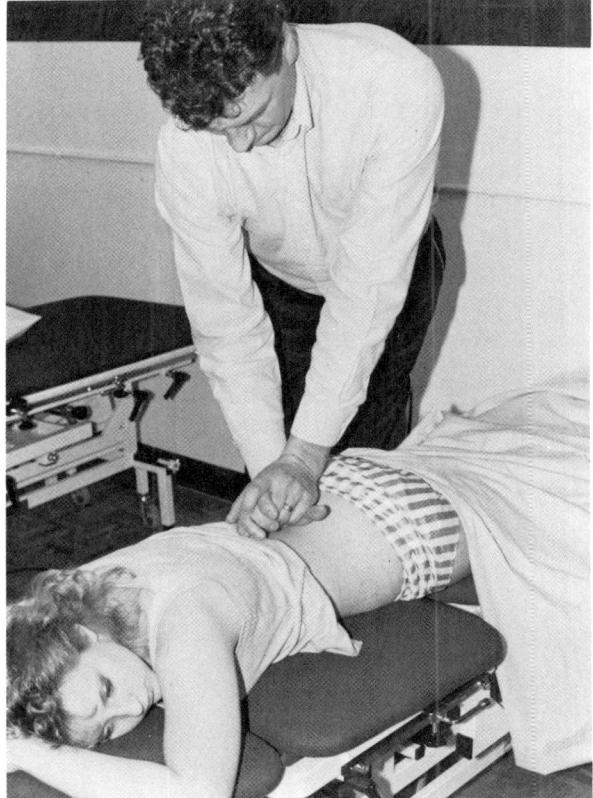

Figure 5 Application of Maitland's mobilization grades III and IV to L4 vertebra—posteroanterior central vertebral pressure technique.

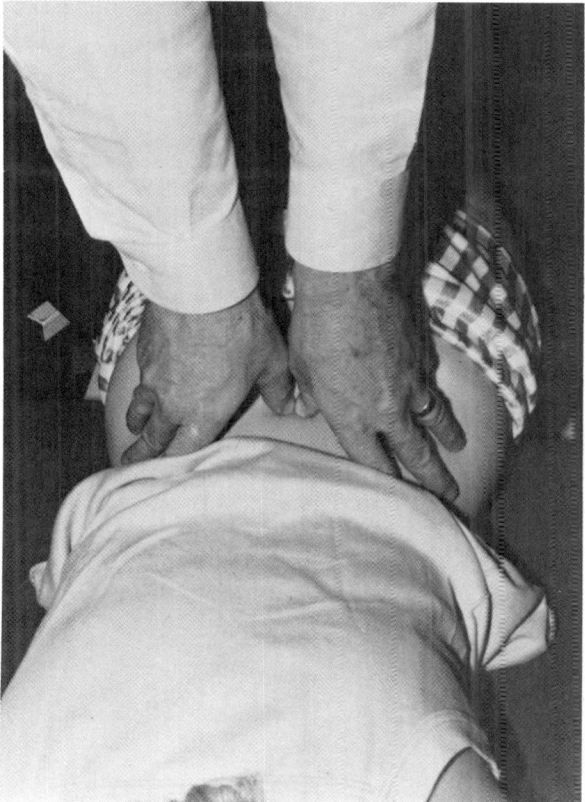

Figure 6 Application of Maitland's mobilization grades I and II to L4 vertebra—posteroanterior central vertebral pressure technique.

treatment on the basis of progress and repeated assessments.

TREATMENT TECHNIQUES

Posteroanterior Central Vertebral Pressure to L4 Vertebra

The patient lies prone on the treatment table with arms by the side and head turned comfortably to one side. To apply a grade III or grade IV technique, the therapist's hands are positioned as shown in Figure 4. The therapist stands at the patient's side with the ulnar border of the hand between the pisiform and hook of hamate resting on the spinous process of L4 vertebra. The therapist positions his or her shoulders directly above the hands with the elbows slightly flexed (Fig. 5). An oscillatory movement in the appropriate grade (III or IV) is obtained by a rocking movement of the trunk up and down in a vertical axis. Pressure is transmitted through the shoulders, elbows, and hands to the vertebra. This technique is primarily used when pain is evenly distributed to both sides of the body. For grades I and II mobilization, the hand position is changed and the thumbs are used instead of the ulnar aspect of the hand (Fig. 6).

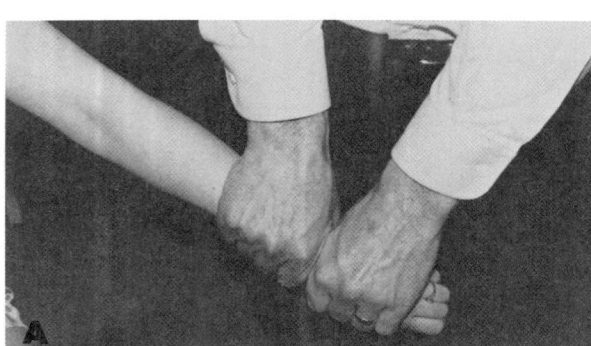
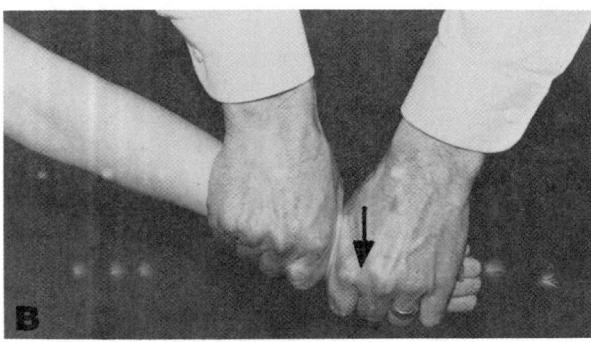

Figure 7 *A*, Lateral transverse mobilization of the wrist; *B*, arrow shows direction of mobilization.

Lateral Transverse Movement to the Wrist

The patient lies on the treatment table with arm abducted so that the wrist lies at the edge of the table. The hand lies over the table and the thumb faces the floor. The therapist stabilizes the radius and ulna with the right hand by holding the bones just proximal to

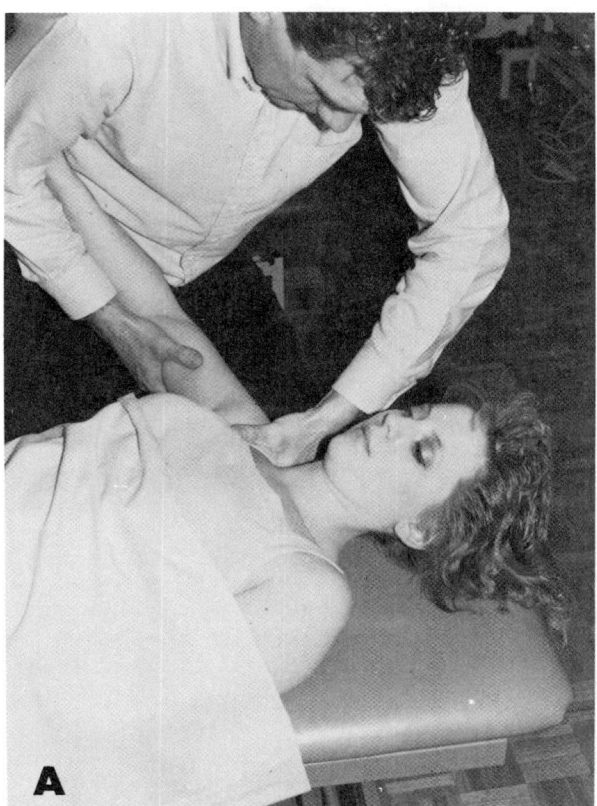
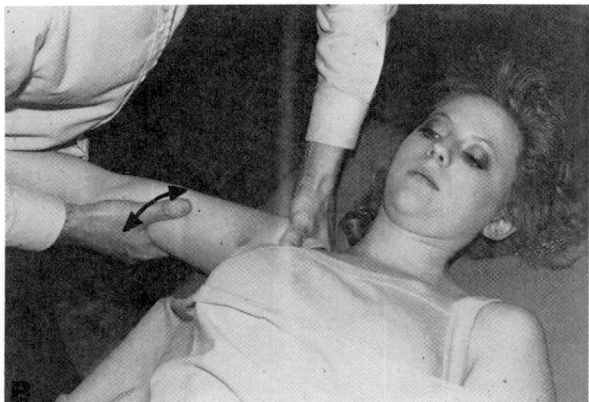

Figure 8 *A*, Maitland's grade IV mobilization of the glenohumeral joint into abduction; *B*, arrow shows direction of mobilization.

their distal end near the styloid processes. The therapist's knuckles "pad" the patient's arm by lying between it and the treatment table (Fig. 7). The therapist's left hand holds the posterior aspect of the patient's hand with the thumb and index finger around the proximal row of carpal bones. The therapist's left hand then oscillates the patient's hand laterally (in a radial direction) at the appropriate grade (usually III or IV) and applies force through the shoulder and the arm. The therapist's left hand and the patient's hand must move as a single unit.

Grade IV Mobilization of the Glenohumeral Joint into Abduction

The patient lies supine on the treatment table. The therapist faces the patient and crouches over the patient's arm placing the left hand over the acromion process and the right hand under the patient's elbow (Fig. 8). The patient's arm is abducted to a position just short of pain or to the position in which the os-

cillations are to be performed. The therapist's right hand is used to perform the appropriate grade of mobilization (in this case, grade IV) into abduction, performing the oscillations by abducting and adducting the patient's arm. The therapist's left arm should not fully restrict movement of the clavicle and scapula.

These techniques are given as examples of Maitland's techniques and as illustrations of the primary concepts of his treatment methods.

SUGGESTED READING

Maitland GD. Treatment of the glenohumeral joint by passive movement. Physiother 1983; 69:3–7.
Maitland GD. Peripheral manipulation. London:Butterworths. 1977.
Maitland GD. Relating passive movement treatment to some diagnosis. Austral J Physiother 1974; 20:129–135.
Maitland GD. The peripheral joints—examination and recording guide. Adelaide:Virgo Press, 1973.
Maitland GD. The treatment of joints by passive movement. Austral J Physiother 1973; 19:65–72.
Maitland GD. Vertebral manipulation. London:Butterworths, 1986.

ORTHOPAEDIC MANUAL THERAPY: MENNELL APPROACH

DAVID J. MAGEE, B.A., Dip. P.T., B.P.T., M.Sc., Ph.D.

The assessment and treatment techniques of American physician John McM. Mennell evolve around the concept of joint dysfunction. Mennell and his father, J. B. Mennell, define joint dysfunction as "a loss of one or more movements of an involuntary nature, which occurs at any synovial joint." These involuntary movements are also known as accessory movements or joint play.

It was Mennell who first put forward the idea of joint play movements and joint play treatment. He defined joint play as a movement that occurred in a normal synovial joint, which enabled the joint to go through a full range of motion, but could not be produced by voluntary muscle action. In most joints, this movement is less than an eighth of an inch in any one direction. It cannot be done actively by the patient, but can be performed by somebody else stabilizing one bone and moving the other bone on it. Normally, this type of movement is pain free. However, with pathology, it can become painful.

ASSESSMENT

Dr. Mennell's assessment technique has the stated purpose of determining whether there is fault in the joint, not necessarily in the surrounding soft tissues (muscles, tendons, fascia, etc.). With this assessment, Mennell attempts to rule out all other problems except joint problems so that he can determine if a treatable joint dysfunction is present. For a joint dysfunction to be present, Mennell feels that the onset of joint pain is sudden and traumatic. This joint pain is aggravated by activity and relieved by rest. Joint pain ceases as soon as the stress ceases, and it is not present as a primary cause when the joint is swollen. If the onset of symptoms is insidious, it is unlikely that joint dysfunction is the primary cause (although it may result secondarily from immobilization or disease). Seldom is joint dysfunction present if several joints are affected unless they have been traumatized or immobilized at the same time.

According to Mennell, joint dysfunction is caused by intrinsic trauma from an extrinsic or external force, immobilization including disease and aging, and finally, following serious pathology to the joint. Mennell feels that the joint could lock as a result of an unreduced subclinical subluxation or a seizing of the joint. The subluxation is a torsional injury, which results in a pinching or stretching of the soft tissues, whereras the seizure is the result of the joint surfaces binding together. It is towards this subluxation and "seizing up" that Dr. Mennell directs his treatment.

Examination of Joint Play Movement

In his assessment techniques, Dr. Mennell describes several rules for examining joint play movements. Although he makes them specific to joint play, the rules may just as easily be applied to any assessment technique for maximum effectiveness. The rules are as follows:

1. The examiner must be relaxed, must use a grasp that is comfortable for himself (herself) and the patient and must impart a feeling of confidence and competence.

2. The patient must be relaxed and fully supported, especially the joint being assessed. This relaxation is enhanced by the examiner explaining what will be done and assessing the opposite uninjured limb first.

3. Only one joint should be assessed at a time; start with the uninjured side and then proceed to the injured side.

4. When assessing a joint, examine one movement at a time and make the movement as pure as possible (for example, flexion or abduction, not both together). Perform patterned movements only if confident about what the problem is.

5. When examining a joint, especially for joint play, one bone is fixed or stabilized while the other bone is moved in different directions relative to the fixed bone.

6. By examining the unaffected limb first, the examiner is able to determine both the normal joint play for that individual and the end feel of that directional movement.

7. Only normal movement patterns (either physiologic or joint play) should be performed and no movements should be forced.

8. When examining any joint, the examiner should never "push through the pain."

9. When it is obvious that there are signs of acute joint or bone disease, examination should be carried

out with care and no irritative joint play movements should be performed.

TREATMENT

Although Dr. Mennell is advocating the assessment of joint play in the examination, he is also advocating the use of joint play as a treatment technique. To perform this technique, he advocates the use of a "fractional therapeutic movement" to restore normal joint play and hence normal range of motion.

He describes this fractional therapeutic movement as a quick thrust that moves the joint rapidly just beyond the physiologic limit of the range of motion, but within the normal anatomic limit. It is a sharp springing thrust that is not forceful. It is important that the individual applying the technique take up the slack first. The movement is repeated several times so that it may take several minute "thrusts" to produce a noticeable increase in joint play range of motion and hence in physiologic range of motion.

To perform these joint play techniques, the same rules are used as were used for the examination. It must be remembered that the treatment movement is a springing movement and is not a forced movement. The treatment movement is performed at the limit of the available range of motion or at the point of pain so that slack is taken up before the technique is performed. The treatment technique is performed in one direction at a time.

Mennell points out an important concept, which is applicable to any joint play, mobilization, or treatment technique regardless of who advocates it. Once the treatment technique has restored joint play and physiologic ranges of motion, it is essential that the patient be properly instructed in therapeutic exercise and other muscle reeducation techniques to maintain the newly restored range of motion. If this part of the treatment is left out, the joint soon regresses—if not back to its original state, then nearly so—and the treatment process must be repeated. It is extremely important to explain the patient's role in treatment and how to prevent recurrence of the condition.

TREATMENT TECHNIQUES

Mobilization of the Metacarpophalangeal Joint

Mennell advocates four joint play movements for the metacarpophalangeal joints—long axis extension, anteroposterior tilt, side tilt, and rotation. These same techniques may also be applied to the interphalangeal joints.

For long axis extension, the metacarpal bone is stabilized with one hand while the phalanx is moved. This same arrangement is also used for the other three techniques. The metacarpal bone is held near its head with the thumb and index finger of the therapist. The other hand grasps the proximal phalanx with the fingers and thumb (Fig. 1). The joint is positioned at the end of the available range of motion or where pain begins and the slack is taken up in the joint. The phalanx is then pulled away from the head of the metacarpal bone using several small thrusts. The process is repeated several times. One must be sure to have the correct starting position each time.

Anteroposterior tilt is performed from the same starting position except the thumb and finger of the moving hand are placed with the thumb posteriorly (anatomic position) and the finger anteriorly distal to the base of the first phalanx. Pressure is applied alternately to the thumb and finger, tilting the base of the phalanx backward using the thumb as a fulcrum and anteriorly using the finger as a fulcrum. As with the previous technique, this technique is performed in only one direction at a time and the joint is positioned and the slack taken up before small thrusts are performed. The movement performed is a tilting movement and not a parallel movement (the two joint surfaces parallel). Attempt to "open up" the joint anteriorly or posteriorly; the anterior technique is used to enhance flexion, whereas the posterior technique is used to enhance extension.

Side or lateral tilt is performed in the same fashion as anteroposterior tilt except the thumb and finger of the movement hand are placed along the two sides of the phalanx. Again, the thumb or finger is used as a fulcrum, opening the joint medially or laterally. The medial tilt (in the anatomical position) is used to enhance adduction at the metacarpophalangeal joint, whereas lateral tilt is used to enhance abduction.

Rotation of the proximal phalanx on the metacarpal involves grasping the phalanx with the finger and thumb of one hand while stabilizing the meta-

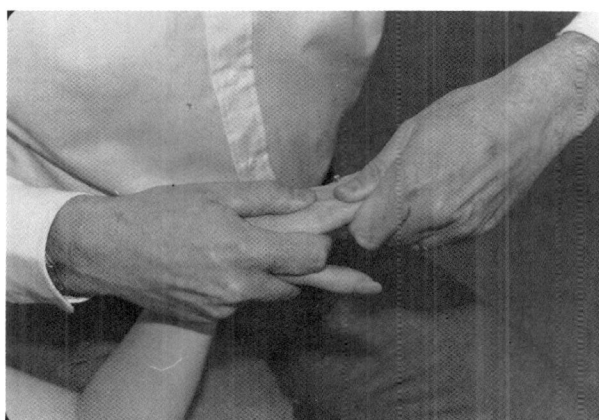

Figure 1 Positioning for joint play mobilization of the metacarpophalangeal joint.

carpal bone with the finger and thumb of the opposite hand. The joint is again positioned at the end of the available range of motion, or where pain begins, and the slack is taken up in the joint. The phalanx is then rotated, using several small thrusts, clockwise or counterclockwise on its long axis in relation to the metacarpal head.

Mennell feels that once normal joint play has been restored in the metacarpophalangeal joint(s), it is necessary to restore the normal gliding movement of the base of the phalanx around the head of the metacarpal bone because the joint is not a "true" hinge. The movement performed is a large amplitude movement with the joint surfaces parallel throughout the physiologic range of motion.

To perform the movement (example illustrates technique to improve flexion), the therapist places the thumb of one hand proximal to the anterior surface of the head of the metacarpal bone and the thumb of the other hand distal to the base of the proximal phalanx. While the one thumb stabilizes the metacarpal bone,

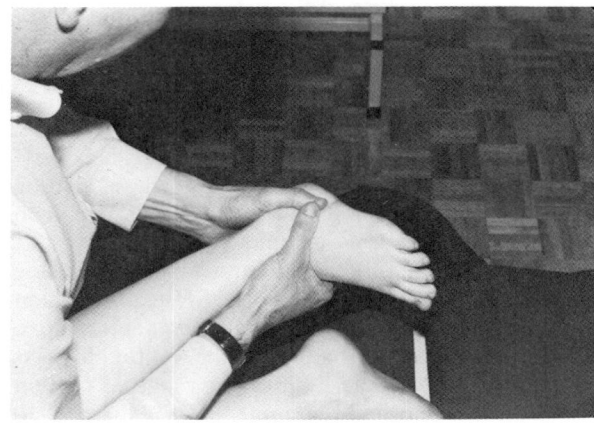

Figure 3 Joint play mobilization of the subtalar joint.

the other thumb pushes the base of the proximal phalanx around the head of the metacarpal bone, keeping the thrust at a right angle throughout the movement (Fig. 2). A similar technique in the opposite direction may be used to improve extension at the metacarpophalangeal joints.

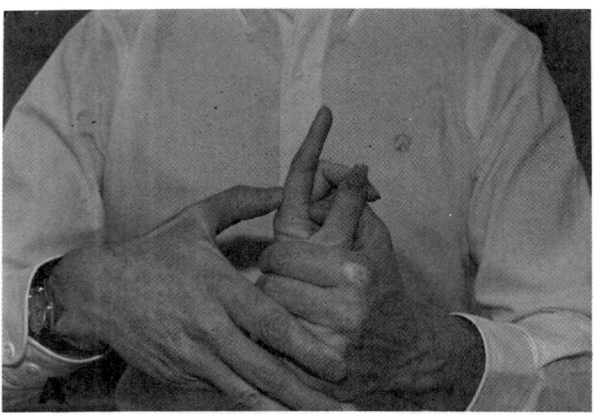

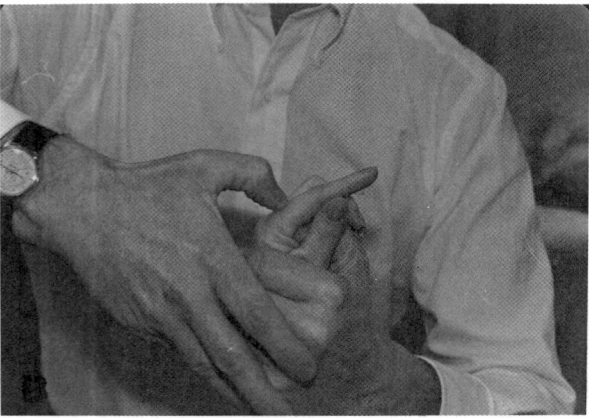

Figure 2 Large amplitude movement to restore normal gliding into flexion at the metacarpophalangeal joint. *A*, starting position; *B*, end position.

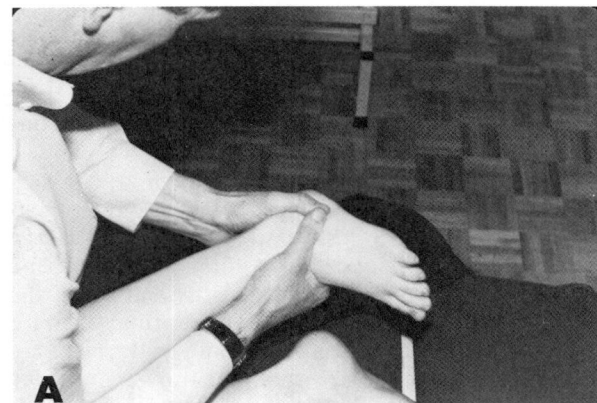

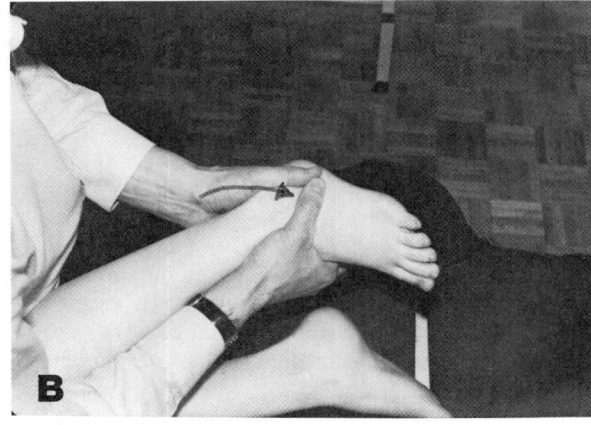

Figure 4 Talar rock. *A*, thrusting calcaneus anteriorly, *B*, arrow indicates direction of movement.

Joint Play Mobilization of the Subtalar Joint

The joint play movements possible for the subtalar joint are long axis extension, side tilt, and rotation of the talus on the calcaneus (talar rock).

The first two techniques are similar to the techniques performed at the metacarpophalangeal joints. Because bigger joints are involved, more force is involved for the thrusts to have the desired effect. For all three techniques, the positioning of the therapist and the patient are the same. The therapist sits on the treatment table with his or her back to the patient, who lies supine with hip and knee flexed so that foot lies in front of therapist as shown in Figure 3. One of the examiner's hands (web space) is placed posteriorly to the achilles tendon while the web space of the other hand is placed over the dorsum of the foot as close to the ankle as possible. For long axis extension, the foot is positioned at the end of the range of motion or at the point of pain, slack is taken up and the small thrusts are applied by the therapist leaning backward over the thigh while he or she pushes the patient's foot away on the long axis. The amount

of movement occurring in this case is the summation of the movement at the talocrural and subtalar joints.

Side tilt, medially or laterally, is performed in a similar fashion. The joint is positioned at the end of the available range or at the point of pain, tension is taken up, and the examiner's thumbs are used to impact the medial thrust, or the fingers are used to impact a lateral thrust using the fingers (in the first case) or the thumbs (second case) as the pivot point. Be sure that the calcaneus is tilting on the talus and that inversion or eversion is not occurring.

Talar rocking is performed from the same starting position as long axis extension. The bones of the joint are properly positioned, and the therapist, using the hand around the achilles tendon, thrusts upwards and forward several times causing the calcaneus to rock forward on the talus (for an anterior rock) while stabilizing and directing the movement with the opposite hand, which lies over the talus and the navicular anteriorly (Fig. 4). For the posterior rock (Fig. 5), the therapist uses the hand over the dorsum of the foot. Thrusting backward and downward results in the posterior rock. The movement is a rocking movement and not simply dorsiflexion or plantar flexion.

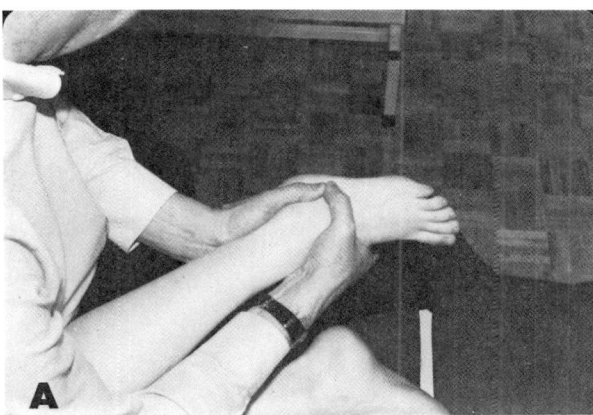

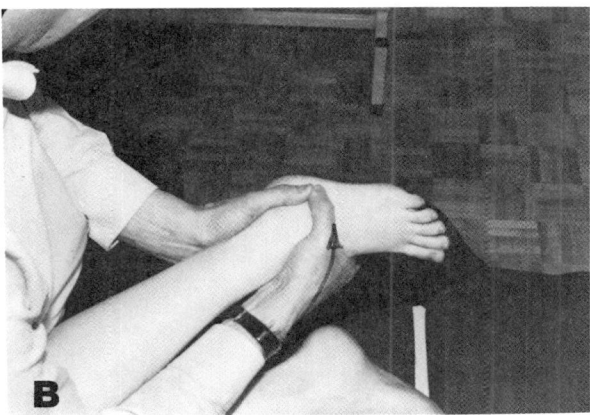

Figure 5 *A*, thrusting talus posteriorly; *B*, arrow indicates direction of movement.

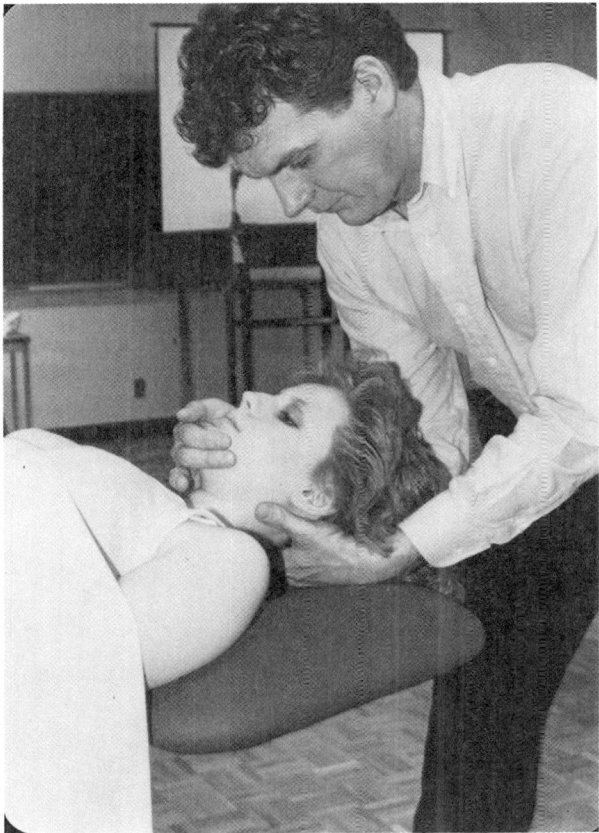

Figure 6 Long axis extension to the cervical spine.

Mobilization of the Cervical Spine

Mennell's techniques for the spine may be classed as general and specific techniques, which means the techniques may involve more than one joint at a time or may be isolated primarily to one level. The three techniques demonstrated are called long axis extension, anteroposterior glide, and side glide.

For all three techniques, the patient lies supine with the therapist at the head. For long axis extension, the therapist flattens the cervical lordosis by pushing or dropping the chin to the neck. The therapist's nondominant hand is placed under the patient's occiput while the dominant hand is placed around the chin to prevent flexion or extension of the head during the mobilization technique (Fig. 6). A steady "long axis" pull is applied primarily through the occiput until just before the patient's body begins to move. The therapist then applies small thrusts in this position. This technique is classed as a general technique.

To perform anteroposterior glide, the patient and therapist are in the same position as for the previous technique as are the therapist's hands. The index finger of the nondominant hand is placed over the spinous process of the level to be treated (for example,

C4). Thus, this technique is a specific technique for the treatment of C4 vertebra. To mobilize anteriorly, the head and neck are carried anteriorly (Fig. 7) through their full arc of movement with the face kept parallel to the treatment table. Both facet joints are treated at the same time by applying the small thrusting movements following the direction of the facet joint surfaces. The thrusting movements are applied through the spinous process by the index finger of the nondominant hand.

To perform the posterior movement, the head is returned to the treatment table. To mobilize in a posterior direction, the therapist stabilizes the spinous process of the level to be treated (for example, C4) by holding it still with the index finger of the nondominant hand. The vertebra above is then allowed to fall back (in the example sited C3 falls back on C4). The "thrusts" are in effect supplied by the weight of the head.

During the side gliding movement (right or left), the two facets at the same level are being treated at the same time. The patient and therapist are in the same positions as previously described. The therapist's hands are placed along side the head to control it and to keep the chin tucked in. The neck is sup-

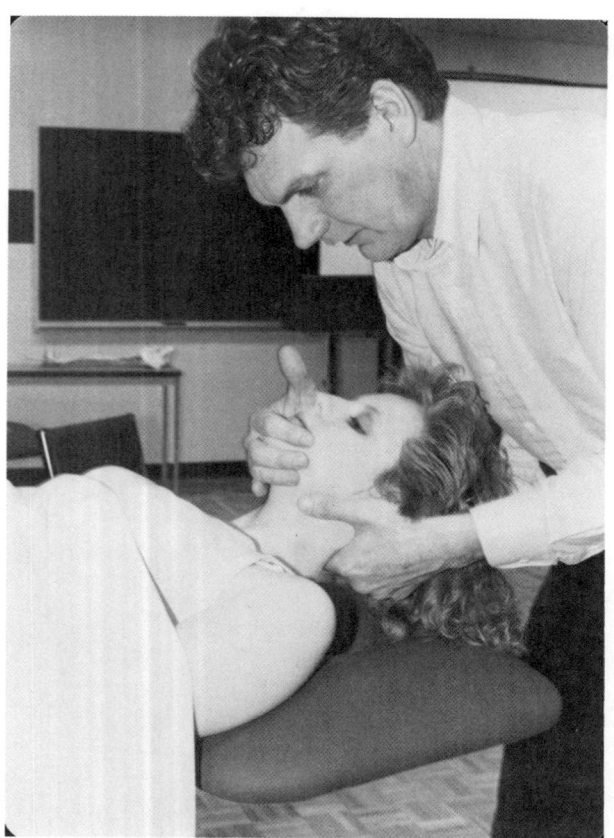

Figure 7   Anterior glide to C4 vertebra.

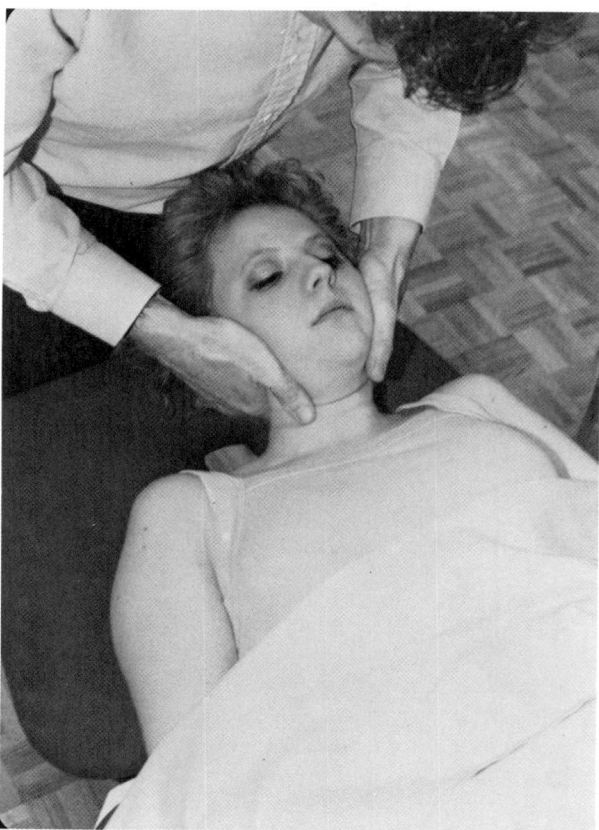

Figure 8   Side gliding mobilization of the cervical spine.

ported by the palm and the third to fifth fingers. The head is then carried to the left (or right) keeping the chin and head parallel to the long axis of the body (Fig. 8); the distal interphalangeal joint of the index finger is over the spinous process of the level to be treated; and the proximal interphalangeal joint is over the right transverse process. This hand positioning makes the technique specific. The head and neck are properly positioned and small thrusts are applied through the proximal interphalangeal joint of the index finger. The same method may be used for each vertebrae for both the left and right sides.

The above techniques are given as examples of Mennell's techniques and how they might be applied. His techniques for the peripheral joints are more com-

monly used than are those for the spinal joints. If one keeps in mind Mennell's rules for assessment and treatment the therapist finds the techniques useful and effective.

SUGGESTED READING

Mennell JM. Back pain—diagnosis and treatment using manipulative techniques. Boston: Little, Brown, 1960.
Mennell JM. Foot pain. Boston: Little, Brown, 1969.
Mennell JM. Joint pain—diagnosis and treatment using manipulative techniques. Boston: Little, Brown, 1964.
Mennell JM. Manipulation of the joints of the wrist. Physiother 1971; 246–254.
Zohn DA, Mennell JM. Musculoskeletal pain—diagnosis and physical treatment. Boston: Little, Brown, 1976.

McKENZIE APPROACH FOR LOW BACK PAIN

RIKI YAMADA, Dip. P. & O.T., M.C.P.A.

Low back pain afflicts a large sector of the population and is the number one cause of lost time in industry. Most episodes of pain are self-limiting in nature, although it is common to find recurrences. Each exacerbation tends to be worse than the previous one.

Although many approaches to treatment are available, (i.e., various manipulative therapy techniques, electrotherapy, acupuncture, and hydrotherapy among others), Robin McKenzie has developed a protocol that addresses the need to control the recurrent nature of low back pain and allows or even demands that patients take active control of their problem. Self treatment and prophylaxis are the keys to management of spinal pain using this approach. McKenzie has managed to divide patients into two main groups; those with pain derived from a mechanical lesion within the spine and those with pain attributable to inflammatory or other nonmechanical causes. It is the former in which the McKenzie approach is applicable. The principles and concepts he has developed can be used in the treatment of pain, which originates from any part of the spine, and need not be isolated to lumbar lesions.

CRITERIA FOR THE SELECTION OF PATIENTS

In order to select patients who are appropriate for this approach, McKenzie has defined principles that are useful in identifying spinal pain syndromes. He has emphasized the clinical significance of identifying mechanical and nonmechanical pain, the use of repeated movements and the concept of centralization and peripheralization of pain as an assessment and treatment tool.

The recognition of mechanical pain is established by close questioning during the subjective examination, in addition to observing the objective signs. The comparable characteristics are listed in Table 1 as follows.

Traumatic lesions are a mixture of both chemical and mechanical pain. Initially, there is an inflammatory reaction (substrate phase) causing nonmechanical pain, followed by a mixture of chemical and mechanical pain during the fibroblastic phase. In the maturation phase, when collagen remodelling takes place, there is purely mechanical pain caused by the physical deformation of nociceptors.

It must be noted that a large disc derangement is also capable of producing constant pain. The pain remains as long as the derangement continues to produce mechanical deformation of pain sensitive structures, such as the posterior longitudinal ligament and the dural sleeve.

Chemical pain is best dealt with by modalities or medication that reduce or eliminate the chemical irritants. Once the chemical pain has resolved, any mechanical pain must be dealt with by mechanical means. This may include exercises, mobilizations, and manipulations or traction.

A thorough subjective examination must be performed to rule out conditions that are contraindications for physical therapy. In addition, questions about aggravating and easing factors of the patients symptoms often give clues as to the direction the therapeutic exercises or techniques should take. For instance, if a patient has low back and leg pain which is aggravated by bending or sitting but eased by standing or walking, then it is quite likely that the symptoms will be eased by exercises or techniques that utilize lumbar extension since the lumbar spine comes into extension during standing and walking.

Having concluded from the subjective examination that we are dealing with a mechanical pain, the objective assessment serves to confirm the subjective findings. The objective examination incorporates familiar tools, i.e., observation of contours, posture, asymmetries, range of movement, and neurologic signs. Most importantly, it also incorporates the use of repeated movements and the observation of centralization and peripheralization to get a fuller understanding of the relationship between the symptoms and spinal movement.

Repeated movements are useful in assessing the spine under repeated stress and more specifically the behavior of the disc under repeated loading. This type of loading should affect the movement of the nucleus within the disc if the hydrostatic mechanism of the disc is still intact. Discography has shown that the nucleus is capable of migrating in the opposite direction of spinal movement. During flexion, the nucleus shifts towards the posterior part of the disc, whereas it moves anteriorly during extension. Should a lesion of the annulus be present, repeated loading may further enhance the derangement, whereas repeated loading in the opposite direction may reduce the derangement.

TABLE 1 Characteristics of Mechanical versus Nonmechanical Pain

Mechanical	Nonmechanical
Constancy	
Intermittent	Constant
Nature	
Sharp/sudden/twinging pain	Pulsing/throbbing ache
Behavior	Position/movement worsened
Altered by position/movement may be either eased or worsened	but not eased
Better after prolonged rest worsens the longer mechanical; not eased by anti-inflammatory agents	Stiff and sore after prolonged rest eased with anti-inflammatory agents
Signs	Often heat, redness, or
No heat, redness or swelling	swelling detectable

Peripheralization is a term used to describe the referral of symptoms away from the midline and towards the extremities. The hypothesis for this phenomenon may be explained in anatomic terms. A small derangement may only press against central pain sensitive structures, thereby causing central pain. As the prolapse increases, other structures may become affected such as the dural sleeve and nerve root. This results in pain in the relevant dermatome of the leg with or without sensory or motor changes. Cyriax also noted that the stronger the stimulus, the more distal the extent of referral. Centralization is merely a reversal of this process. This behavior is characteristic of a derangement syndrome, but may also be seen in a nerve root adhesion. Treatments should produce a centralization of symptoms *not* peripheralization (except in the treatment of nerve root adhesions).

SYNDROMES

By analyzing the assessment findings, patients may be divided into three syndromes as described by McKenzie. For a full description of the syndromes, the reader is urged to refer to his textbook *The Lumbar Spine—Mechanical Diagnosis and Therapy*. The following is a brief synopsis of each syndrome.

Postural Syndrome

Patients are usually under the age of 30, with poor posture and poor body awareness.

The pain appears to arise from overstretching of normal tissues due to poor posture; hence the lack of physical signs during objective examination. An analogy may be made to the pain that is felt when one keeps the metacarpophalangeal (MCP) joint of a finger extended at maximum range for a prolonged period. The pain is intermittent and may be felt in several areas of the spine (i.e., cervical, upper thoracic, and lumbar) after prolonged stress such as sitting. There

is no centralization or peripheralization on repeated movements.

Dysfunction Syndrome

Patients with this syndrome tend to be over the age of 30, especially those with a history of insidious onset of pain. Patients may be of a younger age group if trauma has been involved—this includes those involved in lifting injuries. These patients are frequently under exercised.

Pain from this syndrome is usually felt adjacent to the midline of the spine and is *never* referred below the knee unless it is caused by a nerve root adhesion. A sharp or pulling pain is felt at the end of the available range of motion, *not during* the movement. It is eased by rest or avoidance of maximum range. A definite loss of range is noted on examination. Repeated movements do not cause centralization or peripheralization of pain. There are no neurologic signs unless they are residual from a previous derangement.

The pain arises from stretching of abnormally tight tissues. This may be a result of adaptive shortening following years of poor posture in which case the history is that of an insidious onset. It may also be caused by stress of inextensible scar tissue formation following trauma (this includes patients with a history of previous derangement).

Derangement Syndrome

Patients with this syndrome are typically between 20 to 55 years of age. The history is usually one of a sudden onset, i.e., pain within hours or days in a patient who was otherwise asymptomatic. Often the onset is insidious, but the patient may also be able to recall a specific incident such as an awkward lift. It is very common to have a previous history of similar or progressively worsening episodes, especially in patients at the older end of the spectrum.

The pain may be felt local to the midline of the

spine or slightly lateral to the spinal column. It may or may not be associated with locking of the back. Frequently, there is some radiation of pain into the leg and foot. The patient may also complain of paresthesia or sensory and/or motor deficit. Symptoms may cross the midline and refer down the opposite leg. Certain movements or maintenance of certain positions may aggravate symptoms, whereas other movements ease symptoms. Pain may be intermittent or constant depending on the constancy of mechanical deformation of pain sensitive structures.

Objectively, a deformity such as a marked lumbar kyphosis or a lateral shift of the trunk may or may not be seen. Since most derangements are posterolateral or posterior, there is often a loss of the normal lumbar lordosis. An accentuated lordosis may be seen in an anterior derangement. Repetition of movements in certain directions increases or peripheralizes symptoms, whereas repetition of movements usually in the opposite direction decreases or centralizes symptoms. Pain is reproduced during the test movement, not at the end of range as in the dysfunction syndrome. Neurologic signs may be present.

The pain felt in the derangement syndrome is thought to be attributable to a derangement within the mobile segment. The most commonly affected structure is the intervertebral disc (IVD). Herniations of the IVD produce pain via the disruption of the annular wall, as well as the mechanical deformation of pain sensitive structures, such as the posterior longitudinal ligament, dura, dural sleeve, and blood vessels.

ESSENTIAL CHARACTERISTICS OF THE THERAPEUTIC APPROACH

Prevention of recurrences and, failing prevention, self-treatment of the condition are goals that are of the utmost importance in the McKenzie approach. In order to achieve these goals, the patient must become a partner in the effort to understand and manage his back pain. Education is on a very basic level; it deals with anatomy and biomechanics and the hypothetical causes of pain. This leads to education about prophylaxis. The necessity of maintaining proper posture, the use of correct body mechanics in activities of daily living as well as in lifting. The use of McKenzie's patient booklets *Treat Your Own Back* and *Treat Your Own Neck* are invaluable tools in reinforcing understanding and compliance. Failing that, some type of written information is an asset for patients to use as future reference once consultation with the therapist has been completed.

The patient is encouraged from the first visit to strive for self-reliance in the management of pain. The patient is given at least the first 24 hours to try and control the symptoms by the use of corrective postures or exercises. It is important to educate the pa-

tient about peripheralization and centralization so that the symptoms are not made worse. The therapist does not intervene at this point with hands on techniques, in order to give the patient a chance to see that he can treat himself and need not become a passive recipient and dependent of treatment. If it becomes apparent on reassessment that the correct advice and exercises have been given, the therapist need only to continue in the role of consultant, refining the program according to progress. The patients are advised to try and regain full range of motion (ROM) in all directions in order to restore optimum function and to decrease the chance of recurrence. The majority of patients are able to become self-reliant. Approximately 30 to 35 percent require manual techniques in order to resolve the pain.

TREATMENT PROTOCOLS

Each syndrome is treated by a specific protocol. In order to become thoroughly familiar with them and with the specific exercise techniques the reader should refer to the text *The Lumbar Spine—Mechanical Diagnosis and Therapy* by Robin McKenzie. The following will be a highlight of the treatment protocols as interpreted by this author.

Postural Syndrome

Postural correction is all that is required here. The patient is reassured that the pain is not caused by tissue pathology, but rather by excessive stress on normal tissue. The bent finger analogy is brought in to illustrate this point. Once the patient is aware that the pain is self-induced, correct posture in standing, sitting, and sleeping is taught. In order to find the natural balance of the spine, the patient must be taken into the extreme of poor posture (if pain is felt there, the point is easier to teach), then brought out to 100 percent correct posture then allowed to relax 10 percent.

The correct standing posture is achieved by restoring the normal spinal curves. If a plumb line were dropped beside the patient, it should fall through the ear lobe, through the shoulder joint (arms hanging at the side), approximately midway between the front and back of the trunk, through the greater trochanter of the femur, slightly anterior to the midline of the knee, and slightly anterior to the lateral malleolus. The apex of the lumbar lordosis should be at the third lumbar level, not the fifth. In order to achieve this posture, the patient may be taught to tilt the pelvis backwards and to move the upper spine forwards by raising the chest. If the patient fails to understand this, pulling up gently by the hair on the crown of the head usually achieves the desired posture.

Poor sitting posture is the most frequent cause of postural pain. The use of a lumbar roll is essential when sitting. The support not only decreases the intradiscal pressure in the lumbar spine, but also places the thoracic and cervical vertebrae into proper alignment. The inclination of the backrest is important in aligning the thoracic and cervical spine. An upright position is the best angle to decrease the stress of a forward head posture—the culprit of much upper thoracic and neck pain as well as headaches. This upright position is of particular importance during driving, and it may well be worthwhile for patients to have a mechanic reposition the seat if it is not easily adjustable. The sitting position at work should be such that the trunk is sandwiched in between the desk and lumbar roll, thus maintaining the lumbar lordosis. An inclined desk surface is of great benefit in reducing strain on the neck. A desk top drafting board may be of use for people with desk jobs.

Sleeping posture is often helped by the use of a lumbar roll. A simple procedure is to fold a large bath towel length-wise and fasten it around the waist line. This is very useful when there is a large discrepancy between waist and pelvic width. The roll stops the spine from falling into extreme side bending when sleeping on the side, and also supports the normal lordosis in the supine position. Patients are discouraged from sleeping prone as it places rotational stress on the cervical spine and allows the lumbar spine to fall into an extreme of extension for excessive periods.

Patients must be warned that new aches and pains may appear as a result of adjustments to new postural habits. These should not last more than 4 to 5 days. Patients are asked to practice the slouch to overcorrected posture several times a day especially when they feel the onset of their pain. Daily follow-up may be required for 2 or 3 days until posture can be consistently controlled. The intervals are then gradually lengthened as better posture is practiced.

Young patients, particularly in their teens are difficult to treat since they do not want to appear different from their slouching peers. Enrollment into sports such as ballet or gymnastics, which encourage body awareness and total body exercise, may be of benefit in reinforcing the therapeutic training.

Dysfunction Syndrome

Patients with dysfunction syndrome must follow the same postural advice as in the postural syndrome. In addition, passive exercises are given to stretch shortened tissues. The exercises are done in the direction of the painful restriction. The forcefullness of the stretch depends upon the stage of healing. This procedure is used only in the fibroblastic and maturation phases of tissue repair.

It is during the fibroblastic phase that care must be taken in paying heed to the relationship of pain and resistance. Cyriax's concepts of readiness to stretch are the easiest to explain to patients. If pain precedes

resistance, no stretch is given. Gentle painless movement may be used to decrease pain and to influence the orderly laying down of collagen tissue. When pain and resistance come together, gentle stretching may begin. Once the maturation stage has been reached, stretch should be taken to the point of a "strain" pain. Again, the bent finger analogy illustrates the desired degree of discomfort. In order to maintain tissue remodeling, McKenzie recommends at least 10 repetitions 10 times per day. Postexercise pain should not last longer than 10 to 20 minutes after cessation of the exercises. If pain persists, the frequency and/or number of repetitions should be reduced.

Expected results include marked improvement of function and range of movement within 4 to 6 weeks. As ROM is improved, exercises are decreased to four times a day. When maximum ROM is achieved, the exercises are decreased to twice daily and performed routinely as a prophylactic measure. Range of movement is deemed to be full in extension if the spine can be extended against a pelvis, which maintains contact with the table, while the arms are fully extended. Flexion is full if the knees can be hugged to the chest, and if the patient is able to reach the ankle during flexion in standing.

Pain should not peripheralize except in the treatment of nerve root adhesions. In this case, the dural sleeve and nerve root are stressed, symptoms may be reproduced. However, once the stress is stopped the symptoms should quickly subside. The protocol for this treatment utilizes flexion exercises which are performed first in lying and progressed to standing. Two important considerations must be followed.

1. Flexion exercises should not be done during the first 4 to 5 hours after rising. McKenzie hypothesizes that during this time the disc is more likely to be under increased pressure as a result of nocturnal imbibation and reabsorption of fluid. This may then increase the risk of derangement should additional loading be allowed to occur.
2. Extension exercises preferably in lying should be performed after the flexion exercises to counteract any stresses which may have been placed on the disc wall.

The same precautions apply in the treatment of limitation of spinal flexion, but without root adhesion.

The prevention of scar tissue adhesion following surgery is of great importance. To this end, the introduction of passive straight leg raising postsurgically every 2 hours is recommended. This can be done with the use of slings and pulleys or the help of nurses and relatives. Once the surgical site has stabilized, gentle ROM exercises in all directions may be started. It is recommended that extension be the last exercise performed in order to counteract any stresses on the posterior wall of the discs adjacent to the surgical site.

Derangement Syndrome

The main aims of treatment are to reduce the derangement, to teach the patient how to maintain this reduction, and to restore maximum function and mobility to prevent recurrence.

McKenzie has described seven different types of derangements that are recognizable in the lumbar spine. Although the majority of these types respond to the extension principle, i.e., extension exercises and the maintenance of the lumbar lordosis, the direction for treatment depends on the assessment findings. The correct direction is one in which the pain centralizes. In the case of an anterior derangement, flexion may be the direction of choice.

If the direction selected is the correct therapeutic direction, a reduction or resolution of symptoms is noted, in addition to an increase in the previously restricted movement. If self treatment is applicable, reduction of the derangement should be achieved during the first treatment session. It is not unusual to perform extension in prone lying in two to three sets of 10 repetitions in the first session before complete relief of pain is achieved. As long as the symptoms continue to centralize, the exercise should be continued. The patient should be warned that as it approaches the center of the back, the pain (often described as a tremendous pressure) may increase in intensity for a short while, but is relieved with continued extension.

The patient should be left for 24 hours to continue his exercise program—usually prone lying, prone lying in extension (elbow propping) and passive extension exercises performed in prone—a repetition of 10 every hour, and should then be reassessed. If the patient is able to remain asymptomatic, the frequency of the extension exercises are then reduced to every 2 hours and gradually to three times a day, if the patient remains painfree for 3 days. Flexion exercises in lying and later in standing may then be introduced (if this movement does not reproduce symptoms) in order to restore maximum function. The precautions for flexion as discussed in the Nerve Root Adhesion section must be followed.

It is imperative that the patient be taught to maintain lumbar lordosis especially in the first 24 to 48 hours so that reduction is not lost. Advise against sitting unless it is absolutely necessary; and then only with a lumbar roll in firm chairs. Teach the patient to rise maintaining a lordosis and to sleep with a towel support around the waist.

The author has found that the use of a lumbosacral belt may be beneficial for a day or two following reduction of a large derangement. These patients often are relieved of their pain, but the back may feel weak or the reduction may be temporary. The belt gives them a little added support in the early phase of treatment, but should be weaned off as quickly as possible.

Once the patient has regained full or maximal ROM and remained asymptomatic, advise continuation of a routine of extension in lying in the morning and flexion in lying followed by extension in lying in the evening for 6 weeks. He is thoroughly educated on prophylactic measures and advised to perform extension exercises in standing during the day when faced with situations that require prolonged flexion of the spine. He is also taken step by step through the self-treatment program in case of a relapse.

Failure of the extension regime may be attributable to the following:

1. The patient does not perform the exercises correctly. The extension should be done passively with the pelvis resting on the floor or table and the arms pushing the spine into extension. It is not unusual to feel strain discomfort in the upper back or arms due to this effort. Daily reassessment in the first 24 to 48 hours of treatment prevents the needless continuation of any incorrect exercises.

2. Insufficient time allowed for the reversal of the nuclear fluids to take place. A constant low back pain or loss of lordosis may be the result of accumulation of intradiscal material posteriorly, which causes a physical widening of the posterior margins of the vertebral bodies and allows mechanical deformation of pain sensitive structures. A period of prone lying (about 5 to 10 minutes) with progression to prone lying with lumbar extension is helpful in starting to reduce the derangement. If the deformity is large, several pillows may be required in order to accommodate the protrusion. Gradual easing into the neutral position is achieved by slowly removing the support, one pillow at a time. Then gradual positioning into extension is begun. Once extension is introduced, further reduction is brought about by repeated passive extension exercises in lying.

3. An undetected lateral shift; this is the most common cause for failure. McKenzie has found that 52 percent of patients with low back pain have a relevant lateral shift. A shift is relevant if alterations of it cause a change in the intensity and/or site of the symptoms. Small shifts may be detected only when testing the side of the trunk during standing. One side gliding direction may be restricted and may affect the symptoms. If extension is forced on this type of deformity, the result is often a peripheralization of symptoms. The lateral shift must be corrected to a point of overcorrection, then extension exercises may be applied in this position. Most shifts can be corrected in the standing positions, but occasionally patients may need to have the lumbar spine in some degree of flexion before the shift can be corrected. The patient is perched on the bed or stool and the trunk is shifted in the direction that centralizes the symptoms. Once overcorrection is achieved, the patient is taught to ex-

tend gradually by repeated movements in standing then in lying.

4. A combined lesion may be involved; there may be a derangement with an underlying dysfunction. In this case, the pain may become centralized, but the patient may continue to complain of a central low back ache during and following passive extension exercises. Upon questioning, most patients are able to distinguish the strain type pain of dysfunction as opposed to the nagging pressure ache typical of a derangement.

IF SELF TREATMENT FAILS

Self treatment, though a large part of the protocol is not the entire McKenzie approach. A rational system of mobilization and manipulative techniques is used to ensure that maximal function is regained.

The addition of manual techniques may be required if (a) there is a plateau in progress which has not changed over a period of 1 to 2 days; (b) there is some improvement, but it is so slow that the patient is becoming noncompliant; (c) the reduction of symptoms using the self-treatment regime is inadequate; or (d) if total relief is short-lived.

CONTRAINDICATIONS

Absolute

1. Patients with signs or symptoms of serious pathology or disease, i.e., neoplasms, aneurysms, active inflammatory diseases, infections, fractures or dislocations, or diseases of the bone.
2. Patients with signs of central nervous system lesions or cauda equina lesions.
3. Gross neurologic signs especially if they are worsening.
4. Severe pain, or constant pain with no position or movement that eases it. If pain is diagnosed as

having a mechanical cause, it may be worthwhile to reassess after a period of bed rest to see if signs become favorable to treatment.
5. Structural faults of the bone, which produce instability.

Qualified Contraindications

Strong or forceful techniques are absolutely contraindicated in following situations, but gentle and cautious movements may be attempted.

1. If structural anomalies or defects are stable, i.e., mild spondylolisthesis/spondylolysis in which a derangement is superimposed.
2. In mild osteoporosis.
3. In mild neurologic signs that are improving.

The McKenzie self-treatment approach may not be as dramatic as relieving pain with manipulation, but it does allow the patient to learn and gain self-confidence in treating pain. The benefit of working with and through the pain enables the patient to gain insight into the nuances of treatment and the purpose of prophylaxis.

SUGGESTED READING

Adams MA, Hutton WC. Gradual disc prolapse. Spine 1985; 10:(6):524–531.
Joyson MI, ed. The lumbar spine and back pain. 2nd ed. Tunbridge Wells, England: Pitman Medical, 1980.
McKenzie RA. The lumbar spine. Mechanical diagnosis & therapy. Wellington, New Zealand: Spinal publications, 1985.
McKenzie RA. Treat your own back. 3rd ed. Wellington, New Zealand: Spinal publications, 1985.
Nachemson AL. The lumbar spine: an orthopaedic challenge. Spine 1976; 1(1):59–71.
Ponte PJ, et al. A preliminary report on the use of the McKenzie protocol versus Williams protocol in treatment of low back pain. J Sports Phys Ther 1984; 6(2):130–139.

ISOMETRIC EXERCISE

ELIZABETH C. HENLEY, B.P.T., M.Cl.Sc.

Muscle strengthening techniques are of fundamental importance in the rehabilitation of injured individuals. The specific techniques employed by physical therapists are dependent on a variety of factors. Of primary importance is the underlying pathology and the stage of recovery from the causative trauma. One of the most common techniques employed, particularly in the early stages of recovery, is that of isometric exercise.

A muscle contraction is isometric when the muscle contracts and produces force with no change in the joint angle. An isometric contraction may also be described as that point in a contraction when the load becomes great enough to exceed the ability of the muscle to lift it. An isometric contraction is sometimes termed a static contraction.

When using isometric exercise for strengthening muscles, there are a number of exercise properties that must be considered. These include tension, speed of maximum tension development, frequency of contraction (session and repetition), duration of the contraction, inter-repetition interval (or rest period), and muscle length and joint angle.

PROPERTIES OF THE STRENGTHENING STIMULUS

Tension

The isometric tension needed to secure a strengthening effect is generally associated with training at muscle tensions of 50 to 100 percent of maximum. However, in some instances, the tension may be very low because of the overlying pain, edema, etc., which limits the patient's ability to perform a voluntary contraction.

Speed of Maximum Tension Development

The speed with which a given muscle reaches a specific level of tension requires a finite amount of time, which differs with the muscle. For example, the finger flexors can complete the process quickly, whereas the larger quadriceps femoris muscles are considerably slower. Differences in contraction times should therefore be considered when selecting the duration of the isometric contraction.

Duration

Greater than 40 percent of maximum tension is generally developed in the first 200 milliseconds of muscle contraction, even for larger muscles such as the quadriceps femoris. Therefore, 1-second maximum muscle contractions generate increases in strength. The most commonly used therapeutic duration tends to be 3 to 5 seconds. Unnecessarily long contraction times appear to be counterproductive.

Frequency

Both session frequency and repetition frequency need to be addressed as properties of the strengthening stimulus. Generally, significant strength improvements have been produced with the use of twice-daily exercise sessions. However, the beneficial effects of multiple sessions level off at about the 3-week stage. Whether this is due to boredom, fatigue, initial skill learning, or some other factor is difficult to determine.

Increasing the number of repetitions or "sets" of repetitions per session is considered to be advantageous for increases in strength. The repetition set tends to be multiples of five, either five or ten being the standard number.

Inter-Repetition Rest Period

The recovery period is another factor that must be considered in the application of isometric exercise. This interval is usually arbitrarily chosen and usually varies from 2 to 3 seconds to 1 minute. As a general rule, the more intense contractions (80 to 100 percent of maximum) with high repetitions require greater rest periods to minimize the effects of fatigue.

Muscle Length-Joint Angle Relationship

Joint angles determine muscle length and, consequently, the amount of force that can be generated at different joint angles. There is some transference of strength gain by isometric training at one joint position to different joint positions, usually limited to a 20 to 30 degree radius. This fact supports the concept of isometric training at different points throughout the available range of motion.

Clinical Application

Clinically, isometric exercise techniques are employed under a variety of conditions. With immediate postoperative patients, static exercise is commonly the first technique introduced. Following surgical repair of fractures that have been stabilized with fixation devices, isometric exercises are performed to help maintain the strength of the muscles surrounding the fracture site, as well as to stimulate circulation. Initially, the exercises entail voluntary static contractions of 2 to 3 seconds in duration. Minimal resistance is provided by the therapist's hands, primarily to guide the patient as to which muscle is being contracted. Similar guidelines are used for any stable fracture or fractures immobilized in casts. In the situation where postoperative pain is severe, when joint range is permitted but painful, isometric exercise would also be initiated.

With simple operative procedures, such as most of the work performed under arthroscopy, isometric exercises commence within 1 to 3 days of surgery. The exercises are performed with repetitions that are determined by the amount of pain and swelling present. For example, with a lateral retinacular release at the knee, exercises do not commence until the third day because of the amount of bleeding during the procedure and the risk of restarting that bleeding as a result of intense contractions. Generally all progression of programmes in early postoperative patients, especially for exceptional cases, are performed in consultation with the surgeon.

In late postoperative patients, isometric exercise can continue to be employed by systematic progressive resistance. Strengthening can be performed at different points throughout the available range of movement. Similarly, static strengthening can be used when exercising through range is painful (for example, in patients with chondromalacia patella). Gradually, as strength improves, the painful points within the range diminish and eventually disappear.

Isometric exercises are commonly the exercise technique of choice in the treatment of arthritic conditions. Use of isometric exercise allows increases in strength, without aggravating the pain or inflammatory process. The literature certainly supports isometric exercise as the preferred method of increasing muscle strength in addition to the endurance of the rheumatoid individual.

Isometric exercises are introduced in the subacute phase of the disease process. The exercises are recommended to be done once daily, ten repetitions for each exercise. The resistance application point is always distal to the involved joint, but not extending below two joints; for example, with hip abductor strengthening, the resistance is applied proximal to the knee joint rather than proximal to the ankle. Patient compliance is a limiting factor with exercise programmes for the arthritic patient because of the number of joints involved and, hence, the large extent of

the exercise programme. For this reason, in the short term it is recommended that the exercises be performed five times weekly—well motivated patients perform daily. In the long term, for maintenance of strength gains, the recommended programme is at least four times weekly. Isometric exercises in the arthritic patient are generally confined to the large group muscles; in fact, they are contraindicated in the small muscles of the wrist and hand.

Most commonly, pain is the major factor that dictates the time at which progression of exercises is made. Progression of the programme initially entails increasing the number of repetitions or sets of repetitions. As pain and fatigue diminish, resistance is added. Sufficient resistance is applied to attain near maximum tension without causing pain in the joint.

There are circumstances where isometric exercises are contraindicated. These conditions include infection in the area, unstable fractures, early tendon repairs, and large rotator cuff repairs. With unstable fractures, increasing the muscle tension across the fracture may cause disruption of the fracture site, such as with fractures of the surgical neck of the humerus or fractures of the patella. Increase in pain during or following isometric exercise indicates the need for review of the programme. The intensity of contraction, the number of repetitions and the position of the joint during the performance are a few of the factors that may cause or contribute to the increase in pain.

Isometric exercise is a valuable tool in the battery of techniques that are available in the development of an appropriate rehabilitation programme. Some of the conditions for which isometric exercise can be used and the appropriate timing of introduction of this form of exercise are outlined here. One distinct advantage of isometric exercise is that it is easily performed by the patient at home, with equipment no more elaborate than a seatbelt and a towel.

SUGGEST READING

Atha J. Strengthening muscle. In: Miller DI, ed. Exercise and sports sciences reviews. Franklin Institute Press, 1981:1-73.

Knapik JJ, Ramos MV. Isokinetic and isometric torque relationships in the human body. Arch Phys Med Rehabil 1980; 61:64-67.

Knapik JJ, Wright JE, Mawdsley RH, Braun J. Isometric, isotonic and isokinetic torque variations in four muscle groups through a range of joint motion. Phys Ther 1983; 63(6):938-947.

Knapik JJ, Mawdsley RH, Ramos MV. Angular specificity and test mode specificity of isometric and isokinetic strength training. J Orthopaedic Sports Phys Ther 1983; 5(2):58-65.

Lehmkuhl LD, Smith LK, eds. Interaction of mechanical and physiological factors in function. In: Brunnstrom's clinical kinesiology. 4th ed. Philadelphia: FA Davis, 1983: Chapter Four.

Nosse LJ. Assessment of selected reports on the strength relationship of the knee musculature. J Orthop Sports Phys Ther 1983; 4(2):85-87.

Soderberg GL, Cook TM. An electromyographic analysis of quadriceps femoris muscle setting and straight leg raising. Phys Ther 1983; 63(9):1434-1438.

SACROILIAC PAIN

NANCY S. MICK JONES, B.Sc. (PT), M.Sc.

Sacroiliac joint (SI joint) integrity is an important aspect of trunk and lower limb function. Any interruption of this joint can result in marked disability and pain. Because of its close proximity to the lumbar spine, pain arising from the SI joint is sometimes confused with lumbogenic pain and vice versa. It is currently believed that true SI joint pain is rare and that low back pain is generally not derived from this origin. However, SI joint dysfunction can and does occur and is a disorder likely to be encountered by a physical therapist in the clinical setting. Therefore, the first objective is to discriminate between true SI joint pain and pain arising from other sources. This is accomplished by a careful and detailed history and examination and by the elimination of other possible diagnoses.

The "typical" patient with SI joint dysfunction is female, between 25 and 45 years of age, sedentary to moderately active, and slightly obese. Usually, she has been required to perform a repetitive asymmetrical type of activity either at the home or in the work place. Increased lumbar lordosis also produces a higher risk for SI joint strain.

ASSESSMENT

Pertinent Functional Anatomy

Several factors regarding SI joint anatomy and function should be kept in mind during the assessment. The SI joint is a plane, synovial joint and as such is biaxial in a very limited range of motion. The articular surfaces are grooved reciprocally, thereby adding to the stability of the joint. There are no muscles intrinsically responsible for its support and, therefore, the SI joint relies heavily on a number of strong ligaments for maintenance of normal opposition. With forward flexion of the trunk or flexion of the hips, the ilium rotates posteriorly on the sacrum. The opposite action occurs with trunk and hip extension. There is also a slight superior glide of the left sacrum on the ilium with right trunk side flexion and vice versa.

The primary function of the SI joint is to disperse forces from the upper body via the vertebral column to the lower limbs and ground via the ilium and femoral heads. However, forces can also travel cranially to converge on one or both SI joints. These opposing forces acting on the SI joints often give rise to injury.

Mechanisms of Injury

Possible mechanisms include simple bending, lifting, and torsion movements. More forceful sudden jolts or direct trauma may be involved, whereas leg length discrepancy and spinal fusion place additional demands on SI joint mobility. Decreased movement in the lumbar spine (from whatever cause) tends to place excess stress on the SI joints during movement of the trunk. Normally, the SI joints are involved in all trunk movements, but with very small amplitudes in comparison to the lumbar segments.

EXAMINATION

Subjective

The history should include the patient's perception of the pain and what factors aggravate or relieve it. Commonly, pain arising from the SI joint is manifested as a dull ache over the involved joint and occasionally into the buttock, hip, or posterior thigh area. There is also point tenderness directly over the joint. More acute injuries are accompanied by sharper types of pain. Pain usually comes on with various trunk movements, stair climbing, running, jumping, and walking while carrying any kind of weight.

Objective

The physical examination should include a general scan of the spine and lower extremities; particular attention should be paid to postural alignment. Specific tests for the SI joint include (1) stress testing of the ligaments around the joint; (2) palpation and observation of the SI joints in standing, during flexion and extension of the trunk (sitting and standing), and during alternate hip and knee flexion in standing; and (3) palpation of the sacrotuberous ligament. Levels of anterior superior iliac spines (ASISs), posterior superior iliac spines (PSISs), iliac crests, and pubic tubercles should also be noted. From the results of these tests and the general scan, the diagnosis of mechanical SI joint dysfunction is made.

CLINICAL SYNDROMES

On the basis of onset, location of pain, and alignment, SI joint dysfunction can be divided into one of the following three catagories:

type 1—Rapid onset of SI joint pain with normal alignment;

type 2—Rapid onset of SI joint pain with abnormal alignment;

type 3—Slow onset of SI joint pain with abnormal alignment.

All categories may show an alteration in normal SI joint movement; this alteration being a more consistent finding in the latter two.

TREATMENT

Testing and mobilizing techniques are very similar in dysfunctional SI joint management. The following are several available techniques.

Technique 1

With the patient prone, stand on the nonaffected side facing the SI joints. Place the heel of your cranial hand just above the PSIS on the far ilium, while placing your caudal hand in the same area on the near ilium. With extended arms, exert a gentle anterolateral pressure in an oscillating manner; this glides the ilium anteriorly on the sacrum and stresses the dorsal sacroiliac ligaments.

Technique 2

Maintaining the same position as described above, place the heel of your cranial hand on the apex of the sacrum and the heel of your caudal hand directly over it. Exert a gentle anterior pressure in an oscillating manner. This rotates the sacrum posteriorly on the ilium.

Technique 3

With the patient supine, stand facing the patient's pelvis. Place the heel of your cranial hand on the far ASIS and the heel of your caudal hand on the near ASIS. Apply gentle oscillating pressure with extended arms, in a posterolateral direction. This glides the ilium posteriorly on the sacrum and stresses the ventral sacroiliac ligaments.

Technique 4

With the patient supine, passively flex the hip and knee to an angle of 90 degrees or slightly greater. Grasp the medial side of the leg and support the thigh while moving the leg into full adduction. Apply gentle pressure at the end of the movement. This rocks the ilium on the sacrum.

There are numerous other techniques that can be applied to the SI joint based on a thorough understanding of the functional movements. In addition, a combination of techniques can be used, i.e., techniques 1 and 2 can be combined such that one hand applies anterolateral pressure on the ilium while the other hand applies anterior pressure over the sacral apex, thus simultaneously rotating the sacrum posteriorly and the ilium anteriorly.

Any findings from the history and assessment that may indicate a causative factor for SI joint dysfunction should be dealt with. These factors may include postural abnormalities, weak or shortened muscle groups, or incorrect resting and working positions and contribute to all SI joint clinical syndromes. In addition, women should be aware of the increased SI joint strain caused by high-heeled footwear.

Generally, *type I* can be considered the acute SI joint strain. The main objective in the initial stage of treatment is pain reduction. This can be accomplished by a number of modalities including ice, ultrasonography, transcutaneous nerve stimulation (TNS), and interferential therapy. The need for proper resting positions and adequate rest periods should be stressed. In the subacute stage, attention should focus on ensuring the return of normal movement patterns between the sacrum and the ilium.

Type 2 SI joint dysfunctions are not as common as the others described. A patient with a rapid onset of pain from SI joint origin is generally able to identify a mechanism of injury. This may include a fall, a blow to the area, or a major trauma such as a motor vehicle accident. With these patients, as with all types of SI joint dysfunction cases, pain reduction and education are important objectives, and can be dealt with as described under type I treatment.

With the type 2 patient, it is important to ascertain the degree and direction of abnormal alignment. If the ilium is fixed in anterior rotation, the findings include a hypomobile joint, superior PSIS and inferior ASIS when compared to the other side, and an inferior pubic tubercle on the affected side. Due to the rotation component of this position, the PSIS also appears deeper on the affected side. The sacrotuberous ligament is stressed and may be tender on palpation. A pure cranial shift of the ilium on the sacrum may also occur (sometimes referred to as an 'upslip") without the rotation component. If the ilium is fixed in posterior rotation, the opposite findings are true.

This type of patient (i.e., fixed in anterior ilium rotation or upslip) responds well to a manipulative technique as follows: with the patient prone and the sacrum stabilized (easiest to have another therapist apply cranial pressure through sacral apex), stand at the foot of the plinth and grasp the leg on the affected side, just above the ankle; lean backwards and slowly take up the "slack." Once full tension is felt and the patient is relaxed, apply a sharp caudal pull. This maneuver should not be uncomfortable and may be repeated if necessary. Check alignment immediately after maneuver in both prone and standing positions. This treatment technique may be required over two or three visits and, when applied correctly, is successful.

The general principles and techniques described under type 1 treatment are also applicable to types 2 and 3.

The *type 3* problems are probably the most common of the SI joint dysfunction syndromes. The asymmetry seen in this patient is most likely due to soft tissue adaptive shortening. An example of this may be a shortened quadratus lumborum holding the ilium in anterior rotation. This condition responds best to slow steady stretching techniques such as contract-relax (muscle energy techniques). Again it is important to find and correct the cause of the asymmetry.

GENERAL COMMENTS

A SI joint problem not responding to treatment should be reassessed to determine if the diagnosis is correct and if the treatment techniques are appropriate. A true SI joint injury gives some positive findings (pain) with one or more stress tests of the surrounding ligaments. In addition, the possibility of concurrent involvement of other areas should be considered. Exercise should be encouraged in the patient who is symptom-free. A simple exercise done on a daily basis puts the SI joint through its range of motion and is as follows: lying supine (or sitting if more comfortable) the leg is flexed to a 90-degree angle at the hip and knee and rotated laterally to approximately 45 degrees. This is most appropriate for the patient whose objective is to maintain normal sacropelvic movement.

PRECAUTIONS

There are several circumstances where caution should be exercised in regard to SI joint treatment. They include the following:

1. The acutely painful, hot swollen joint—this may indicate an active disease process and discussion with the referring physician should precede any treatment.

2. Severe muscle spasm—as with any type of mobilization, the use of excessive force (i.e., manipulation) through muscle spasm is contraindicated. Mobilizing techniques such as types 1, 3, or 4 can be done at a gentle level initially and can be increased as spasm decreases.

3. The older SI joint—after the age of 50, the SI joints are prone to anterior fusing, to some extent, particularily in men. Because of this potential occurrence, any excessive forces (i.e., manipulation) is not indicated.

4. Pregnancy and menstruation—during pregnancy, the ligaments around the SI joint become gradually more lax (secondary to hormonal changes), which may lead to abnormal movement (hypermobility) and pain. Treatment includes instruction on proper resting positions, corrective exercises and avoidance of activities that may strain the susceptible joints. Some women experience a similar problem in their SI joints towards the end of the menstrual cycle. If the problem is severe, an SI support or belt may be considered.

The SI joint dysfunction syndrome responds well to physiotherapeutic techniques providing proper patient and treatment selection criteria are applied. It is therefore very important to complete a thorough history and assessment on the patient to ascertain the source of pain and, if SI joint in origin, the type of syndrome.

SUGGESTED READING

Cyriax J. Textbook of orthopaedic medicine—Vol. 1. Diagnosis of soft tissue lesions. London: Bailliere Tindall, 1978.

Hoppenfeld S. Physical examination of the spine and extremites. East Norwalk. CT: Appleton-Century-Crofts, 1976.

Kaltenborn FM. Mobilization of the spinal column. Translated by R. Mckenzie. Aukland, New Zealand: University Press, 1970.

Kapandji IA. The physiology of the joints—Vol. 3. The trunk and vertebral column. New York: Churchill Livingstone, 1976.

Maitland GD. Vertebral manipulation. London: Butterworths, 1977.

RHEUMATOID ARTHRITIS IN THE GENERAL HOSPITAL SETTING

JENNIFER INGLIS ELLIS, Dip. P.T., M.A.P.A., M.C.P.A.
MARY ORTI, P.T.

Rheumatoid arthritis (RA) is a chronic systemic inflammatory disease of unknown origin. It is characterized by its extensive joint involvement. Patients with RA are usually admitted to the Rheumatic Diseases Unit (RDU) of a large general hospital. This unit is headed by a rheumatologist. The members of the unit may include a specialty resident, nurse, physical therapist, occupational therapist, social worker, pharmacist, and dietician. A complete medical work-up by the physician at admission includes a history of the presenting problems, past and current drug management, a review of systems, and a musculoskeletal examination.

Physical therapy involvement should begin as soon as it is determined that the patient has joint problems. Early involvement allows for a more accurate assessment of the stage of the disease.

ASSESSMENT

The physical therapy assessment should include the following:

1. History of the disease
2. Joint examination
3. Morning stiffness
4. Grip strength measurement
5. Timed 50-ft walk
6. Duration of morning stiffness
7. Functional inquiry
8. Extra-articular features

History of the Disease. History should include the course of the disease from the time of onset, the extent of joint(s) involved, previous admissions, as well as a history of drug management. The presenting problems should be clearly defined, including any problems related to coping at home or at work.

Joint Examination. Each joint is assessed based on the criteria of the American Rheumatism Association (ARA) classification of an active joint(s). A joint is described as active if it has one or more of the following: (1) tenderness on pressure over the joint line, (2) stress pain at the end of passive range, or (3) joint effusion. It is important to note the number of joints that show an active synovitis. Special note is made of loss of joint range of motion (ROM) and any loss of muscle strength.

The therapist should be aware that the patient who has pain on joint stress only, without any other objective findings, may be a patient with low pain tolerance, rather than one with active disease. The therapist must be able to differentiate between an active synovitis and a chronic "boggy" synovitis.

Duration of Morning Stiffness. The actual amount of morning stiffness is recorded. Stiffness may last from minutes to all day. It is usually in direct proportion to the acuteness of the disease.

Grip Strength Measurement. An average of three readings using a modified sphygmomanometer inflated to 20 mm Hg is recorded.

50-ft Walk. The patient is timed walking at normal pace in regular footwear and without the use of any walking aid if possible.

Functional Inquiry. The patient is classified according to the ARA classification of functional capacity—class 1 being completely independent, and class 4 being largely or wholly bedridden or confined to a wheelchair.

Special note is made of the patient's occupation and specific difficulties at home, work, or during recreation.

Extra-Articular Features. These include rheumatoid nodules, vasculitis, and neuropathies such as carpal tunnel syndrome.

TREATMENT STRATEGY

The Acute Stage

Rest. During this stage, joints are painful, hot, and swollen, morning stiffness may last 3 hours or more, grip strength may be only 40 mm Hg, and a 50-ft walk may take 20 seconds. The main treatment is rest. Rest may be local or general. Local rest for a single joint involves using resting splints. Bed rest is recommended when there is extensive upper and lower extremity involvement. This period may last from a few days to a week. Patients are encouraged to rest in a prone position for 2 half-hour periods twice daily. This helps to prevent hip and knee flexion contractures. Physical therapy treatment at this stage consists of patient education, local ice for the swollen joint(s), splinting, and ROM exercise(s).

Patient Education. This is an extremely important part of any treatment plan. Patients experiencing their first flare-up of arthritis are often frightened, depressed, worried about their job, and the long-term effects of the disease on their lifestyle. Long-term patients may have the same feelings, and may in fact have to face a definite change in lifestyle. A formal patient education program should be an integral part of any rheumatology service, with all team members contributing. Most patients are very interested in their disease process. Often the role of educating the patient is left to the therapist. An education program should include the following:

1. A brief outline of the pathology of the disease
2. The role of rest
3. The importance of a balanced exercise routine
4. Energy conservation and joint protection
5. An explanation of the hospital routine
6. Guidelines for recreational activities.

Ice Packs. Ice packs are used to assist in the management of joint pain and swelling caused by the inflammation. Ice can be used two to three times daily on a joint. Care must be taken to check the patient's sensation prior to treatment. Some patients who are experiencing a severe flare may not be able to tolerate the weight of the ice pack, or in some instances patients complain of increased pain following treatment. Ice should be discontinued in either case.

Splinting. Resting splints may be used at this time. Splints are recommended to reduce and prevent contractures, and to reduce protective muscle spasm. Splinting at this hospital is the responsibility of the occupational therapist, although at other centers it is the physical therapist's responsibility. The therapist must monitor the patient's tolerance for wearing splints and must state how often they should be worn. Splints should be removed at least once a day and the joints put through an active or assisted range of motion. If at all possible, resting splints should be worn through the night.

Range of Motion (ROM) Exercise. During this stage the aim of the exercise routine is to maintain normal joint range, to prevent joint stiffness, and to increase joint range. Each joint is put through an active range of motion at least once a day. This may be an assisted movement if the joint is too painful. Passive movements are not recommended at this stage, and the joint is not moved beyond the limits of pain. The number of exercise repetitions is monitored daily, and increased only when there is no increase in morning stiffness or evidence of increased synovitis. This stage may last anywhere from a number of days or weeks; however, in most cases most patients show a positive response to the team approach after a few days.

The Subacute Stage

At this stage all of the indicators of an acute joint may be present, however, there is objective and subjective evidence of improvement in disease activity (e.g., less morning stiffness and a decrease in joint synovitis). An increase in the grip strength and a decrease in time over a 50-ft walk will also have taken place.

Aims. The aims of physical therapy management at this stage are to maintain or increase ROM, to increase exercise tolerance, and to decrease pain.

Repetition of ROM can now be increased. The range of repetitions during this stage is usually between three and five. Variation of these numbers is possible, the guiding factors remain the same, i.e., the degree of morning stiffness and evidence of acute synovitis.

Exercises. Exercises at this stage should be active, although in some instances some joints may require assistance. It is quite usual to find a combined picture of acute and subacute joints. The patient at this stage is generally more active and may now attend the department for therapy. A typical schedule may include a hydrotherapy session in the morning, followed by a class exercise session in the afternoon.

Modalities. These play an important role in the management of RA. The most commonly used modalities are hydrotherapy, hot packs, wax, and transcutaneous electrical nerve stimulation (TENS) type stimulation. Care must be taken to test the patient's skin condition and sensation prior to the application of heat or ice. Hydrotherapy helps to decrease pain, and increase ROM. Hubbard tank or pool sessions are popular with most patients and provide the ideal treatment medium for multiple joint involvement. Hot packs are used to help decrease local joint pain and stiffness. Wax is used to decrease hand stiffness. TENS and interferential therapy may assist in relieving pain. Ultrasonography is used to treat local tendinitis.

Education. Education is an ongoing activity. Group sessions provide the opportunity for patients to share their problems as well as being a means of providing mutual support.

The need for a formal rest period continues throughout the sessions. This is usually after lunch for an hour. Again the patient is encouraged to rest lying prone. The rest period means that every effort is made to avoid scheduling any activity during this time including visiting hours.

With modern day medical costs putting pressure on acute hospital beds, patients may be discharged at this stage. The follow-up therapy is provided by the therapists from the Arthritis Society or is continued on an outpatient basis. In instances where there is a recognized need for prolonged intensive therapy, the patient may be transferred to a rehabilitation center.

Prior to discharge the patient should be reassessed, and results of this reassessment should be compared to those of the admission assessment in order to record accurately the changes in the patient's condition.

The Chronic Stage

Patients in a general hospital at this stage of their disease may be admitted for a number of reasons, perhaps for drug management, systemic problems such as anemia, or vasculitis, or as is very often the case, for surgical intervention. Whatever the reason, the patient should be assessed by the physical therapist. The evaluation this time differs from the acute stage assessment. Chronic stage disease is characterized by the amount of damage to the musculoskeletal system. A joint is classified as damaged if it shows any of the following findings:

1. Loss of 15 degrees or more of ROM
2. Ligamentous laxity
3. Gross crepitus
4. Joint deformity.

Patients at this stage may also have significant functional disuse and may need ambulatory assistance.

Aims

The aims of treatment at this stage are to decrease pain, to increase ROM, to increase muscle strength, and to improve functional capacity.

Decrease Pain. Modalities can be used as indicated. The choice is similar to the subacute stage. TENS type stimulation is being used successfully to decrease and to control pain in the chronic stage. Many patients have their own home units. Interferential therapy is also effective in pain management. Acu-stimulation is very effective around the cervical spine and shoulder regions.

Increase ROM. The guidelines for determining repetition of ROM will depend on the degree of joint damage. Joints that show evidence of subluxation should not be forced passively. This can cause further subluxation and possible ligament damage. The degree of joint crepitus also determines how much exercise a patient can tolerate without a significant increase in pain. Generally exercises should be assisted active or active. It is better to start conservatively, and repetitions of five are unlikely to cause further increase in joint discomfort.

Joint contractures are very common at this stage. The common causes are joint destruction, ligament laxity, a tight joint capsule, or chronic joint swelling. Every effort should be taken to try to reduce the contracture. Treatment choices can include gentle passive stretching, splinting, possibly using serial splinting and/or mobilization techniques.

Increase Muscle Strength. It is sometimes difficult to load a muscle effectively without putting undue strain on surrounding joint structures, especially ligaments. Isometric type contractions are safe and effective. The resisted movement can be performed at different ranges and at different starting points. Resistance through range must be carefully monitored and should not be performed at the expense of joint stability and pain. Pain that lasts for more than 2 hours after an exercise routine is due to too much stress on the joint(s). Resisted exercises through range should never be performed if the joint is swollen or if there is coarse crepitus. Hydrotherapy is a safe, effective, and enjoyable medium to increase muscle strength and can be continued on a regular basis making use of community resources.

Improve Functional Capacity. Loss of functional independence is very distressing to the patient. Methods of improving function demand that the physical therapist and occupational therapist work together to develop a specific program to improve function. A careful assessment of the problem should lead to an individual exercise program aimed at strengthening weak muscles. There may be a need to assess the use of particular walking aids. Energy conservation should be reviewed with the patient at this time. A home exercise program is given to the patient. Follow-up therapy is coordinated with the Arthritis Society therapist to ensure that the patient can maintain an active role at home.

The Role of Manual Therapy

Manual therapy has certainly become a useful and powerful tool in the management of RA; however, like all powerful tools it must be used cautiously and only in experienced hands. Its use should be considered only after a careful assessment of the joint(s) and after examining recent x-ray studies. This cannot be stressed too much, especially when dealing with the cervical spine with particular reference to the atlantoaxial joint. Maitland type mobilizations can be used to increase joint range, bearing in mind that the pathology of a rheumatoid joint warrants special consideration in order to avoid irreversible joint damage. Grade I and grade II mobilizations can be performed on peripheral joints with minimum risk of damage. However, when a joint is acute these grades, even a grade 1, can cause an increase in pain. Manual therapy techniques are best perfected on nonrheumatoid patients and modified as required for the rheumatoid patient. Passive stretching techniques also play a role in the rehabilitation of the patient. It is best to assume that manual therapy techniques will only be performed by therapists who have perfected the techniques under careful supervision.

THE JUVENILE RHEUMATOID ARTHRITIC (JRA)

The same principles of treatment apply when treating the JRA patient. Family participation is important to ensure continuity of treatment. A daily exercise routine is necessary to prevent loss of joint range, and to prevent contractures. Special attention must be paid to posture. Some children may develop leg length discrepancy with hip involvement. Back problems are also quite common among children, and every assessment should include a back assessment. Back extension exercises should be included in the daily exercise routine. Splinting may be required at times, for the same reasons as with the adult patient. Patience and encouragement on the part of the therapist and family are required to help the child through this difficult and painful stage. Children also need to have regular rest periods and should be encouraged to rest in a prone position.

Most children respond well to a hydrotherapy program. This is an excellent medium to help maintain joint range, and improve muscle strength. In the subacute and chronic stage, this program can be expanded to become a family recreation time.

The cooperation of the school teacher is important. In many instances it is the teacher's first encounter with arthritis, and the therapist and/or parents will need to inform the teacher as to the child's limitations in certain programs, especially those involving physical activity.

GAIT TRAINING OF THE LOWER EXTREMITY AMPUTEE

DAVID F. M. COONEY, M.Sc., P.T., C.P.O.

Lower extremity amputations result from a variety of etiologies. Vascular disease and its concomitant sequelae are the primary causative factors seen in most practices today. Knowledge of the associated psychological and physiological aspects of this systemic involvement can only serve to support successful ambulatory management of the older lower extremity amputee. It is understood that there are other pathologies leading to amputation, but understanding current thought and practice in this older population lends itself equally to rehabilitative intervention as a result of other causes.

Intervention by therapeutic means is not an absolute necessity for successful ambulation by the amputee. Many amputees attain a functional gait despite their physical obstacles, and often without the benefit of professional guidance. A well-designed systematic approach aimed both at educating the patient and at creating an objectively sound foundation can instil a greater confidence, reduce setbacks (by minimizing patient trial and error), and promote independence.

Determining the candidacy of a patient for the rehabilitative process engenders a number of preferred criteria. Where feasible, preprosthetic evaluations and the necessary preparations should be made to obtain trust, to establish a professional rapport, and to ensure the best physical climate for the postsurgical course. The following are some primary areas of concern: Motivation—this is undeniably the greatest indicator for success, without which your program is destined to fail in a functional sense—regardless of the strength of the other parameters. It can and should be instilled prior to program institution; Cognition—this is certainly preferred, but not an absolute necessity with companion attendance; Presence of contractures—include involved and uninvolved extremity; Current medical status—include cardiovascular, nephrologic (if dialyzed, volume fluctuations can be expected), vision, etc.; Muscle, range of motion, and sensory testing—baseline values and anticipated areas of concern; Nutrition—establishing well-defined sets of blood test values can help to better ensure primary wound closure without extended delays; Premorbid functional status—can provide a target level of program achievement.

A thorough evaluation using these guidelines can serve as a good barometer for success. A program that targets improvements in deficient areas and maintains or strengthens sound areas should be initiated as soon as possible. Indeed, the better received the patient's condition, the greater the potential for success.

It is also imperative that an open line of communication and professional relationship exist between the physical therapist and prosthetist. A prosthetist's knowledge and expertise in providing an intimate fit of the residual limb within the socket, in addition to understanding the biomechanics of gait and the principles of prosthetic alignment, should be a frequently tapped resource. While gait training, a prosthetically comfortable patient is a happy patient; an amputee in pain is a "no win" situation.

Another factor that has been well documented in the literature and should be mentioned in this context is the use of postsurgical ambulatory devices. Whether the methodology used incorporates rigid dressings with removable pylon or pneumatic systems utilizing nonarticulated cones, the advantages of these postsurgical ambulation systems have distinct positive features. They prevent edema, protect the wound, and thereby promote healing; they also assist in residual limb maturation and shaping. The amputee's ability to see progress quickly after surgery can have a positive influence on the prosthetic and rehabilitative process.

Gait training with the above devices, while allowing for bilateral weight bearing and reciprocal gait, do not generally allow for more than rudimentary ambulation. Not until the patient is cast for and fit with a preparatory prosthesis can gait training along more normal guidelines be pursued. Only when the residual limb tissues have been determined by the clinical team to be capable of tolerating increased weight-bearing pressures is more advanced gait training pursued

PRE-GAIT TRAINING

Pre-gait training consists of instructing the amputee in the proper donning method for their respective level of amputation. For the below-the-knee amputee, the prosthesis is donned while the patient is seated and in the following sequence:

1. Removal of compression stocking or elastic wrap;
2. Inspection of limb for any areas of erythema or abrasion;

3. Application of prosthetic socks with visual and tactile insurance of wrinkle-free application-education and continued reinforcement regarding proper sock ply number cannot be underestimated, as one ply of sock can be the difference between comfortable and painful ambulation even in a well-designed prosthesis.

4. Don the insert—most amputees utilize a soft insert. Once donned over the socks, palpation of the distal end should confirm total contact with no air space between the insert and the residual limb (especially the distal end).

5. The knee is flexed with the prosthesis on the floor. The limb is inserted into the prosthesis from a posterior superior angle. Patient must be instructed to maintain knee flexion both to facilitate donning and to prevent distal anterior tibial compromise.

6. Initial confirmation of proper donning can be determined via landmark indicators. These are as follows:

- Patella centered in anterior cut out;
- Distal pole of patella at proximal anterior border of socket;
- Adductor tubercle at level of proximal medial trim line.

Definitive ascertainment of proper fit cannot be made until patient has ambulated on the prosthesis.

7. Secure selected suspension method.

For the above-knee amputee, there are generally two methods of suspension with separate donning methods. One method utilizes a suspension strap, or belt; the other utilizes suction. In the first, the amputee dons the appropriate sock play number to maintain ischial seat weight bearing with total contact distally (too few ply cause "bottoming out" with distal femur and ramus pressure; too many ply render the prosthesis functionally tall and unstable, creating a void at the distal end with subsequent weight bearing). While seated, the amputee pulls the socket onto the residual limb, heeding proper alignment by matching the adductor longus tendon with the anteromedial corner of the socket. Keeping the residual limb-sock interface intimate by holding the socket on the leg, the amputee rises from the chair and fastens the suspension apparatus, maintaining weight bearing in a proper toe out position. In a standard quadrilateral socket, the ischium should evidence purchase on the ischial seat of the prosthesis, and palpation of the distal end through the valve seat should also display total contact. On a narrow medial-lateral (ML) designed socket, the ischium should be contained within the medial posterior corner of the socket, with equally evident total contact distally. There are variations outside these parameters, about which your prosthetist should be consulted.

Donning the suction socket requires adequate standing balance to pull the tissues of the residual limb into the socket using a "pumping" motion. Patients either wrap their residual limb with an elastic wrap, pull a length of tubular stockinette over the limb, or use a silk scarf to pull the tissues into the socket by gradually pulling the material out through the valve seat. As one hand applies tension to the material, the amputee slightly hikes the hip on the involved side. As the material slowly yields, weight is again borne on the socket. With these reciprocal motions, progressive seating of the tissues of the residual limb occur. Once the material is evacuated from the socket, the valve is replaced and suction suspends the prosthesis. Many above-the-knee patients devise their own peculiar methodologies for donning the socket, but the results should all afford comfort with weight bearing without excessive pistoning when lifted during the swing phase.

Patients unable to develop proper technique can easily become discouraged and choose to forego prosthetic use. Therefore, repetition and attention to detail in donning the prosthesis is of paramount importance for optimal gait training benefit and, ultimately, ambulatory independence. Inadequate technique or improper alignment of the stump-socket interface can create gait deviations and can lead to pressure on the limb that can challenge tissue integrity.

Preambulatory exercises in preparation for gait training should target those muscle groups responsible for stance phase stability and swing phase fluidity. The hip flexors, extensors, abductors, and adductors should all be addressed throughout the training period. Because of their importance in creating pelvic stability and upright trunk control, the hip extensors and hip abductors need to be challenged to a greater degree than the flexors and adductors. Quadriceps and hamstring strengthening are also targeted for the below-the-knee amputee. Weakness in any group can result in compensatory mechanisms that can be difficult to correct if not addressed early.

All of the following procedures are applicable to either the above-knee or below-knee amputee. Modification of intensity or number of repetitions should mirror the clinical need. Except in extraordinary cases, the parallel bars are usually the first staging area for gait training.

WEIGHT BEARING AND GAIT

Standing balance exercises are initiated to establish a level of confidence and trust of the prosthesis by the amputee, whose biggest fears are pain and falling. Selective, positional control of the biomechanics necessary to ensure safe and stable posture must first be approached. The primary target is to establish equal weight bearing through both extremities, while maintaining a stable prosthetic base. The trunk is kept erect, via hip and knee extension, and weight is shifted in an anterior-posterior and lateral to lateral direction. Joint motions should only occur at the ankle. Deviations, majoritively forward and/or lateral trunk bending, should be corrected manually using counteractive force at the pelvis and hip, with resistance also provided at the shoulders to facilitate an upright posture if necessary.

Once the patient is confident on a stable base, movement about this base can proceed. Stance phase prosthetic control is addressed first, as the patient tends to feel more stable, starting from a position of stance. The amputee is instructed to advance the sound limb from a heel off position to a heel strike position without advancement of the prosthesis. It is very important during this period that a level pelvis is maintained, and smooth weight shifting and pelvic progression over the prosthesis occur. Manual resistance to those movements the patient has difficulty with helps to facilitate preferred motion. Hip extension throughout this stance phase, to ensure a stable knee, is of utmost importance in the above-knee amputee. The below-knee amputee does not usually evidence a lack of stance-phase knee control. If such is identified, reexamination of the initial alignment of the prosthesis, in addition to muscle testing, may reveal the cause, which can then be addressed. Achieving stance-phase stability can only come with continued repetition and practice.

Swing-phase control commences next. Beginning from a position of double limb support with the sound limb forward of the prosthesis, forward pelvic movement is initiated through an extension force created by the residual limb hip extensors. Prosthetic heel rise and toe off occur as weight is shifted to the forward foot, and hip flexion on the prosthetic side initiates the swing through. Adequate hip flexion force to reach full prosthetic knee extension has to be practiced repeatedly to ensure a stable alignment for initial contact without causing an excessive heel rise in initial swing or a forceful extension impact at terminal swing. Again, an erect posture and maintaining a level pelvis help prevent early formation of bad gait habits.

Reciprocal gait should not be pursued until the amputee demonstrates control and a functional understanding of the described components of prosthetic gait. Knee control—via hip extension in the above-knee amputee and via hip and knee extension in the below-knee amputee—is the key to a fluid, symmetrical gait, and to establishing confidence in the amputee. Without adequate control, the knee can buckle with weight bearing or evidence a "double bump" as the patient reaches midstance.

Once a confident level of ambulation has been reached in the parallel bars, the patient progresses to an appropriate assistive device, consistent with the clinical level. Many older amputees have difficulty utilizing crutches safely and may opt for the security of a walker. Initially, this should not be challenged and the patient should be allowed to walk with a walker in open areas to get used to being out of the parallel bars; however, progression to greater levels of independence using crutches or canes should be pursued directly, as ambulation with a walker can hide many deviations and can retard the preferred fluidity of amputee gait. Again, deviations noted with each training progression should be addressed and corrected immediately, even if it entails a return to the initial sequences.

Training Modalities

Throughout the training period, all available modalities should be utilized to optimize the gait training sessions. During the initial parallel bar sequences, consistent verbal cueing, in conjunction with hands-on corrective or facilitative resistance to the preferred motions, is of paramount importance in establishing a sound gait base. Affixed at each end of the parallel bars, mirrors assist in maintaining correct posture and weight-bearing symmetry while providing immediate feedback when corrective measures are taken. These are the minimum requirements needed in order to derive benefit from gait training sessions. As prosthetics becomes more provocative and varied, and as clinical settings become more sophisticated, the arsenal of mechanisms available to the clinician increases.

Biofeedback, using surface EMG electrodes, can assist the therapist and patient throughout the training period. Using the device over those muscle groups requiring reeducation and strengthening prior to prosthetic intervention can provide for follow-through by the patient once fitting has occurred. EMG can also be used during the gait training sequence providing audible feedback to the amputee while monitoring target muscle groups for dynamic reeducation at specific periods during the gait cycle (i.e., hip abductors at midstance).

Videotaping the gait sessions has also proved valuable. Both therapist and patient can identify deviations in gait from both frontal and sagittal views. The tape serves as a learning tool so that after corrective measures have been taken, the patient can see the difference objectively, thereby reinforcing the proper mechanics. Other advantages of the videotape are the record keeping capabilities that a video library provides. New patients can be shown the natural progression of amputee gait that can help to allay any fears they may initially have and to dispel any preconceived notions they might have. The videotape also supplies a comparative yardstick, should the patient begin to have difficulties in the future. Deviations noted from the previous video can help to identify any potential causative factors in an objective manner.

Gait training the lower extremity amputee provides a challenge to the therapist to duplicate as near normal a gait as prosthetically possible. As a means toward this end, it is adamant that the therapist have a thorough understanding of the biomechanics of normal gait and the prosthetic alignment parameters that can affect the amputee's gait. There are a multitude of deviations that can evidence themselves in the course of amputee gait training. Causes of these deviations can be attributed to many factors—initial prosthetic alignment, skeletal anomalies, pain, poor fitting, or suspending prosthesis—with many more too exhaustive to address in this forum. It is the responsibility of the therapist to become familiar with these variations in order to appreciate fully an optimal gait for the amputee. In addition to harboring a knowledge of the mechanics affecting amputee gait, the therapist is well-advised to become familiar with the ever-changing field of prosthetics relative to componentry and application of new methods and materials, so that patients can glean the best benefit from the available prosthetics.

SUGGESTED READING

American Academy of Orthopedic Surgeons. Atlas of limb prosthetics—surgical & prosthetic principles. St. Louis, MO: CV Mosby, 1981.

Cooney DFM, Vinnecour K. An advanced approach toward improved prosthetic fittings. Clin Prosth & Orth 1985 (Summer); 9(3).

Mensch L, Ellis PM. Physical therapy management of lower extremity amputations. Rockville, MD: Aspen, 1986.

Rehabilitation Institute of Chicago, Procedure Manual. Lower extremity amputation: a guide to functional outcomes in physical therapy management. Rockville, MD: 1986.

Sanders GT. Lower limb amputations: a guide to rehabilitation. Philadelphia, PA: Davis, 1986.

FLEXOR TENDON REPAIR

JOHN B. JOHNSON, B.A., D p. P.T.

Flexor tendon repairs are one of the more common operations referred to our Physiotherapy Hand Unit. Because the surgical techniques used for primary and secondary tendon repairs in the hand have been developed only over the past 15 to 20 years, and because the technology for these repairs is improving dramatically each year, physical therapists, occupational therapists, and hand therapists must be flexible in their treatment regimes and be ready to change as surgical techniques improve.

In the past, it was believed that following flexor tendon repair, one should not stress or even move the tendon for as much as 6 to 8 weeks to allow the poorly vascularized tendon to form the solid union necessary to withstand the tremendous forces that would transmit through the tendon during activity and work. Observance of this delayed movement philosophy led to several problems for the hand therapist. The patient was often placed in a plaster of Paris cast or heavy dressings during the 6-week recovery. When the cast or dressings were removed, the therapist would be faced with very limited range of motion due to tight joint capsules, very weak extrinsic and intrinsic muscles, and, the most difficult problem, adhesions that had developed between the healing tendon and the tendon sheath that would make smooth gliding nearly impossible. Tendolysis was often needed before full movement could be achieved.

Now, early movement is possible because of better sutures and suturing techniques as well as the form of protection that can be provided to the tendon through proper splinting and appropriate exercises. The aim of early movement is to maintain range of motion in all joints of the affected digit or digits and to minimize the number of adhesions that are allowed to develop between the tendon and the tendon sheath.

The early motion treatment technique can be used on nearly all flexor tendon repairs, whether they be single or multiple, primary or secondary tendon repairs. Primary repairs are those done within the first 3 or 4 days after the injury and secondary (or delayed) repairs are those repairs done at a later date. Generally, the patients selected for early motion technique have had a fairly tidy laceration(s) without other complications, such as a crush, burn, or degloving injury.

The essential characteristics of the early motion technique are as follows:

1. Maintain wrist in 20 to 30 degrees of flexion, the metacarpal phalangeal (MCP) joint in 80 to 90 degrees of flexion and the proximal interphalangeal (PIP) and the distal interphalangeal (DIP) joints are in 70 degrees and 30 degrees of flexion respectively, with room in the splint to take the PIP and DIP joints (actively or passively) to full extension while maintaining the MCP joint in flexion.
2. Within the first couple of days following surgery, establish an exercise regime that incorporates active extension and passive flexion at the PIP and DIP to maintain joint range of motion and to establish gentle tendon gliding. No active flexion or passive extension should be allowed.

Occasionally some assisted extension is necessary to regain full extension at the PIP and DIP joints, but this need not be pushed too vigorously as this range usually shows a constant improvement over the first 2 weeks and pushing the range manually may cause pain and swelling, which does in fact, delay recovery.

The technique we employ is as follows: while the patient is still in the operating room, the surgeon places a heavy gauge (2–0 monofilament nylon) suture through the distal end of the fingernail leaving a loop about 2 inches in length. The patient's hand is placed in a heavy dressing with a back slab that maintains the wrist in 20 to 30 degrees of flexion, the MCP joints in 80 to 90 degrees of flexion and protects the PIP and DIP joints from being forcefully extended. The day following the surgery, providing there are no complications, the patient comes to physical therapy where we fashion a thermo plastic splint that is designed to maintain the above position. However, there are two notable design features in this splint that were not incorporated into the operating room dressings. First, the splint is made so that the patient can remove it to shower or gently wash his or her hand (while maintaining the protected position). The second feature is a hook that is placed approximately 3 inches proximal from the distal carpal crease. This hook is placed so that it lies in the plane formed by flexion-extension of the affected finger thus allowing for a pull, through the suture which is attached to the fingernail, that does not put lateral pressure on the MCP or PIP joints. An elastic band connecting the hook to the suture (Fig. 1) should be taut and strong enough, when it has been placed on the wrist hook, to maintain the MCP joint in 80 degrees of flexion and the PIP joint in 80 to 90 degrees of flexion (the DIP joint is in full extension when the splint is in place), but flexible enough to allow the patient to begin to extend the PIP joint against the elastic band's resistance. The goal at this stage is to achieve full active extension at the PIP joint.

The splint is held in place by soft velcro straps; one strap across the palm—positioned so it does not impede flexion of the MCP or PIP joints; one strap over the wrist—allowing for free movement of the elastic band; and one strap at the proximal end of the splint for stability. Figure 2 provides an illustration of the overall design and position of the splint.

For the first 3 weeks the patient is instructed to extend actively the PIP and DIP joints against the resistance of the elastic band. Another elastic band can be substituted to increase resistance as the extensor strength improves. Each time the patient actively extends and passively flexes the PIP and DIP joints, the repaired tendon glides up to as much as 3 cm. This glide is the main objective of the early passive motion technique. Adhesion formation is decreased considerably and it is also believed that the strength of the tendon is improved with the slight tension that the movement places on the healing site.

During weeks 4 through 6 postsurgery, the patient is instructed to remove the elastic band and gently begin to flex the affected finger actively. It is very important to stress that even though the skin wound may be well healed, thus giving the illusion that the entire injury is healed, the tendon itself, because of poor blood supply, is not yet solid and can be easily ruptured if aggressive exercise is attempted. Also dur-

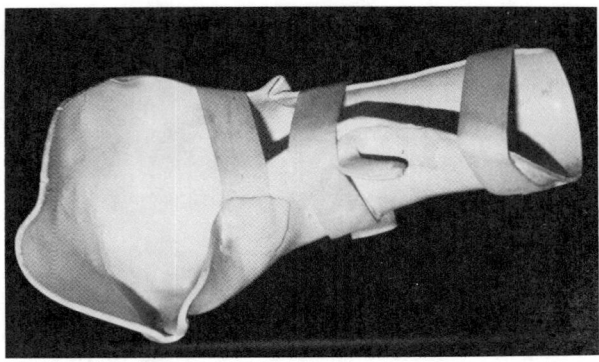

Figure 2 Overall design of protective dynamic splint used following flexor tendon repair.

ing this stage, the splint can be adjusted to allow the wrist to come to neutral and the MCPs to be held in 50 degrees of flexion. This starts to stretch the muscle-tendon complex gently, with the goal being to achieve full extension at the wrist and all fingers by about 8 weeks postsurgery. During the sixth and seventh week, the splint can be removed several times daily and both wrist and fingers can be actively exercised into flexion and extension as able. Gentle progressive resistance can be given during the flexion phase of the exercises; full resistance during extension.

By week 8 the patient should have full range of motion throughout the hand. Commercial hand exercisers can be used at this stage to give controlled resistance, but heavy work should not yet be attempted. From week 8 the splint can be totally discarded and aggressive range of motion and strengthening exercises can be encouraged. Occasionally, during this time, a small extension splint may be needed to gain the last degrees of extension at the PIP and MCP joints.

By week 12 the patient should be able to go back to his or her regular job with full confidence that the tendon is totally healed and able to withstand the load that will be placed upon it.

The early-motion technique of treatment for flexor tendon repairs has very few complications or side effects. The splint, when it is first made, may cause some discomfort, but this is easily remedied by simply adjusting the shape of the thermoplastic or by padding the appropriate area. In addition, the elastic band must be of the right strength (resistance) in order to protect the healing tendon from sudden stretch or tension, while still allowing active extension of the finger to the splint with the elastic acting as the resistance.

If the patient has an area of paresthesia due to nerve damage, care must be taken to control the amount of pressure placed on any bony prominences to ensure that no skin breakdown occurs. A well-made splint

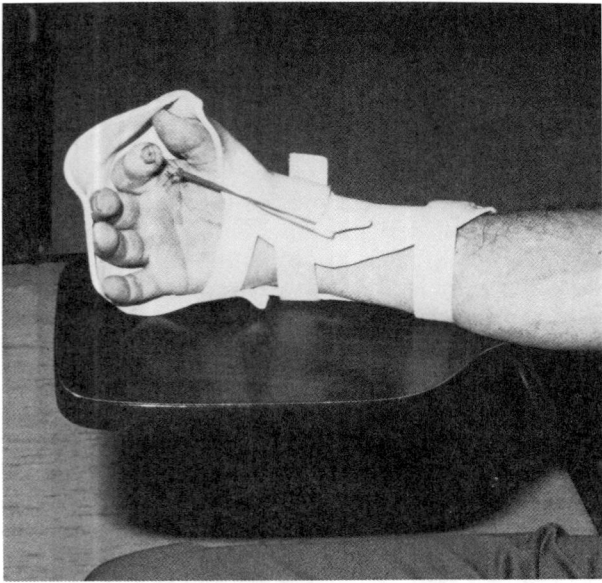

Figure 1 Note elastic band connecting suture to hook. For greater flexion of DIP and PIP, the elastic can be directed through a pulley attached to the velcro strap across the palm.

should be comfortable and should not cause any adverse affects. Often patients live considerable distances from the hospital so that specific instructions must be given to ensure that the patient understands that one need not 'suffer' through any pain caused by the splint. If pain is felt, the splint should be padded, and the patient should return to the clinic as soon as possible to have the necessary adjustments made.

BIVALVED CASTS FOR NEUROLOGICALLY INVOLVED CHILDREN

MARILYN J. WRIGHT, B.Sc.P.T.

Feet provide a base for upright stability and mobility. The structural and functional development of a child's feet are dependent upon neuromuscular development. Children with neurologic conditions causing abnormal foot postures and weight-bearing patterns have no stable base upon which to develop the proximal stability and normal patterns of movement required for efficient functional activities. Prolonged abnormal positioning and weight bearing can result in contractures and deformity.

Pediatric neuromuscular conditions can cause hypotonia or hypertonia in the muscles acting on the feet. Children with hypotonia have inadequate muscle tone to provide the stability necessary to maintain the bones of the feet in a properly aligned position. This, often compounded by ligamentous laxity, results in joint hypermobility. When the child begins to bear weight through the lower extremities, the feet assume a calcaneovalgus and pronated position in association with knee flexion or hyperextension, hip flexion, abduction, and external rotation, pelvic instability, and abdominal weakness.

Children with hypertonicity generally present with increased tone in their plantarflexors and primitive reflex activity such as a positive supporting reaction and plantar grasp. This results in the child standing in an equinus position. The feet get minimal or no weight bearing through the calcaneus. Abnormal muscle pull may also result in valgus or varus positioning in addition to the equinus. Prolonged abnormal stresses through the feet may result in subluxation of the midtarsal joints. These patterns are often associated with abnormal extensor positioning throughout the lower extremities and abnormal tone or compensatory postures in the pelvis, trunk, neck, and upper extremities.

As a result of these abnormal forces acting upon the feet and body, hypo- and hypertonic children receive abnormal sensory input from their feet, develop poor movement patterns, and are subject to potentially damaging biomechanical stresses.

Bivalved casts, also known as inhibitive or tone-reducing casts, are used as an adjunct to therapy for neurologically involved children to minimize these interrelated problems. The casts align the feet in an optimal position to provide a stable base upon which desirable movement components can be developed and experienced, and help to maintain the muscular and bony integrity of the feet (Fig. 1).

The aims of therapy are to inhibit abnormal movements and postures, while facilitating normal and efficient movement patterns, and to prevent deformity. The goals of bivalved casting are analogous. The casts provide a more normal sensory input as the children do not continually experience abnormal positioning of the feet. Excessive weight bearing through the metatarsal heads, medial or lateral structures and toes is inhibited. Weight is taken evenly throughout the whole foot, particularly through a properly aligned calcaneous.

Casts help to direct certain motor components into desired postures and movement patterns. In all users, proper foot alignment decreases compensatory tone, abnormal postures, and undesirable movement patterns throughout the body. In hypertonic children, positioning of the toes inhibits a plantar grasp, and fixing the ankle at 90 degrees prevents a positive supporting reaction, thereby allowing better motor patterns to develop. The casts promote tone reduction by imposing a prolonged stretch to the plantar and toe flexors and overall relaxation by allowing weight bearing through the lower extremities and breaking up total extensor patterning.

Casting can also benefit the bony and soft tissue integrity of the foot. Properly aligned weight bearing can protect lax or vulnerable ligaments from being overstretched or damaged. Sustained positioning in the casts helps to maintain or increase range of motion in the foot muscles that are prone to contractures and to promote elongation of the hip and knee musculature. Well-aligned weight bearing through the joints promotes normal formation of bones and articulating surfaces in the lower extremities. Nonremovable casts have been used in the past; however, the bivalved cast ensures better hygiene, permits monitoring of the skin, and allows mobility for certain situations.

USES

The most common users are children who are ready to stand and to progress to ambulation. Casting at this stage allows standing and gait patterns to be developed with the feet in a neutral position.

For more severely involved children with significant, dynamic hypertonia, casts may be indicated for general relaxation of tone or positioning in equipment such as prone standers.

The casts can provide a readily available and relatively inexpensive assessment tool to ascertain whether bracing would improve the function of a particular child.

Surgery may be avoided or postponed by maintaining adequate muscle length. Although avoidance is optimal, in many cases surgery is the correct approach. However, timing is very important. Postponing surgery by casting can allow children to achieve an optimal gross motor stage, making postoperative rehabilitation more effective and easier for all involved. Postponing heelcord-lengthening surgery may prevent the need for repeated lengthenings, as children who have this operation before the age of 5 often require repeat lengthenings. In some cases, the casts have been used specifically for postoperative rehabilitation after lower extremity surgery.

PATIENT SELECTION

Bivalved casts are indicated for a child whose feet can be held in a neutral position and whose treatment objectives are consistent with the goals of casting.

Most of the children who are casted have cerebral palsy. Those with mildly to moderately involved spastic diplegia, hemiplegia, and quadriplegia, causing a dynamic equinus stance or gait, benefit most. The casts are particularly effective in children with compensatory hypertonicity, that is, tone that is reduced at rest or with handling, but increases with independent activity. Some spastic athetoids have been successfully casted; however, they are more susceptible to skin breakdown because of their fluctuating tone.

The casts are used for moderately low toned children with conditions such as hypotonic cerebral palsy and congenital hypotonia. They have also been used in the treatment of head injuries, spina bifida, and idiopathic toewalking.

The best results are achieved in the 1 to 5 year old age group as their feet are usually still mobile, and they are progressing through the developmental stages of standing and walking. The technique has also proved useful in certain older children and in adults. Occasionally children under 1 year of age have been casted to decrease extensor tone or if they or their parents are anxious for them to be standing.

Specific indications or contraindications for patients to have casting incorporated into their treatment include the following

1. Contractures: The joints of the foot should be able to be mobilized into and held in a neutral position with the knee flexed or extended. There should be no hip or knee contractures such that the joints

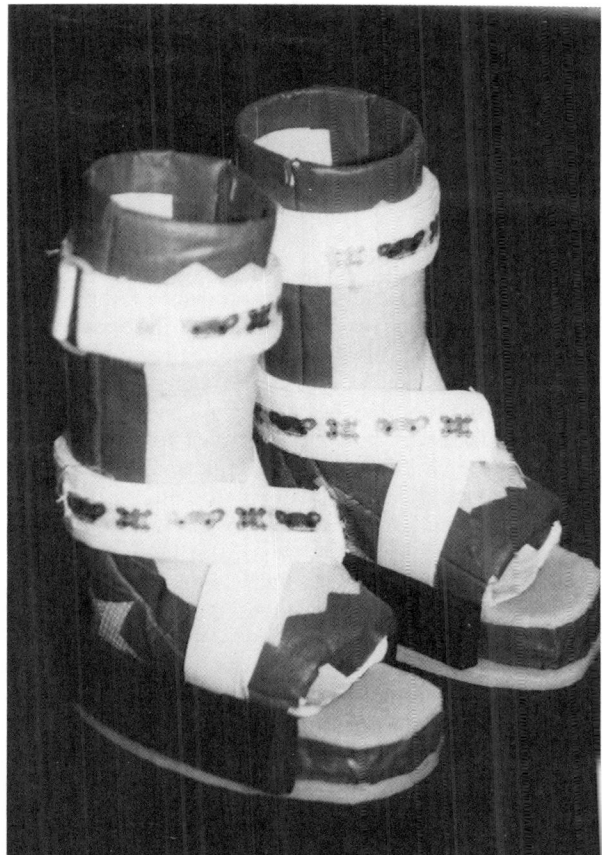

Figure 1   Bivalved casts.

would be in a flexed position when standing with the ankles fixed.
2. Rotational problems: Children who would exhibit exaggerated internal or external rotation due to the weight or torque of the casts are not good candidates as they would be subjected to unnecessary stress on their joints.
3. Parental compliance. Those caring for and working with the children must be reliable in using the casts appropriately and in promptly reporting any problems.
4. Availability of therapy: Children should receive regular therapy to work on an active exercise program, to have the fit of the casts monitored, and to allow continued assessment of function.

TECHNIQUE

The process of fabricating the casts should be learned from an experienced therapist in a practical teaching situation or in a course specific to the technique. The therapist must have an understanding of the mechanisms of normal and abnormal foot development and a knowledge of functional foot anatomy.

Specific techniques and materials have continually changed over the past years and tend to vary among centers, but general principles are consistent. Presently the most commonly used techniques are selected from those presented in the TRAFO (Tone Reducing Ankle Foot Orthoses) workshops taught by the Langer Biomechanical Group from Deer Park, New York.

The atmosphere should be as comfortable as possible for optimal patient relaxation and compliance. Parents or familiar people should be in close proximity, and distractions such as food, music, and toys that do not cause excessive movement should be available. Sedation has been used in cases of extreme behavior problems, but only as a last resort.

With the child sitting, in a seat or on a lap, with hips and knees flexed, a layer of stockinette is put on the foot and calf to allow space for wearing socks under the completed casts. A strip of leather is taped to the stockinette to act as a guard when removing the cast. A second stockinette layer is applied over the first layer and the leather strip to line the inside of the cast. T-foam pads are put over the malleoli for added skin protection. The foot is held by one person while a second wraps it in a roll of flexible fibreglass based casting tape from slightly below the knee to the base of the toes. This is then wrapped in a tensor bandage and carefully molded into a position with a neutral subtalar joint, 0 degrees dorsiflexion, and a properly stabilized and aligned forefoot. When the casting tape is dry the tensor is removed and the cast cut off with an exacto knife. This inner shell is covered with a roll of stronger casting tape, a lightweight but durable material. The cast is bivalved, so that more support is left medially for valgus feet and more laterally for varus feet. Edges are sanded and taped and velcro straps are made to hold the casts together. These steps can be done by an aide to save in therapist time. The shells are then aligned and secured on a base of shoe rubber. This step is important as malaligned casts can cause joint stress, change the center of gravity, or alter body posture. Leg length discrepancies can be compensated for and a crepe sole is applied. A toe platform of rubber or dense foam is placed under the toes to hold them in neutral or slight metatarsal phalangeal extension depending on the amount of plantar grasp. Experimentation with toe positioning and angulation can be done with minimal modifications. Colored tape and decorative trim is chosen by the children for cosmesis and acceptability. Casts are always made bilaterally to promote symmetry and balance.

TREATMENT

Success in using the casts is dependent upon proper use and well-planned therapy programs. The goals for treatment should be consistent with the individual child's total program. Initially the wearing time should be short, often only during exercise sessions. The feet must be carefully checked for areas of irritation, and problems must be remedied. As tolerance increases the wearing time can be lengthened. Casts should not be worn when sleeping as this can result in exaggerated rotational forces being exerted on the hips and knees. W-sitting, or other positions in which the casts act as levers to increase torsion, should be discouraged.

The casts provide inhibition of abnormal foot positions and movements, thereby allowing the therapist to concentrate facilitation of stability and mobility more proximally. Overall relaxation can ease handling and positioning.

In weight-bearing activities, attention should be paid to proper alignment of all body parts to encourage more normal postures. The therapist can work on antigravity movements in appropriate patterns. Facilitation of the hips, pelvis, and trunk works towards improved mobility, strength, weight shifting, and righting and equilibrium responses. These provide the components necessary for the functional activities set as goals for the patient.

Children should always receive some therapy out of their casts to allow for mobility and variations in sensory awareness. Wearing the casts during occupational and speech and language therapy can also be advantageous as a stable base, and relaxation can improve body position and control of upper extremities, respiration, and oral motor structures.

Continuity of treatment is imperative for optimal benefit from the therapy. All involved in the child's care should have an understanding of and skill in using the casts. Parents are very receptive to casting as the casts provide them and other caregivers with more ease in handling the child and with assurance that the feet are in an optimal position when bearing weight. Parents should be warned that initially some skills, such as floor sitting, may be awkward as the child must learn to cope with the added weight and restricted ankle movement imposed by the casts.

Treatment Progression

Through continuous evaluation of the child's progress, appropriate decisions regarding progression to less restricting foot orthoses can be made. The aim is to decrease the amount of immobilization required while maintaining optimal weight bearing, alignment, and quality of movement in functional activities.

Some children can be gradually weaned from the casts to regular footwear. Continuing treatment and monitoring is necessary as movement patterns can deteriorate quickly with changes in activities or growth spurts. It may be beneficial to reintroduce casting when such changes necessitate a period of treatment with increased ankle stability.

Certain children can progress to having the casts cut down to shoe level, thereby allowing ankle mobility while maintaining foot stability. In some centers, casts with hinged ankle joints, which allow dorsiflexion, are available.

Another method of providing some stability without limiting active ankle mobility is the use of molded heelcups in regular shoes to stabilize the heel and forefoot. These heelcups are appropriate for children with flexible calcaneal valgus positioning without excessive hypertonicity, equinus, or rigidity. The heelcups prevent excessive pronation of the feet and the associated compensatory postures caused by this foot problem. Heelcups have also been used as initial orthoses in mildly hypotonic children who need some support to prevent weight bearing in a calcaneal valgus position, but do not require the full support of bivalved casting.

Children who are ready to progress from wide-based, fully encompassing orthoses and who are not growing rapidly may benefit from polypropylene ankle foot orthoses. These are necessary if there is instability in the hindfoot, which warrants rigid fixation of the ankle joint. When the orthoses are made, therapists should work closely with the orthotist to maintain the specific contours and positions found to be beneficial in the casts.

The more severely involved children wearing the casts to reduce generalized hypertonicity or for positioning in equipment may be long-term users of bivalved casts or may be able to progress to well-supporting ankle foot orthoses.

Progressions should ideally take place gradually while regular therapy is continued. This enables the therapist to teach proper movement patterns used with increased foot and ankle mobility (allowed by the less restrictive orthoses) and maintainance of optimal strength, balance, and postural control. In some cases, children may use different orthotic devices for different situations, such as casts for therapy and heelcups for other activities.

ASSESSMENT AND RESEARCH

Many quantitative and qualitative parameters are available for subjectively and objectively assessing the effectiveness of casting.

These include muscle tone, ease of handling, postural alignment, tolerance of maintaining positions, range of motion, primitive and postural reflexes, functional levels, and parental observations. Gait can be evaluated by measures such as stride length, weight-bearing patterns, and videotapes or by gait laboratory analysis of EMG activity, power patterns, joint angles, kinematics, and mechanical energy.

The number and variety of measurements make the treatment approach conducive to research studies. For valid data researchers must ensure standardization of fabrication, treatment programs, patient and family compliance, and patient selection criteria.

SUGGESTED READING

Bertoli DB. Effect of short leg casting on ambulation in children with cerebral palsy. Phys Ther 1986; 66(10):1522–1529.

Carlson SJ. A neurophysiological analysis of inhibitive casting. Phys Occup Ther Pediatr 1984; 4(4):31–41.

Jordan RP, Resseque BA, Cusack JJ, Bly L. Dynamic components of foot function: understanding its role in the management of the patient with neuromotor dysfunction. Deer Park, NY: The Langer Biomechanics Group, 1984.

Salek B. The significance of structural and functional development in the normal foot and therapeutic implications thereof in the child with neuromotor disorder. Bohemia, N.Y: Association for the Help of Retarded Children, Suffolk Chapter.

Watt J, et al. A prospective study of inhibitive casting as an adjunct to physiotherapy for cerebral palsied children. Dev Med Child Neurol 1986; 28:480–488.

NEUROLOGIC PHYSICAL THERAPY

ROOD APPROACH: AN EVALUATION

SUSAN M. ATTERMEIER, M.A., L.P.T.

Basic to the understanding of Rood's approach is the idea that she was constructing a "generic" method for assessing and treating movement problems. In this respect, her approach is similar to proprioceptive neuromuscular facilitation, but dissimilar to Brunnstrom's, which was developed specifically for the adult hemiplegic, and the Bobaths', which was developed specifically for the child with cerebral palsy and later applied to the adult stroke patient. Rood developed her ideas from wide reading in the areas of neurology, anatomy, kinesiology, and psychology. Blessed with a photographic memory, she could retain minute details from all of these fields and could put together a treatment for anything from multiple sclerosis to hiccups. She taught her students to consider central and peripheral nerve tracts, origins and insertions of muscles, autonomic, developmental, cognitive, and emotional factors when analyzing movement deficits. She herself did not refer to a "Rood approach," but rather talked about a "Neurophysiological approach"; nor would she engage in certification of therapists, since her most fundamental premise was that the individual therapist carried the responsibility of self education, problem-identification, and clinical hypothesis testing. What she did offer to her students was a set of general principles and a battery of techniques, whereby the process of applying principles and selecting appropriate techniques was specific to the patient at hand.

SPECIFIC FEATURES

Developmental Sequences

Regardless of the age of the patient, one of the ongoing conflicts in describing abnormal motor function is the level at which the movement problem is being conceptualized. Does one focus on "functional" issues, such as the ability to sit, stand, and walk? Or

is quality of movement the critical point? The literature on therapeutic exercise is replete with differing views, and some of the currently used methodologies tend toward one or the other extreme. However, common sense dictates that both aspects of movement deserve attention and that the level of emphasis varies according to the particular configuration of a problem in addition to the long-term prognosis. One of the unique characteristics of Rood's theory is her concise ways of looking at both function and quality; this is accomplished by presentation of two relatively separate, yet parallel, versions of a developmental sequence.

Key Patterns. By way of an overall guide for assessment and progression of treatment, Rood presented what she referred to as an ontogenetic developmental sequence of "key patterns." This consists of an ordinal series of naturally occurring patterns corresponding to motor milestones. The components of this sequence are supine flexion, rolling, prone extension, neck cocontraction, prone on elbows, prone on hands, quadruped, standing, walking, and squatting in play. Upon examination of this sequence several features can be noted. First, the key patterns do not comprise a complete developmental inventory and, when taken by themselves, consist primarily of static postures. (Oddly, sitting does not appear in the sequence.) Second, the patterns are presented in their fully mature form; therefore, the therapist cannot rely solely on this sequence for guidance and must supplement it with additional patterns as well as the immature and abnormal versions of the original key patterns. Nevertheless, the key patterns are very useful as an initial screening device as well as an ongoing monitor of overall functional level.

Vital and Skeletal Sequences. In order to carry out a detailed and personalized assessment, the therapist needs a set of guidelines that allow analysis of the building blocks of function so that specific and measurable goals can be set. Again, each major approach to therapeutic exercise offers assessment guidelines based on its underlying theory. The paradigm offered by Rood consists of a developmental sequence incorporating both autonomic and somatic functions and stressing their interrelationships. The components of the sequences are presented in Figure 1. With respect to the vital sequence, (with the excep-

SKELETAL SEQUENCE	Interaction ←→ mechanisms	VITAL SEQUENCE

Reciprocal innervation
  • flexion pattern
  • extension pattern
Cocontraction
Mobility on stability with
  distal end fixed
Mobility on stability with
  distal end free (skill)
	Respiration
	  • inspiration
	  • expiration
	Feeding
	  • suck
	  • swallow
	  • chew
	Elimination
		Phonation
		↓
		Articulation

Figure 1 Vital and skeletal sequences described by Rood. Reproduced with permission of publisher from Campbell S, ed. Pediatric neurologic physical therapy. New York: Churchill Livingstone, 1984:40.

tion of chewing and articulation for speech) all of the components are present at the time of birth since they were laid down prenatally. Deficits in any of these areas call for immediate intervention, and treatment takes place in conjunction with work on the flexion or extension patterns. The skeletal sequence consists of four nonordinal overlapping stages that reflect the normal development and interplay of mobilizing and stabilizing functions. The use of the concepts of mobility and stability as guidelines originated with Rood and continues to be theoretically valid, as well as clinically useful, whereas emphasis on reflexes and muscle tone is falling out of favor. The first stage, called **reciprocal innervation,** encompasses the basic total body flexion and extension patterns. The *flexion* pattern is observed in supine and consists of head movements in addition to midline head stabilization, binocular focus for close vision, mouth closure and sucking, a reversible hand to mouth pattern with wrist dorsiflexion maintained throughout, and a midline flexion-extension of the legs with dorsiflexion of the ankle maintained throughout. Anterior trunk musculature provides proximal stability, but does not contract strongly. The muscles used for the limb patterns are primarily pre-axial and multiarthrodial, and the quality of rhythmic reversibility is critical. The *extension* pattern is observed in prone and consists of symmetrical lifting of the head, upper trunk and legs, with the arms flexed at the elbows and lifted from the surface in a scapular retraction pattern. The eyes are focused for distant vision, and the mouth may be open; the wrists are dorsiflexed, and the fingers are extended. The hips are extended with slight abduction and external rotation, the knees are slightly flexed, and the ankles are held in midline plantarflexion. This pattern has been noted by virtually every observer of motor development and is considered to form the basis of upright function. The trunk, shoulder, hip, and ankle musculature involved in the extension pattern is postaxial and both uni- and multi-arthrodial. The critical qualities are bilateral symmetry and tonic holding.

Cocontraction, the second stage, is observed in a variety of positions. The patterns are neck cocontraction (in prone), prone on elbows, prone on hands, quadruped, standing, and semi-squat position. In observing these patterns, the examiner looks for a balance of muscular contraction on both sides of the joints so that antigravity weight bearing can occur with the joints in proper anatomical alignment.

The third stage is called **mobility on stability with the distal end fixed** and consists of oscillations and weight shifting in prone on elbows, prone on hands, quadruped, and standing. Smooth and easily reversible midrange motions are the hallmark of this stage.

The final stage, **mobility on stability with the distal end free,** is also called the **skill** stage and evolves from the previous stage as weight bearing in each position becomes unilateral. The emergence of rotational components is the indicator that this level of control has been achieved.

These developmental sequences are extremely valuable as a template against which to assess movement and to progress treatment in any type of patient at any age. The sequences supplement rather than conflict with other approaches to evaluation and treatment. However, because of the general nature of the developmental sequences, it is up to the therapist to be familiar with normal age variations. For example, an infant would not be expected to perform midline hip flexion or to maintain consistent wrist extension during a hand-to-mouth pattern. Furthermore, as with the key pattern sequence, familiarity with immature and abnormal versions of the patterns, as well as with transitional movements, is essential.

An assessment would involve careful documentation of functional abilities and needs in the context of daily living skills, followed by examination of performance of the patterns in the sequence. This allows the therapist to pinpoint the basis of the movement problem. In most cases deficits are found in the basic flexion and extension patterns; thus, treatment begins at this level.

Use of Sensory Stimulation

The most widely held misperception of Rood's work concerns her use of sensory stimulation. It was she who introduced icing, brushing, and vibration as clinical tools, and somehow a mystique arose regarding the "magical" qualities of these tools. For some reason, they were also considered the primary elements of Rood's method. Their inappropriate use, which was out of the context of specific movement patterns, led to poor results; subsequently, they came to be regarded as ineffective, and many therapists rejected all of Rood's ideas. This is most unfortunate, since Rood's method of sensory stimulation is effective if done correctly.

Rood originally based her system on a hierarchical view of the nervous system, which she described as follows in an article published in the *PT Review* in 1954:

> Motor patterns are developed from fundamental reflex patterns present at birth, which are utilized and gradually modified through sensory stimuli until the highest control is gained on the conscious cortical level. It seemed to me that if it were possible to apply the proper sensory stimuli to the appropriate receptor as it is utilized in the normal sequential development, it might be possible to elicit the motor responses reflexly and, by following neurophysiological principles, establish proper motor engrams. The movement that results in response to a summation of various reflexes is "boosted" up to higher centers for final reception at the sensory cortical level.

Contemporary theoreticians in the field of motor control are abandoning this strict hierarchical model in favor of other more flexible models, and it is likely that Rood was also in the process of updating her theory. However, since her writings are so sparse, there is no way of knowing this. Regardless of underlying theory, the guidelines that she developed for the application of sensory stimuli have an inherent logic, which makes them clinically very useful. These principles are as follows:

1. Brief, fast stimuli give rise to big-burst (i.e., large but short-lived) responses, with rebound effects.
2. Fast, repetitive stimuli give rise to maintained responses with arousal.
3. Rhythmic, repetitive stimuli lead to inactivation of mind and body.
4. Maintained stimuli give rise to maintained responses with little or no arousal.

Based on these principles, a wide variety of techniques was devised; these include icing, brushing, and vibration as well as different types of exteroceptive and proprioceptive stimuli applied with the hands. Rood herself—with degrees in occupational as well as physical therapy—was exceedingly creative in her use of available materials, frequently improvised sensory-

motor treatment strategies, and was always receptive to the ideas of others. Stimulation (regardless of type) was applied with a specific motor response in mind and was followed by observation of effect. If the patient showed aversion to the stimulus, or if there was no effect after a reasonable trial, the stimulus was not used. In no case was the application of a stimulus considered a treatment in and of itself.

CONCLUSIONS

As with all of the models of therapeutic exercise developed in the last 40 years, there are elements of Rood's theory and technique that are worthy of retention, elements to be taken with a grain of salt, and elements that can no longer be considered valid. In the latter category, the use of a strict hierarchical model as a basis for thinking about evaluation and treatment is out of date. Although this model is well entrenched in much of the literature, the systems and information-processing models hold much more promise for therapists; this is exemplified by current research on posture control, which makes use of a systems model and leads directly to specific and measurable treatment protocols. In the category of "questionable" elements, would fall precise statements regarding which nerve pathways and central nervous system structures are being activated during a particular activity. For example, it may be true that light touch is only detected by Meissner's corpuscles, but it is also possible that a wide variety of endings can detect the stimulus.

However, numerous elements of Rood's approach remain valuable. The developmental sequences, principles of stimulation, and consideration of autonomic and emotional as well as motoric factors present an approach to patient care that is simultaneously global and specific. Her emphasis on functional motor patterns lays a foundation for evaluation, goal-setting, and measurement of efficacy that is more meaningful than a system that emphasizes reflexes or muscle tone. But, aside from these particulars, her students were forced (sometimes against their will) to become independent thinkers and problem solvers, to resist mistaking hypothesis for fact, and to become consumers of literature as well as being clinicians. In the context of current advances in theory and technology, this may be the best advice of all.

SUGGESTED READING

Attermeier S. Evaluation of motor function from a Rood perspective. In: Campbell S, ed. Pediatric neurologic physical therapy. New York: Churchill Livingstone, 1984:37–54.

Cromwell F. In memorium: Margaret Rood. Am J Occup Ther 1985; 39(1):54–55.

Farber S. Neurorehabilitation: a multisensory approach. Philadelphia: WB Saunders, 1982.

Rood M. The use of sensory receptors to activate, facilitate and inhibit motor response, autonomic and somatic, in developmental sequence. In: Approaches to treatment of patients with neuromuscular dysfunction. Course IV, Third International Congress, World Federation of Occupational Therapists. Dubuque, IA: Wm C Brown, 1962:26-37.

Stockmeyer S. A sensori-motor approach to treatment. In: Pearson P, Williams C, eds. Physical therapy in the developmental disabilities. Springfield, IL: Charles C Thomas, 1972:186-222.

Stockmeyer S. An interpretation of the approach of Rood to the treatment of neuromuscular dysfunction. Am J Phys Med 1967; 46:900-956.

ADULT HEMIPLEGIA: ROOD APPROACH

MARILYN F. HUMPHREY, B.Sc. (PT)
MARY ELLEN McLEAN, B.Sc. (PT)

The Rood approach to assessment and treatment is based on sensorimotor learning and involves the selective use of sensory receptors to either activate, facilitate, or inhibit somatic or autonomic motor responses in a sequential order based on pre- and postnatal developmental patterns.

Normal movement occurs as a result of sensory feedback or sensory feedforward. The appropriate sensory input is necessary to achieve the desired motor response. This sensory input need not be a conscious sensation. In assessment, the input that produces and controls motor output is carefully analyzed. In treatment, naturally occurring sensory stimuli, such as touch, stretch from gravity and joint compression, or therapeutically devised stimuli, which closely resemble natural stimuli, are utilized. Exercise is not therapeutic unless the pattern of muscle activity in the motor response is correct and results in a sensory feedback that enhances the learning of that response.

The Rood approach considers that movement is automatic and, for the most part, noncognitive. In treatment, "automatic" motor responses should be elicited from patients, thereby providing sensory feedback.

Restoration of homeostasis or steady state between autonomic, somatic, and psychic functions is an essential element of the Rood approach. In assessment, it is important to evaluate the state of the autonomic nervous system. People under stress react differently to environmental stimuli. An assault to the central nervous system is considered a stress. Some hemiplegic patients demonstrate a constant sympathetic reaction and an inability to tolerate environmental stimuli. In treatment, it is necessary to restore homeostasis between sympathetic and parasympathetic functions. If the sympathetic influence is dominant, specific sensory stimuli are used to inhibit the dominant response.

Techniques to calm the base and to restore homeostasis include perioral stimulation, slow rhythmic stroking, maintained pressure, and neutral warmth. Perioral stimulation is a maintained pressure to the upper lip in the area of sensory innervation of the trigeminal nerve. Slow rhythmic stroking is repetitive stroking from the crown to the buttocks in the area of sensory innervation of the posterior primary rami. Maintained pressure to the abdomen, the palms of the hands, or the soles of the feet results in a maintained response. Neutral warmth results in calming as it is nonthreatening and does not result in activation of the sympathetic nervous system. In treatment, the state of the entire nervous system is considered and balance is restored to ensure that the desired motor response is obtained from specific sensory input.

Rood has based her hypothesis and treatment approach on the concept of the developmental sequence. Motor responses are sought in the order of pre- and postnatal development. Four levels of function are recognized in the developmental sequence—mobility, stability, mobility superimposed on stability, and skill. Individual muscles, patterns of movement, and functional activities all have a developmental sequence. The components of the developmental sequence form the building blocks of skilled movement. The most complex patterns (i.e., skill level activities) are not restored unless the more elementary patterns are first reactivated as a foundation.

Rood emphasized that the developmental sequence differs for the neck, the trunk, and the extremities. In development, the neck and the trunk are initially involved in heavy work, that is, work against gravity and against resistance. From a developmental standpoint, the proprioceptors are activated first. Light work (i.e., work without resistance) is the first to occur in the extremities and, the exteroceptors are initially activated. To restore normal patterns of movement, movement is reeducated in the same manner in which it occurs through development. Initially, we work to gain heavy work in the neck and trunk, to develop proximal stability, and light work in the extremities, to develop reciprocal movement.

Rood identified two major sequences in motor development, the Skeletal Function sequence and the Vital Function sequence. The Vital Function sequence develops three primary functions, respiration, feeding, and communication. The Vital Function sequence consists of inspiration, expiration, sucking, swallowing fluids, phonation, chewing, swallowing solids, and speech articulation—the skill-level activity. In treatment, the abilities to suck, swallow and chew must be restored as these activities are motor requirements for the skill-level activity of speech articulation. Through development, the Vital Function sequence occurs concurrently with and is interactive with the Skeletal Function sequence. In treatment, they are approached as two interacting mechanisms, and both are dependent in terms of the degree and the distribution of proximal tone.

The Skeletal Function sequence involves the neck, trunk, and extremities and develops two primary functions, mobility and stability. The Skeletal Function sequence consists of withdrawal supine, roll over, pivot prone, cocontraction of the neck, on elbows, on all fours, standing, and walking. In the Skeletal Function sequence the first pattern to restore is the withdrawal supine or total flexion pattern. This pattern involves heavy work in the neck and trunk with light work in the extremities. All movement occurs towards the midline. In this pattern, the head flexes, the mouth closes, and the hands move towards the midline. The second pattern is the roll over pattern. A component of this pattern is flexion of the topmost extremities. This pattern is useful in restoring body-righting reflexes and encouraging integration of postural reflexes.

The Pivot Prone Pattern is a total extension pattern perceived by Rood as centred at T10. In this pattern, all the major postural muscles are activated in their shortened range. This pattern of muscle activation is an essential prerequisite for normal postural alignment in weight bearing. The pivot prone pattern is facilitated in treatment through the tonic labyrinthine reflex and by stretch from gravity or resistance to the major postural extensors. The pivot prone pattern is a prerequisite for cocontraction. Neck cocontraction is a cocontraction pattern in which the postural muscles are activated. The remainder of the developmental sequence is used in treatment for the refinement of motor activity.

Movement is evaluated closely to determine if specific muscles are activated in the total movement pattern. Facilitation or inhibition techniques are utilized to activate or inhibit specific muscles within the pattern. Tactile stimulation, or touch, is used to activate normal patterns of movement "towards" the stimulus and to inhibit abnormal motor responses. Rood regarded tactility as the beginning of reflex behavior. Light-moving touch to the mouth affects movement in the extremities by reflex connections in the trigeminal complex and the cervical plexus. In the upper extremities, midline light touch activates the components necessary for automatic movement towards the touch. In adults, a movement response may not be seen, but muscle tone and range of motion are affected. Quick-moving touch around the level of the umbilicus activates movement patterns in the lower extremities. In hemiplegia, it is used to facilitate the pick up pattern in the swing phase of gait.

Other techniques to facilitate a motor response include vibration, brief ice, resistance, quick stretch, slow maintained stretch, joint compression greater than body weight, and fast brushing. Inhibitory techniques include very slow stroking, neutral temperature, and slow rocking.

In the Rood approach, the central nervous system experiences the appropriate sensory input to produce normal patterns of movement. Treatment progression is based on normal motor development.

SUGGESTED READING

Farber FD. Neurorehabilitation: a multisensory approach. Toronto: WB Saunders, 1982.
Stockmeyer SA. An interpretation of the approach of Rood to the treatment of neuromuscular dysfunction. Am J Phys Med 1967; 46(1):900–961.

HEMIPLEGIA: BOBATH APPROACH

DEBORAH A. WILLEMS, B.Sc. (PT)
MARY E. WHEELWRIGHT, B.Sc. (PT)

The Bobath approach to treatment of hemiplegia was developed in the 1940s as a treatment philosophy for cerebral palsy children. These children consistently demonstrated abnormal postural tone and movement patterns. Mrs. Bobath discovered that by inhibiting these patterns it became easier to facilitate normal movement. This philosophy of treatment has evolved over the years into a treatment concept that is applied to neurologically impaired children and adults and is used by both physical therapists and occupational therapists.

The Bobath approach uses functional activities during treatment and teaches methods of managing tone. The emphasis is on quality of movement in all activities, while encouraging the patient to do as much as he can himself. Early intervention is stressed whenever possible. Even immediately following a cerebrovascular accident, proper positioning techniques can be taught, in order to encourage recognition of and use of the affected side. Bed mobility skills are taught as soon as possible, in order to avoid movement patterns that can reinforce abnormal reflexes.

The therapist must provide the necessary control to allow for a normal movement pattern to occur. The patient is taken through the movement to develop a "feel" for it. Gradually, the therapist removes control, allowing the patient to take over. "Key points of control" are used to help facilitate normal movement. Initially, these are proximal, i.e., the trunk or pelvis. As the patient progresses, more distal "key points" are used. The therapist must grade her input, allowing the patient as much control over the movement as he is able to exert.

Reflex-inhibiting postures are used during treatment. These postures are not extremes of positions, but provide a normal dynamic alignment of the body. In sitting, the position is as follows: the pelvis is in a slight anterior tilt, the scapula is protracted, the shoulder is in slight abduction, flexion, and external rotation. The elbow is in front of and away from the body in slight flexion, with the wrist pronated, in neutral or slight extension; the thumb is radially abducted and the metacarpals are spread. The hips, knees, and feet are in a straight line, with the knees slightly lower than the hips.

In standing, the position is much the same for the upper body, but the pelvis is in neutral. This posture provides a dynamic background of tone upon which normal alignment is the beginning of postural control. It is a treatment technique in and of itself, until the patient is able to assume and maintain the position independently.

POSTURAL CONTROL

Normal postural control consists of a tone quality in the supporting musculature that allows maintenance and control of the body in any position. Out of necessity, it is also very dynamic. The tone quality needed for normal postural control is actually a range of tone with a mixture of high and low tone. That range must be high enough to maintain posture against gravity, but low enough to allow movement. Therefore, postural control is both a prerequisite as well as an integral component of movement and function. Functionally, when awake, orientation of normal development is vertical; thus the main emphasis of this treatment is on gaining control in vertical postures (i.e., sitting and standing).

Bobath has divided postural control and movement into five basic components—trunk control, head control, midline orientation, weight shift, and limb control. All five components are interdependent and develop progressively with much overlap. Development of normal trunk control is essential before the other components can be established. In patients who lose dynamic stability in the trunk, attempts to fix and stabilize themselves proximally cause high tone and more distal loss of mobility. Therefore, treatment aimed at facilitating proximal stability reduces tone and allows freer limb control and function.

Head control evolves after trunk control begins to become established and involves attaining and maintaining vertical orientation of the head. Control of the head separately or "in isolation of" trunk movements must be obtained in order to maintain the head vertically as the trunk moves (as in head righting). Midline orientation must be established throughout the development of trunk, head, and limb control as a point of reference and to allow integration of all components of the body used for movement. Weight shift is an essential component of normal postural control that allows postures to be dynamic. Weight shift involves movement on a base of support to provide both equilibrium and balance during function. The limbs are seen as extensions of the trunk—moving with the proximal limb girdle and dependent upon its dynamic stability. Distal fixation, or weight bearing on the hands and feet, helps to establish dynamic stability and precedes use of the limb in a nonweight bearing skilled pattern.

TRANSITIONAL MOVEMENT PATTERNS

Besides being able to control the body in postures, it is also necessary to be able to move from one posture to another. Disassociation or isolated movement of the head, two shoulder girdles, and lower trunk is essential to transitional movements. Not only must each segment be able to rotate in isolation of the other segments, but also the patient must be able to move in a diagonal direction, which requires a combination of lengthening of one side and shortening of the other occurring simultaneously with rotation. All of these components must be assessed and, if not present, facilitated during treatment.

In normal development of transitional movements, postural control, essentially isometric activity, is accomplished first. Next, movements from a posture into gravity, or eccentric movement, can be achieved. Last, moving concentrically into a posture against gravity can be controlled. When teaching transitional movement patterns the same sequence is used to facilitate control.

Function in Postures

Although postural control and the components necessary for transitional movements are essential, improving the patient's function is the main aim of treatment. Therefore, it is important to be aware of and to consider all of these components when working on control during a functional task. Hence, gait and daily living skills are taught, input is provided and control of the trunk and limbs is established during movement. Thus, it is essential for the therapist to analyze the components of movement for each task and for each patient individually because of the normal variability in how each person approaches or accomplishes any task.

SUGGESTED READING

Bobath B. Adult hemiplegia: evaluation and treatment. London: William Heinemann Medical Books, 1978.

Davis PM. Steps to follow: a guide to the treatment of adult hemiplegia. New York: Springer Verlag, 1985.

Umphred DA, ed. Neurological rehabilitation. Toronto: CV Mosby, 1985.

STROKE MANAGEMENT: BRUNNSTROM APPROACH

PATRICIA J. CROSS, Dip. P. & O.T., B.Sc. (PT), M.C.P.A.

Management of patients with neurologic conditions forms a major area of practice in physical therapy. One such group of patients presents with the residual effects of cerebral vascular accident. Depending upon the location of the lesion, these residual effects may include hemiplegia or hemiparesis, sensory deficits, perceptual and cognitive dysfunction, and emotional lability. Secondarily, these patients may experience a sudden change in lifestyle, often to the point of complete physical and mental dependence upon others. Timely and appropriate therapeutic intervention can, in almost all cases, minimize these residual effects and restore a measure of independence.

Signe Brunnstrom's approach to the management of hemiplegia is one of several neurophysiologic approaches, each contributing greatly to accurate assessment and appropriate training procedures. The theoretical basis for Brunnstrom's approach is derived from early research into the functioning of the central nervous system, reflexive behavior evoked in laboratory animals, and observation of similar reflexive behavior in stroke patients. The clinical basis is derived from observation of the motor behavior of many stroke patients, development of treatment techniques by 'trial and error' and evaluation of the results. Brunnstrom has not been active in promoting, revising or updating her approach since the early 1970s. However, at that time, she contributed greatly to improved patient care by providing physical therapists with the first potentially quantifiable motor assessment and basic practical text on the subject. Clinical therapists who were introduced to her approach have continued to select, modify, and develop certain aspects of it, thus enriching the chances for a return to more normal motor behavior.

THEORETICAL BASIS

Three closely related theories regarding the process of recovery following a stroke form the basis for Brunnstrom's approach to management. Each theory is supported by contemporary research, particularly that of Twitchell and Reynolds.

The first theory establishes six stages in motor recovery following stroke. These stages range from flaccidity, through development of spasticity and concurrent appearance of primitive reflex behavior, volitional movement within synergic patterns when spasticity is at its peak, decrease in spasticity with increasing control over movement out of synergy, control over isolated, purposeful movement, to almost normal coordination and speed of movement. Brunnstrom postulated that all patients progress through these stages sequentially, not missing any stage, although progress may be stalled for an indeterminant length of time or stop completely at any stage. Change from one stage to the next is gradual and the upper and lower limbs may progress independently of each other.

The second theory establishes the synergic patterns of movement observed in the typical hemiplegic patient. These patterns of movement reflect the degree of spasticity present and so correspond to the stages of recovery. Brunnstrom describes the synergies for the upper and lower extremity to include an extensor pattern with shoulder adduction and internal rotation, elbow extension and forearm pronation. The usually dominant flexor synergy includes shoulder girdle retraction and/or elevation, shoulder abduction to 90 degrees and/or extension, external rotation of the shoulder, elbow flexion to 90 degrees, and forearm supination. Components of the lower extremity flexor pattern are flexion of the hip to 90 degrees with abduction and external rotation, flexion of the knee to 90 degrees, dorsiflexion of the ankle and foot inversion. The usually dominant extensor pattern is comprised of hip extension to neutral with adduction and internal rotation, knee extension, ankle plantar flexion and foot inversion. Rarely are all components of one synergy present and rarely is one component present in full range.

These synergic patterns are closely related to the third theory regarding the postural reflex level of the stroke patient. Early researchers attributed the appearance of "primitive" reflex activity to "evolution in reverse." Recent research provides a more sophisticated explanation of how the central nervous system functions, thereby changing this perspective. Current theory denotes the central nervous system as being organized hierarchically, with each level contributing to the quantity and/or quality of movement available. Spinal reflex activity forms the foundation of all motor function, and supraspinal and cortical centers inhibit or facilitate this activity to allow increasingly complex motor behavior. When injury occurs to the central nervous system, afferent-efferent mechanisms are disturbed and control over centers below the lesion is lessened, thereby allowing lower level reflex activity to influence the quantity and quality of movement. Brunnstrom did recognize the impact of unintegrated reflex activity on motor behavior, and the importance of inhibition and facilitation to coordinated movement. Brunnstrom also felt that both afferent and efferent mechanisms were necessary to perform skilled movement and developed her approach on a sensorimotor concept.

ASSESSMENT

A Brunnstrom sensorimotor assessment corresponds to the stages of recovery. Motor behavior characteristic of each stage is tested and graded for the upper and lower extremity. For instance, if the upper limb is completely flaccid with no voluntary movement and if no changes in tone can be reflexly elicited, it would be classified as being in stage one. In stage two, changes in tone may be elicited reflexly without producing actual movement. One or more components of a synergy may appear as an associated reaction in response to a stimulus. Voluntary initiation of movement within synergy is representative of stage three. This movement may involve one or several components in partial range, for example, slight elbow flexion or one-quarter range of shoulder girdle elevation. Full range is rarely seen. Stage four is represented by movement patterns deviating from basic synergies, such as hand to sacrum, which involves use of both synergic patterns in one movement, or knee flexion past 90 degrees, which is not a component of either synergy. Stage five is reached when the patient gains enough control to be able to perform more isolated movements, such as knee extension with the hip flexed or ankle dorsiflexion with the knee extended. Classification in stage six indicates near normal coordination and speed of alternate movements in the limb. A scoring system can be applied readily to this motor assessment, making it potentially useful as a research tool.

Brunnstrom's assessment of sensory status, balance, and gait compare closely with other neurophysiologic assessments.

This assessment can be administered in a brief time, in combination with treatment procedures, and forms a baseline for continuing reassessment throughout training. In many centers, therapists have adapted or combined selected parts of existing assessment forms to develop an appropriate assessment for their situation. The Brunnstrom motor assessment gives the therapist a reliable indication of the severity of hypertonus in the stroke patient and the degree of control that the patient has over this tone.

TREATMENT

Psychological Aspects

Each person who suffers a stroke is unique, with differing psychological perspectives and physical problems. Brunnstrom understood the overriding influence of the psychological aspects of treatment on the patient's progress. This is a very strong component of her treatment philosophy. The importance of establishing a working partnership between therapist and patient cannot be stressed enough. The approach of the therapist sets the stage for a cooperative adventure and determines, to a great extent, whether this adventure is a success or failure. A positive but realistic attitude assists the patient and family to adjust to their changed lifestyle. A confident therapist who can convey this confidence helps the patient overcome fear of falling, which is probably the most common problem following a stroke. Once rapport is established, then the technical aspects of training become important.

Sensory Facilitation

Brunnstrom's sensorimotor approach involves the use of sensory stimuli through auditory, tactile, visual and proprioceptive pathways in order to facilitate motor responses.

Auditory Input

The ability to communicate effectively is fundamental to the practice of physical therapy. Brunnstrom recognized the influence of the therapist's intonation, vocabulary, volume, speed and delivery of a command on motor responses. For instance, if the patient is expected to relax, the "relax" must be spoken in a relaxing manner. When trying to encourage movement, the therapist is more successful if energy is injected into the command. Rhythmic delivery of commands encourages rhythmic movement. This is of particular value in facilitating change of direction in movement. The auditory quality of the surroundings is also important. Too much background noise is distracting, and may cause increased tone as the patient struggles to concentrate on the task at hand.

Tactile Input

Brunnstrom was of the opinion that touch is a great facilitator of tone and, therefore, should be used with caution and only as necessary. The same principles apply to other forms of exteroceptive stimuli. As soon as the desired response is evoked, the facilitatory stimulus should be withdrawn. She recommended that in handling a limb, contact should be on less stimulatory or nonstimulatory areas and changed only if necessary. For example, the upper limb can be supported through range quite adequately at the medial and lateral aspects of the elbow and with a V-hold at the wrist contacting only the thenar and hypothenar eminences, which are nonstimulatory.

Visual Input

Many of Brunnstrom's training procedures are carried out in sitting, not only because sitting is a functional position, but also because it encourages eye contact between patient and therapist. By sitting facing the patient, the therapist is in an advantageous position to gain and maintain the patient's attention and concentration. Visual cues can be taken from the surroundings to assist orientation to the vertical and the horizontal. Upper extremity activities can be combined with balance activities in the sitting position to take advantage of visual feedback.

Proprioceptive Input

As the name of Brunnstrom's text *Movement Therapy in Hemiplegia* indicates, proprioceptive input is involved in all technical aspects of her approach. Repetition of active-assisted or resisted movement of the limb contributes to the "feel" of where it is in space. Quick stretch, resulting in a localized increase in tone may predispose the muscle towards active contraction. Resisted muscle work, which reflexly causes more motor units to fire, thereby resulting in a greater contraction of the muscle, certainly contributes to the "feel" of the movement. However, today therapists tend to emphasize other means of increasing proprioceptive input, for example, weight bearing.

Although the use of proprioceptive reflexes is controversial, the influence of these reflexes on tone and volitional movement is undeniable. It is important that therapists be aware of the reflex activity that may appear following a stroke, but to consciously use it or feed into its development is to encourage abnormal movement. However, it is interesting to note that some neurophysiological techniques, not necessarily originating with Brunnstrom, may inadvertently take advantage of reflex activity, while stressing other forms of facilitation (for instance, elbow extension is frequently elicited initially in supine lying). The therapist asks the patient to look at the arm. Although giving visual feedback, this activity may also be making use of the asymmetrical tonic neck reflex.

Inhibition

One of Brunnstrom's treatment principles is to inhibit unwanted reflex activity. She believed that at least 50 percent of treatment is inhibition and suggested various inhibitory techniques.

The most obvious inhibitory technique is positioning. For instance, when in supine lying, a small firm roll under the knee inhibits extensor tone in the lower extremity. The sitting position, with hips at no less than 90 degrees flexion, minimizes the effect of most abnormal reflex activity.

The therapist's intonation and manner in approaching the patient and the handling techniques used, may inhibit or facilitate tone. Brunnstrom also suggested the use of reciprocal inhibition as a means of preparing a limb for functional movement. For example, if the patient has strong spasticity in pectoralis major, which interferes with normal movement patterns, strong active retraction of the shoulder girdle might inhibit this tone, thereby allowing the patient to perform activities that involve a degree of abduction at the shoulder.

The use of resistance to reinforce muscle activity is not accepted by many therapists. If used, resistance must be carefully graded, so that unwanted reflex activity is not stimulated. Resistance increases tone in a muscle as more and more motor units are activated. Therefore, resisted activity would not be desirable in a muscle that already has too much tone. However, a hypotonic muscle may respond to an eccentric type of muscle work, for example, holding against resistance.

Closely related to the grading of resistance is the grading of effort demanded of the patient. The more resistance applied, the greater effort required. This effort may cause irradiation of increased tone to other muscle groups or raise general tone throughout the body. This increased tone takes a long time to dissipate, thus interfering with further training procedures during a treatment session. The amount of effort expended also depends upon the difficulty of the task. Therefore, it is essential that the complexity of an activity be carefully analyzed and adapted or simplified so that the patient has a chance to master it without undue effort.

Progression of Treatment

This area of Brunnstrom's approach has been controversial, depending upon the interpretation of her philosophy. Her goal of management is to progress through the stages of recovery toward functional, controlled movement. The synergic patterns of movement representative of stage three are nonfunctional. Therefore, it would seem purposeless to train control of these synergic patterns. It is more logical that once the limb has been classified as in stage three (indicating the quality of movement available), the aim of treatment would be to introduce stage four types of activity, thereby making use of the synergies in the following manner. If the flexor synergy is dominant in the upper extremity, working on a component of the extensor synergy (for example elbow extension), perhaps in a weight-bearing activity would be appropriate. This weight-bearing activity could initially incorporate positioning of the shoulder to take advantage of the strongest component of the extensor pattern (shoulder adduction). When at least a small range of active elbow extension is present, progressing to elbow extension with the shoulder in more abduction would be appropriate. Another example to illustrate use of the synergic components while not actually contributing to its development, is the facilitation of ankle dorsiflexion first with the knee and hip flexed, progressing to the same movement with the leg more extended.

Use of Associated Reactions

Brunnstrom described associated reactions and the related neurophysiology in detail and suggested use of these reactions to facilitate a reflex contraction in a specific muscle group. Since the amount of effort required to elicit an associated reaction is maximal, the idea of using these reactions in treatment is contrary to the previously discussed principles of inhibition. Present concepts in treatment focus on avoidance of associated reactions. The level of tone serves

as a barometer in judging the appropriateness of an activity.

Face and Hand

Brunnstrom provided a functional assessment of the hemiplegic face and hand. The activities tested also serve as training activities. She investigated tone in the hand and suggested techniques for handling this tone and for releasing tension in the fingers. She also stressed that the hand was an integral part of the upper limb, was influenced by activity in the rest of the limb, and should be receiving specific training at the same time as more proximal muscle groups. Her observations on grasp reactions in the hand alerted therapists to the potential influence of these reactions on hand function.

SUGGESTED READING

Brunnstrom S. Movement therapy in hemiplegia. A neurophysiological approach. New York: Harper and Row, 1970.

Brunnstrom S. Recording gait pattern of adult hemiplegic patients. J Am Phys Ther Assoc 1964; 44(1):11–17.

Carr J, Shepherd R. A motor relearning programme for stroke. London: William Heinemann Medical Books, 1982.

Lavigne J. Hemiplegia sensorimotor assessment form. Physiotherapy 1974; 54(2):128–134.

Leo K, Soderberg G. Relationship between perception of joint position sense and limb synergies in patients with hemiplegia. Phys Ther 1981; 61(10):1433–1437.

MOTOR RELEARNING

PATRICIA J. CROSS, Dip. P. & O.T., B.Sc. (PT), M.C.P.A.

Stroke rehabilitation is a major area of specialization in physical therapy, and there are many approaches to follow. Knott and Voss, Brunnstrom, Bobath, Rood, and Johnstone each have a slightly different perspective, and each contributes to the overall rehabilitation outcome. However, there is an aura of mysticism surrounding these approaches, in that therapists do not necessarily feel comfortable or confident applying the principles in their treatment programs unless they have undergone special training. Once trained in one approach, there may be a tendency to restrict practice to a set way of managing the stroke patient. In the meantime, ongoing research continues to change and to add to our understanding of the central nervous system. It is questionable whether physical therapy management of the stroke patient is keeping pace with this changing knowledge base. Motor relearning, a program for stroke management, was developed in an effort to stimulate therapists to examine the effectiveness of their methods and to apply new concepts based on current knowledge of brain function.

THEORETICAL BASIS

Mechanisms of Recovery

Various theories have been proposed in recent literature regarding the mechanisms of recovery following a cerebrovascular accident. There is anatomic evidence to support assumptions that changes take place in neural organization, although how this reorganization takes place is not as yet ascertained. Researchers agree that the brain has a degree of plasticity. Recent animal studies suggest that adaptation and reorganization take place to a great extent during early recovery and are enhanced by functional training. Carr and Shepherd suggest that therapists must take advantage of this theoretical capability for recovery. They may influence recovery by introducing familiar activities to the patient at the earliest moment possible. On the other hand, lack of practice of familiar activities immediately post stroke may discourage this capability and may lead to a feeling of helplessness on the part of the patient.

Human Movement and Muscle Biology

Any functional activity is comprised of essential components of movement that, when linked together properly, constitute a smooth coordinated movement. Studies on human movement have provided therapists with the necessary knowledge to analyze an activity for its essential components and to assess which, if any, components are missing when the patient attempts the activity. This knowledge, coupled with recent theory regarding the optimal conditions for muscle reeducation, increases the probability of success in retraining functional activities. The therapist must know the kinesiology and biomechanics of a particular muscle. Does the muscle normally function as a prime mover or as a fixator in such a position? Effects of gravity, length-tension ratio, temperature, timing, and range are important considerations.

Motor Skill Acquisition

Motor skill acquisition combines formal theories of learning with practical factors, such as the environment in which learning takes place.

The process of motor learning is a cognitive task, which involves gaining a general understanding of the skill to be learned, becoming proficient in the essential components, linking components together while discarding extraneous movement, and practicing the whole skill until it becomes more automatic, that is, until it requires less cognitive effort.

It is the therapist's responsibility to create an environment that promotes learning. Success depends upon many factors.

Problem Solving

The most important factor which influences motor skill acquisition is the ability of the therapist to solve problems, that is, to ascertain correctly the missing components of a skill. Then, the environment must provide opportunity for accurate practice of each missing component within the context of the complete skill, followed by practice of the complete skill. Problem-solving skills continue to sharpen in the process of analyzing performance and of instituting the necessary corrections.

Feedback

Another factor which influences the final result in motor skill acquisition is the type and quality of feedback provided by the environment; visual and verbal feedback are most useful. Visual feedback provides the patient with knowledge of performance and spatial cues. As a source of proprioceptive feedback, vision is being recognized as more sensitive than mechanical proprioceptive feedback via the vestibular system. It orients the body in space and to the midline, thereby assisting the vestibular system in stimulating necessary postural adjustments to maintain alignment during movement. The patient should be encouraged to use visual feedback to participate actively in monitoring performance.

Verbal feedback must be accurate and relevant. The ability to give appropriate feedback depends upon the therapist's verbal skills.

Verbal Skills

Good verbal skills are extremely important in all aspects of physical therapy. They are of particular importance in providing clear explanation, instruction and feedback to the stroke patient. A motor skill must be explained in terms that an individual can understand. Short, goal-oriented instructions, using vocabulary relevant to the activity and to the individual patient give focus to the desired movement. To take advantage of the patient's initial concentration on the instruction, the main point should be expressed in the first few words of the command, such as "touch my hand." Verbal feedback must reflect actual performance. Carr and Shepherd suggest that "good" be erased from therapeutic vocabulary.

Practice

Another factor which influences the final outcome in motor skill acquisition is the type of practice demanded. Accurate motor practice is obviously beneficial. However, of great importance is mental practice, that is, thinking about the desired movement or activity, and verbal practice, that is, talking through the activity. Mental and verbal practice are encouraged not only during training sessions, but also during other times of the day or evening. These forms of practice are ideal homework for the patient who may not be able to practice the actual activity. Family members can participate by encouraging the patient to talk through an activity during a visit.

Motivation

Motivation is the deciding factor in learning a motor skill. Motivation depends upon many factors. Some people are self-motivated. However, when faced with the effects of a catastrophic event such as a stroke, even these people may become passive unless motivated by their environment. The therapist plays a crucial role in creating a motivating climate. The patient is likely to be interested in practicing relevant activities. In this respect, the patient should actively participate in deciding upon both the long-term and short-term goals of training. Each short-term goal must be clearly perceived as contributing to the long-term goals. Short-term goals include not only goals to be achieved in 1 week or 1 month, but also goals to be achieved in one session. Goal-setting leads to another important factor in creating a motivating climate, that is, ensuring a measure of success in each training session. Ensuring success depends upon good problem solving by the therapist, the setting of a goal which is challenging yet attainable, provision of enough guidance and support at first so that the patient experiences successful practice, and introduction of slight variations in the activity as soon as the patient's performance is reasonably correct. In this way, the patient focuses on a new goal, while still practicing the former activity, and feels successful. Success also depends upon the quality of explanation and feedback provided by the therapist.

Another motivating factor is the degree to which the patient is involved in arranging the daily routine. Regular training sessions at prearranged times convenient to both patient and therapist contribute to the reestablishment of responsibility for and control over daily routine by the patient.

MISCONCEPTIONS

As is suggested by the term "motor relearning," the program endeavors to correct several misconceptions regarding the functioning of the brain. Early researchers hypothesized that the brain regressed to immaturity following injury, as evidenced by the appearance of primitive reflex activity. Thus, the patient might be taken through the developmental sequence in treatment in an effort to reintegrate primitive reflex behavior and to redevelop adult motor behavior. However, many of the patterns of movement and positions involved in the developmental sequence may appear irrelevant to the patient and may represent new learning. The stroke population is generally comprised of mature adults, most of whom retain their cognitive abilities following stroke. Therefore, training should use the patient's cognitive abilities in relearning former motor behavior.

Another misconception is that movement can be retrained in mass patterns. Specific muscles are represented in the brain and, therefore, require special reeducation in order to function normally. However, activities involving familiar patterns of movement are easier to learn than unfamiliar activities. Therefore, specific reeducation of muscles should take place within the context of familiar activities.

Spasticity may not be as much a natural phenomenon following stroke as it may be an "overactivity," produced by habitual positioning. Habitual positioning results in some muscles being at a mechanical advantage while other muscles are at a mechanical disadvantage, creating an imbalance in muscle activity. This imbalance can be prevented by frequent change in positioning and by early mobilization; at the very worst, the imbalance should be transitory.

The notion that recovery takes place proximally to distally is also a misconception. Although proximal stability is necessary for skilled movement distally, both should be trained concurrently.

A final misconception is that residual sensory impairment is permanent. Although considered an important prognostic indicator, this impairment is often transitory. The motor relearning program is designed to minimize sensory impairment by early activity, since sensory awareness and movement are interdependent.

ASSESSMENT

The motor assessment scale developed by Carr and Shepherd measures the level of function in everyday activities. It is based on performance of the essential components of these activities and not only serves as an indicator of progress, but also as a guide for training procedures. When Carr and Shepherd researched the scale, it scored high on inter-rater and test-retest reliability. Clinically, it appears to be a realistic and objective measure of progress and can be incorporated into assessment forms used in any facility.

Everyday activities included in the scale are supine to side lying, lying to sitting over the side of the bed, balance in sitting, sitting to standing, walking, upper arm function, hand movements, and advanced hand activities. General tonus is included in the scale; however, it is a subjective observation, and is not included in reliability testing. Detailed guidelines are provided with the assessment scale, and once familiar with the guidelines, the therapist can go through the assessment in a brief period of time, using very little equipment. Patient compliance can be expected because all activities are relevant to daily routine.

APPLICATION OF PROGRAM

Early institution of retraining procedures is necessary, in order to give the patient immediate, positive experience in familiar, everyday activities. These early activities should include sitting and standing. Normal alignment of body parts must be maintained while performing the activity. Extraneous movement or compensatory strategies must not be permitted, and the patient should gradually assume responsibility for maintaining proper alignment independently. Normal alignment is necessary, not only for normal mobility, but also for normal muscle contraction.

As mentioned before, movement should be goal-oriented. Commands such as "touch my hand," "bring your shoulder to my shoulder," and "reach toward the mirror" are most effective. One controversial aspect of this program is a lack of concern for potential stimulation of undesired tone in some muscle groups when giving manual guidance during movement. If excess tone is present in specific muscles, other approaches may stress avoidance of further facilitation of this tone. It is a useful technique to place the overactive muscle in relative disadvantage to the muscle that is required to contract.

Principles of muscle reeducation should be applied. For instance, an eccentric muscle contraction is easier than a concentric contraction. If a muscle does not contract in one segment of its range it may contract in a different segment. Small range movement, for example 1 cm, may be the initial goal. The muscle may be more easily facilitated as a fixator than as a prime mover.

Practice of components of an activity should be followed immediately by practice of the whole activity. This principle forces therapists to break away from traditional routine in treatment, such as mat exercises followed by balance and gait training, which make it difficult for the patient to carry over what was learned on the mat to an activity at a later time. This concept of part-whole practice enables the therapist and patient to accomplish a meaningful goal in the time available, even if only 10 or 15 minutes.

During practice, effective cueing is important. Initially the patient may require tactile cueing as well as verbal and visual cueing. However, tactile cues should be kept to a minimum, verbal cues should be explicit and the patient should be encouraged to use vision, particularly during early training. Too many different cues are confusing. If the patient does not respond to cueing as desired, a change in verbal cueing may facilitate the correct response. For instance, in walking, "swing your leg forward" may result in an immense effort to circumduct, hike the hip, tilt the pelvis, and raise the shoulder, whereas "move your knee forward" may result in exactly the desired response, that is, a smooth step forward with no extraneous movement. It is important that the therapist think about the patient's interpretation of instructions, and make instructions relevant to that interpretation. One more example of faulty verbal cueing is the use of the word "lean." The patient, sitting with feet properly positioned, when instructed to "lean foward" in preparation for standing, might very well curl forward to droop towards the floor. When instructed to "reach forward toward my hand," the patient's weight comes forward, while trunk and neck extension are maintained. Standing up can then be accomplished more readily.

As a last general consideration in applying the program, involvement of the patient's family and other hospital staff is very important in encouraging and reinforcing accurate practice of motor skills outside of the physical therapy department.

PROGRESSION OF TREATMENT

The patient should be constantly challenged to improve performance. This progression can be achieved by decreasing the amount of feedback, manual guidance, or support required, by changing the speed, or by varying the activity. For instance, with the arm supported on a table, the patient may practice wrist extension, then incorporate holding a cup in the hand, progressing to lifting the cup toward the mouth by degrees while maintaining wrist extension. Minor progressions would include increasing or changing the range through which the muscle contracts, the type of contraction or the function of the muscle. Progression demands continual problem solving and imaginative thinking by the therapist.

FATIGUE

Patients are given frequent 'rests' for a number of reasons, which vary from relieving true fatigue to providing the therapist who has a busy caseload a chance to work with more than one patient at a time. Apart from factors such as sedation or other medical conditions, which would cause low activity tolerance, patients who are experiencing success and whose programs are dynamic seldom complain of fatigue. Most patients respond very well to a change of activity.

SOME IMPORTANT ASPECTS OF THE PROGRAM

It is ideal to be able to institute a motor relearning program with every stroke patient in the acute-care hospital. Unfortunately, the ideal is not always possible, and many patients do not begin intensive training until admission to a rehabilitation center. However, application of the principles discussed above gives every patient a chance to recover some functional ability at any point in time following a stroke.

The program is comprised of training that represents the essential activities of daily living. Once familiar with the principles of motor relearning, the therapist should be able to apply these principles to any motor problem faced in stroke rehabilitation. Many of the training procedures originated as 'Bobath types of activities' in so far as alignment, weight bearing, and sequencing are concerned. However, each section offers new concepts and different perspectives on older concepts.

Orofacial Function

In many rehabilitation centers, swallowing activities are managed by the speech pathologist. However, since relearning to initiate swallowing involves specific muscle retraining, as well as proper body alignment, posture, head control, control of respiration and sensory awareness, the physical therapist has a role in these activities. Furthermore, the ability to initiate swallowing is of immediate importance in the management of the acute stroke patient in order to avoid uncomfortable alternatives such as a nasogastric tube. The physical therapist, who should be initiating treatment at the earliest possible moment, can incorporate training of the essential components of the voluntary stage of swallowing into an early mobilization program. One point to be stressed with nursing and dietary staff is that food should be of a definite consistency, such as mashed potatoes, rather than food which becomes liquid in the mouth.

Techniques used to facilitate swallowing are very successful in overcoming two problems of much concern to the stroke patient. One problem is the seemingly excess amount of saliva, which has to be dealt with and which often results in embarrassing drooling. This problem can usually be remedied by reeducation of lip seal and jaw closure, followed by reminders every time drooling occurs. The other problem encountered by the patient is inopportune and embarrassing outbursts of crying. Lip seal and deep breathing may help to control these outbursts if the patient is taught to initiate these techniques at the first sign of becoming emotional.

Facial asymmetry is frequently overlooked by the therapist. Training may require only the conscious relaxation of the intact side of the face to restore symmetry. If specific muscle reeducation is necessary, it should form part of the first and every training session. Facial musculature is important not only for taking in nourishment, but also for communicating normally.

Upper Limb Function

Motor relearning principles are of particular value when applied to upper extremity retraining. Many therapists have become frustrated with the lack of progress in upper limb function, complicated by the frequent development of a painful shoulder and of spasticity. Often, treatment focuses on relief of pain and perhaps on auto-assisted movements within pain-free range. However, relief of pain involves support of the shoulder joint, which is best provided by normal functioning of the muscles surrounding the joint. Thus, early reactivation of this musculature is imperative, and in most instances, some muscle control around the shoulder can be established. It is likely that passive movements are a prime cause of shoulder injury and pain, and that the shoulder should be moved passively only to the position from which it is to work. Active shoulder movements are initiated successfully in supine, a position which places the deltoids at a mechanical advantage. This is one instance in which Carr and Shepherd believe that training in supine is justified. When sitting at a table, the use of a ball for distal fixation of the hand allows controlled, graduated shoulder movements. A broomball provides the appropriate texture and size. Also, the use of this type of ball as support for the hand inhibits flexor spasticity in the fingers and initiates retraining of hand and wrist control while concentrating primarily on more proximal activity. This position is particularly useful in facilitating external rotation of the shoulder. With the elbow supported and the hand on the ball, the patient is instructed to "roll the ball slowly sideways to touch my hand." Extending the elbow so that it is no longer supported progresses the activity.

Hand function is complex and should be included in upper extremity training from the start. A soft paper cup is ideal for retraining the light control required in grasp, that is, grasp without denting the cup. From this initial activity, motor relearning principles should be applied to infinite variation in hand and wrist control, ranging from activities that encourage dexterity to those that require control and strength, such as slicing putty with a knife or using a knife and fork together.

Of particular importance in upper extremity training is proper alignment of body parts and the conscious elimination of extraneous movement or excess tone elsewhere in the body. Use of everyday functional activities provides the optimal chance for recovery of function in the arm and hand.

BALANCE

Carr and Shepherd provide therapists with an enlightened perspective on balance. Although some balance training in the past has involved movement, much time has been spent teaching the patient to respond forcefully to pushing or stabilizations. This technique does not retrain the fine postural adjustments necessary for most normal activities. Recent literature suggests that balance is not a response but occurs in anticipation of movement, in other words, comprises postural set. Carr and Shepherd suggest that balance is dynamic and should be trained within the context of functional activities. They also suggest that balance for one activity cannot be learned in a different activity. Therefore, the patient must experience each activity and practice it in a normal manner, that is, while

maintaining normal alignment and a normal base of support for that activity. Good sitting balance is not a prerequisite for training standing balance because postural alignment is different for each of these activities. Although the patient relearns balance at a cognitive level initially, the goal is for maintenance of balance to become automatic.

OTHER FUNCTIONAL ACTIVITIES

Motor relearning principles in combination with neurodevelopmental treatment principles enhance retraining of functional activities such as supine to sitting, sitting to standing to sitting, and walking. Neurodevelopmental principles of normal alignment, normal weight bearing, and sequencing of the components of these activities form the basis for retraining. Goal-oriented instructions and appropriate verbal feedback during part-whole practice assists in allaying fear of falling, which is frequently a major factor affecting normal function. Conscious relaxation of hypertonic muscles augments inhibitory positioning and weight bearing for control of tone during functional activities.

CONCLUSION

The motor relearning program adds a concrete, new dimension to stroke rehabilitation. Analysis of movement for missing components, followed by retraining of these components, can be applied to any movement disorder in the stroke patient.

Patients respond very well to the cognitive demands of this approach, but success in motor relearning depends upon the problem solving and verbal skills of the therapist. In order to be most successful in the rehabilitation of stroke patients, therapists must be aware of current research findings regarding the function of the central nervous system, and be prepared to incorporate new concepts into their treatment programs.

SUGGESTED READING

Bobath B. Adult hemiplegia: evaluation and treatment. 2nd ed. London: William Heinemann Medical Books, 1978.

Bobath B. Abnormal posture reflex activity caused by brain lesions. 2nd ed. London: William Heinemann Medical Books, 1971.

Carr J, Shepherd R. A motor relearning programme for stroke. London: William Heinemann Medical Books, 1982.

Carr J, Shepherd R, Nordholm L, Lynne D. Investigation of a new motor assessment scale for stroke patients. Phys Ther 1985; 65(2):175–180.

Goldberg M. Motor recovery after lesions. Trends in neurosciences (TINS) Amsterdam, New York, November 1980:288–291.

FUNCTIONAL APPROACH TO MULTIPLE SCLEROSIS

NANCY BUCHHOLZ MOODIE, B.Sc.P.T.
MONIQUE PRENDERGAST, B.Sc., P.T.

Multiple sclerosis (MS) is one of the most common causes of chronic neurologic disability. MS is a significant clinical entity because of its frequency, chronicity, and tendency to attack young adults. The incidence in Canada is 30 to 80 per 100,000. The characteristic plaque lesions of MS have a predilection for certain areas of the nervous system giving rise to the familiar signs and symptoms. These are weakness, paresthesia, diplopia, nystagmus, ataxia of the trunk and/or limbs, sensory impairment, bladder dysfunction, altered emotional state, and fatigue.

The major target areas for physical therapy intervention and management include the following:

1. Truncal instability (central stability is a prerequisite for normal coordinated movement patterns);
2. The presence of abnormal tone;
3. Muscle weakness;
4. Decreased physical endurance;
5. Poor mobility skills (decreased transitional movements, transfer skills, and gait pattern); and
6. Generalized fatigue.

Physical therapy management of these problems includes exercise, positioning, introduction of aids, and patient education. Explaining the pathology of MS, the principles of energy conservation, the importance of exercise and developing a patient-specific home exercise program are essential components of patient education.

Functional abilities are the most significant concern, regardless of the signs and symptoms presented. It is the goal of physical therapy to maximize functional abilities. The therapist evaluates the patient's present physical status with reference to activities of daily living (ADL), home, work, and leisure environments. Practical treatment goals are set based on the patient's concerns and the results from the objective assessment.

ASSESSMENT

The history should contain a description of the first signs and symptoms of the disease, their course, and further exacerbations, in addition to the residual deficits and functional implications. A detailed history of the disease process allows the physical therapist to make a prognostic prediction that is invaluable for appropriate implementation of ambulation devices, transfer, and home modifications. It is important to have the patient relay what the physician has said regarding disease prognosis. Personal and social changes that have occurred over the course of the disease may influence the treatment approach, and therefore, lifestyle changes that affect gait skills, ADL, housing, and employment are noted. Past and present treatments and their outcome are of value to the assessment. Examples include medications, previous therapies, home exercise programs, and exercise regimes implemented by the patient.

The subjective section of the assessment should include a description of the patient's understanding of the overall disease course and prognosis. All misconceptions relating to the disease, either positive or negative must be identified. Motivation is a key area and can be assessed by noting whether the patient voices an interest in treatment and in maintaining functional level. This may be evident by lifestyle adaptations, e.g., moving to a more accessible housing unit, decreasing or increasing social activities, or frequently changing physicians. The therapist should compare the actual level of activity to the level of functional ability as a measure of motivation. It is important for the therapist to evaluate which motivation is greater—that of the patient or of the family members. The effects of fatigue on the patient with MS should be assessed. When is the patient consistently most fatigued? What precedes the fatigue, and how does it interfere with the patient's course of activity? The patient's perception of which physical problem interferes most with his or her mobility is essential for goal setting, in addition to ensuring optimum motivation and participation.

Progressing to the objective part of the assessment, a standard mental status and cranial nerve examination is performed. The results of relevant clinical tests such as a computed tomography (CT) scan cerebrospinal fluid (CSF) oligoclonal banding, auditory evoked responses, cerebrospinal fluid and visual evoked responses should be documented. Medications, such as prednisone, taken for spasticity management or the MS itself, are identified in the assessment. The physical examination includes the assessment of deep tendon reflexes, Babinski's sign, clonus, and sensation. These tests are straightforward, and the results do not directly affect management. Joint position sense is the most important sensory modality to test because of its obvious importance to movement, especially gait.

Thus far, the history, subjective, and observational examination gives the therapist a sense of where the physical presentation will fit. Patients with MS often fit into one of the following categories: hemiparetic, paraparetic, quadriparetic; ataxic; sensory disturbances only; or generalized weakness and/or increased fatigue. These categories help organize and focus both the assessment and treatment.

The next elements of the assessment are key areas—tone, range of motion, strength, coordination, and motor skills. Three questions should be kept in mind when assessing tone either of the upper extremities, lower extremities, or trunk. Where is the abnormal tone? Is it increased or decreased? Is it limiting or preventing movement? Increased tone in the upper extremities is usually present in pectoralis major and minor, biceps, pronators, and the long wrist and finger flexors. Increased tone in the lower extremities occurs in the extensors, gastrocnemii, and the foot intrinsics. The low back extensors may have increased tone triggered by increased lower extremity tone. Conversely, hypotonia is most often generalized and can be more disabling than moderate hypertonia in the trunk as it removes the stable base for extremity movement, sitting, and standing balance.

In the extremities, moderate to severe increased tone may decrease the ability to isolate joint movements. Can the patient flex the elbow with the wrist extended, flex and extend the fingers and thumb in any wrist position, pronate and supinate the forearm with the wrist and elbow in any range of flexion or extension? The patient should be asked how much stiffness or difficulty with movement they notice as well as the methods used to decrease abnormal tone. Is the tone causing or increasing any symptoms of pain, especially in the lower back or at the hamstring insertion site? Is there a potential for loss of range of motion due to increased tone? All of these questions need to be addressed.

Assessment of the articular status is generally straightforward. A functional range is the crucial range of motion required and should be regarded as the norm. Limited areas are often attributable to increased tone in biceps, long flexors of the hand, back extensors, hamstrings, gastrocnemii, and foot intrinsics. Shortening in these groups affects function—hand skills, sitting balance, and gait.

Muscle strength is assessed according to the Oxford muscle scale to set a baseline for the exercise program and for periodic assessment. It is vital not to overlook testing truncal muscles as trunk strength and endurance are essential for mobility skills, sitting, sitting balance, use of the upper extremities, and gait skills. Patients with MS often have problems with generalized fatigue and this should be kept in mind

when assessing strength. Recognizing certain muscles or groups that fatigue over three to ten contractions will identify those that easily fatigue and impair function. Muscles around weakened groups and muscles not used because of decreased mobility often become weak. Identifying these muscles and priorizing them into a treatment program can be of significant value (e.g., back extensor and abdominals following prolonged sitting). The standard tests should be done for coordination; finger-nose, heel-shin, rapid alternating movements, and toe tapping to assess any ataxia or dystonia.

Following these categories of neurologic assessment, the therapist progresses to an evaluation of function, which involves an overall assessment of the ability to perform mobility skills required for home, work, and recreation. This involves an evaluation of bed mobility and the ability to roll from side to side and to prone. Is the patient able to attain a sitting position from lying, to maintain it, and to superimpose movements? The quality of these transitional movements and the level of independence is noted. The standing position is also assessed. Transfers are evaluated—not only bed to chair, but also chair to toilet and chair to floor and up. Type of transfer and level of assistance is documented.

A full gait analysis is subsequently performed. The gait pattern and the aids required are described in detail. Endurance and the ability to perform higher level skills are noted. Wheelchair management or mobie (electric) chair skills with regards to safety and positioning are then assessed. If the patient is ambulatory, the ability to ascend and descend stairs is evaluated and the pattern and level of assistance required is recorded.

Through quick observation, combined with the history and subjective assessment, the therapist can acquire enough information to be able to zero in on the aspects of mobility and function that are most important. These usually center around trunk posture and control, transfers, and method of locomotion.

When planning an appropriate treatment approach for a patient with MS, it is important to keep in mind realistic goals and expectations based on the assessment findings. Multiple sclerosis has a very broad range of clinical features including prognosis; therefore, it is important to establish that there is no universal formula for rehabilitation. Physical therapy exercises aimed at reducing tone and improving strength and range of motion are not enough on their own unless there is carryover into function. The ultimate aim of all exercises should be to maintain and/or improve mobility and level of independence. A functionally oriented approach to treatment also provides the patient with meaning and direction, which in itself is important to increase patient compliance with treatment and any given exercises.

It is important to convey that assessment does not terminate after the initial session. Ongoing assessment is an integral part of treatment and assists the therapist in interpreting treatment effectiveness. Therefore, assessment and treatment go hand in hand.

As identified earlier, the priority target area is the trunk and its effectiveness in controlling posture statically and dynamically. This cannot be underestimated by the therapist since any potential for normal, coordinated activities of the upper extremities cannot be achieved without a stable postural base. For example, an individual with truncal ataxia may be able to control his extremities while supine, but in high sitting all efforts are focused on maintaining truncal stability. Trunk and postural control therefore become the basis for all other control. Mat exercises that include gross motor activities, which result in coactivation of the trunk muscles, are essential in a treatment regime. Examples include bridging and curl-ups with superimposed rolling bilaterally. In sitting, back cocontractions may be achieved by using a ball (approximately 20–25 cm [8–10 in] in diameter) placed between the lower thoracic spine and the back of the chair.

Trunk stability and mobility may be improved by using the stages of the developmental sequence. Rhythmic stabilizations at each stage improve central and proximal stability. Progression through the stages of the developmental sequence allows the therapist to facilitate an individual's ability to move in and out of a given posture (transitional movements) and superimpose movement while maintaining postural stability.

It is important to assess pelvic control in sitting as this control facilitates the ability to stand from sitting and to transfer. Assess ability to perform an anterior and posterior pelvic tilt. If the patient has difficulty tilting the pelvis anteriorly in sitting, this should be considered as an exercise with the therapist guiding the movements. Carryover into function may later be achieved by demonstrating how an anterior pelvic tilt facilitates standing from sitting. In functional activities, upper extremity control may also be associated with inadequate pelvic control.

Displacing body weight beyond the base of support, laterally and in an anterior-posterior plane, is another treatment idea for trunk stabilizing and strengthening activities. Sit-ups in crook lying and upper torso lifts in prone lying, "fly-aways," are effective means of strengthening abdominals and back extensors respectively. The use of a therapeutic (65 cm) ball has proven to be of great benefit when working to improve balance and postural control. The specific effects include the following:

- facilitation of and/or establishment of movement
- encouragement of automatic movements
- establishment of symmetrical movements
- support of body parts i.e., support of a weak, ataxic trunk to encourage use of the extremities
- facilitation of righting and equilibrium reactions and facilitation of weight shifting and automatic postural adjustments.

Spasticity is the second target area for management. Slow passive stretch of the hypertonic muscle groups is an important tone inhibiting technique. Regular stretching of the gastrocnemii, hamstrings, and hip adductor muscles helps to maintain muscle length and to reduce tone. In crook lying, pelvic rocking in a slow, rhythmic motion is an excellent means of reducing lumbar tone. Weight bearing through the heel of the hand to reduce upper extremity tone and the heel of the foot for the lower extremity, is an excellent means of normalizing tone in functional positions. The tilt table may be indicated to reduce tone especially in cases with poor trunk control. Weight bearing through the long bones has the secondary benefit of reducing the development of osteoporosis. Patient education is another aspect in the management of spasticity. Patients and their families should be taught positions that reduce tone, and should understand the nature of tone and the influencing factors. Stimulating the antagonistic muscle groups with a functional electrical stimulator (FES) is also found to be of great benefit in reducing spasticity.

When foot intrinsic hypertonicity is evident, specific mobilizations of the foot are helpful as well as a foam toe spreader. This consists of regular foam approximately 11 cm ($4^1/_2$ in) wide and $2^1/_2$ cm (1 in) thick with slits in it to accommodate each toe. The foam can be worn under the sock and holds the toes in abduction and extension, thereby reducing the effect of the hypertonicity.

Strengthening programs for the patient with MS must be carefully monitored. Weakness may be secondary to nerve conduction block, which is caused by the lesion and cannot be reversed by exercise. With nerve-fiber fatigue, excessive repetitions make the motor action progressively weaker until it can no longer be performed. This type of weakness does not improve with a program of progressive resisted exercises.

Weakness secondary to disuse responds well to progressive strengthening exercises providing the tone remains manageable. It may be necessary to consider functional and tone inhibiting positions for strengthening in order to avoid an increase in the level of tone. Slow controlled squats or step-ups on a bench for quadriceps strengthening are preferable to the standard method of performing isometric quads over a roll. The weight-bearing position with distal fixation helps to inhibit tone and facilitates cocontractions and stability at the hip and knee. Specific strengthening exercises in the presence of near-normal tone may include the use of weights, proprioceptive neuromuscular facilitation (PNF), resisted strengthening, bicycling, rebounding, and swimming. It is important to strengthen proximally to distally to optimize control and functional carryover. The patient with MS should not exercise beyond the point of general fatigue. Following a short rest, planned daily activities should be continued.

Ataxia is perhaps the most difficult problem to treat effectively. Rhythmic stabilizations in sitting, four point kneeling, and standing should be considered in addition to proximal or distal weighting to reduce lateral sway of the trunk and the extremities. Weighting a walker and increasing the base of support while ambulating is also beneficial. When the therapist is considering altering or improving the established gait pattern, the following must be considered: Is the patient's strength adequate for safe, unaided ambulation (antigravity hip abductors)? Does the patient have adequate trunk and postural control to improve gait pattern? Are additional aids and/or orthoses appropriate?

Exercise is of benefit when suited to the individual's functional level and tolerance. The benefits are significant in that problems such as weakness and poor endurance due to inactivity are reduced. Exercise also helps to improve general health and fitness and to stimulate motivation.

Treating the patient with MS is an ongoing challenge for the physical therapist. As MS is a regressive disease, the therapist must anticipate and prepare the patient for each mobility alteration i.e., requiring a cane, walker, or wheelchair.

The goal of physical therapy management of the patient with MS is to maximize mobility and level of independence. A functional approach is an effective way to satisfy this objective.

SUGGESTED READING

Adams R, Victor M. Principles of neurology. New York: McGraw-Hill, 1981.

Baker AB, Baker LH, eds. Clinical neurology. New York: Harper and Row, 1983.

Capildeo R, Maxwell A. Progress in rehabilitation multiple sclerosis. London: Macmillan Press, 1982.

Freal J, Kraft G, Conjell J. Symptomatic fatigue in multiple sclerosis. Arch Phys Med Rehabil 1984; 65:135–138.

Paty DW. Multiple sclerosis. Med North Am 1983; 32:3038–3045.

PHYSICAL MANAGEMENT OF THE UNCONSCIOUS HEAD-INJURED PATIENT

BRIAN R. DURWARD, M.Sc., M.C.S.P.

The physical management of the unconscious severely head-injured patient requires a flexible type of therapeutic intervention by the physical therapist. In the Royal Infirmary of Edinburgh, the acute regional neurosurgical unit for the east of Scotland, a dynamic physical therapy approach has been adopted for the treatment of head-injured patients. This dynamic approach is applied from the time each unconscious patient within the intensive care unit is physiologically stable and is continued over the acute stage of care. Immediately after severe head injury, physical therapy is directed towards achieving two main aims: (1) the promotion of normal motor recovery, and (2) the prevention of secondary neuromuscular complications.

The latter complications are caused by released reflex activity, which can be so dominant as to cause fixed soft-tissue contractures. Heterotopic ossification may also develop, but the cause of this is unclear. By adopting a dynamic approach to treatment, physical therapists have felt that motor recovery has been enhanced and that there has been a more successful management of the secondary neuromuscular problems. This dynamic approach is directed towards stimulating balance control in the functionally important positions of sitting and standing, at the earliest possible stage when the head-injured patient is unconscious.

Following a severe head injury, the problems of unconsciousness, the differing levels of abnormal postural tone, and the complex disturbances to sensorimotor and perceptual organization within the brain, require the physical therapist to assess each individual patient carefully and to apply a problem-solving process to treatment. It follows then that any approach to treatment should consider these problems in order to achieve success.

It has been established that the most common types of brain damage are contusions and lacerations of the polar and basal regions of the cortex and diffuse white-matter damage throughout the brain itself. It is the latter type of brain damage that is now considered to account for severe head injury. Following diffuse trauma to the white matter, there can be prolonged unconsciousness and where there has been gross brain stem damage, a permanent vegetative state can result. Patients with severe head injury can present with differing levels of consciousness and a variety of sensorimotor deficits, which require identification and consideration during planning treatment.

Treatment may be required for the patient who has severely impaired consciousness and is considered in a state of coma. Within this chapter the condition of coma is reserved for patients who do not obey commands, do not utter any comprehensible words, and do not open their eyes, even in response to pain. It may also be the case that less severe levels of unconsciousness are present, and the patient shows signs of agitation, disorientation, and confusion. When adopting a dynamic physical approach, it is necessary to consider this variability in consciousness in order to achieve the therapeutic objectives.

Disorders of movement and motor control are as variable as levels of consciousness following severe head injury and require particular consideration. The released primitive postures that can disturb postural tone and thus prevent normal movement need to be identified in each patient. The presence of decerebrate postures (which result in all four limbs adopting an increase in extensor tone) or decorticate postures (where the forelimbs show an increase in flexor tone and the lower limbs an increase in extensor tone) directly determines the selection of treatment techniques. The release of specific reflexes, such as the symmetric and asymmetric tonic neck reflexes and the tonic labyrinthine reflex, also influences the selection of treatment techniques. The careful assessment of patients, to determine if abnormal reflex activity is present, is essential before dynamic treatment is carried out. Recognition of abnormal reflex activity directs the physical therapist to select treatment techniques that inhibit abnormal postural tone, which has developed as a result of particular patterns of released reflexes.

THERAPEUTIC ALTERNATIVES

Alternative therapeutic procedures that attempt to promote motor recovery and to prevent the development of secondary neuromuscular complications in the severe head-injured patient include the following: positioning the patient in reflex inhibitory postures, passive movements, inhibitory stretching, and passive trunk rotation. Positioning the patient is performed in an attempt to inhibit released reflex activity. The patient is positioned in a semi-prone position, but with pillows placed to support the pelvic and shoulder girdles, and both upper and lower limbs on one side of the patient. Where there is tonic labyrinthine reflex activity then this position minimizes tactile stimuli to either the ventral or dorsal surfaces of the patient. Passive movements have traditionally been used in the management of the unconscious patient. Where there is increased tone, passive movements may cause soft-tissue damage if performed through the full range of a joint. Inhibitory techniques have been developed for the head-injured patient; these techniques involve applying a slow stretch to hypertonic muscles and passively rotating the patient's trunk in order to reduce tone. Attempts at preserving joint range, inhibiting increased postural tone and facilitating motor recovery are made by adopting these conservative approaches during the acute stage. These conservative approaches are particularly appropriate when the patient is ventilator-dependent. At this stage it would be inappropriate to move the patient to an upright position and, therefore, conservative physical therapy is applied. The dynamic therapeutic approach is integrated with the conservative physical therapy practice at a point in the recovery when the patient is considered physiologically stable, following disconnection from a ventilator. The use of a Tilt table has been advocated by workers in this field. The unconscious patient is strapped on to a table, which is then rotated to an upright standing position. Although this technique involves placing the patient in a standing position, I feel that the use of this equipment does not permit a dynamic element because of the restraints which support the patient on the tilt table.

PATIENT SELECTION CRITERIA

The unconscious head-injured patient is treated using dynamic therapeutic techniques unless any of the following complications are present:

1. The patient must have voluntary control of respiratory function and must no longer require the assistance of a ventilator to sustain adequate respiratory function. If the patient is attached to a ventilator it is dangerous to use a technique that might dislodge either an oropharangeal or nasopharangeal tube. Once the patient is able to sustain his breathing without mechanical assistance, even if either of the tubes are in situ, then a more dynamic treatment approach can be adopted—although great care must be taken not to dislodge the tube. If the patient has had a tracheostomy performed, and there is a tube in situ—providing respiratory function can be maintained—then a dynamic treatment can commence with care.

2. The patient must not have an intrapleural chest drain or a severe chest injury, which contraindicates treatment in an upright position.

3. A femoral or pelvic fracture prevents a head-injured patient from being placed in an upright position. Where a stable fracture exists below the knee the patient can be supported in a sitting position. Care is required in moving the patient at the stage when he is considered stable and no longer requires ventilation. There may be an intracranial pressure transducer, intravenous drip, or urine drainage system attached to the patient at the acute stage. Whereas it is not necessary to prevent the patient being positioned upright, particular care is required in applying a dynamic therapeutic approach.

ESSENTIAL CHARACTERISTICS OF THE THERAPEUTIC APPROACH

The essential characteristic of this therapeutic approach is that the body segments are moved and adjusted. These movements and adjustments of body segments are carried out with the patient supported in either a sitting or standing position (Fig. 1).

The external influence of handling produces selected body segment adjustments that are observed

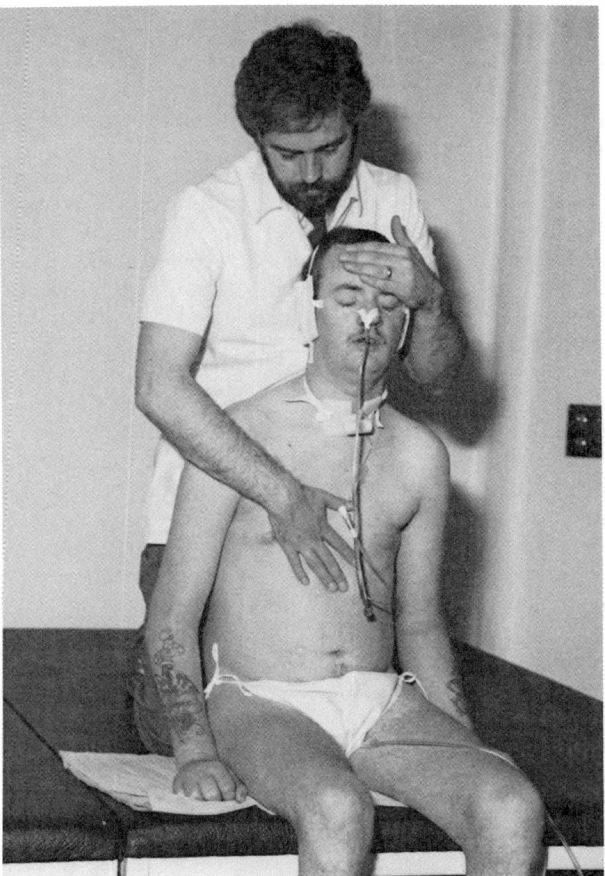

Figure 1   A patient supported in a sitting position.

during normal balance in the positions of sitting or standing. This therapeutic technique is an adaptation of the Bobath concept of "facilitation of movement," which is interpreted as the production of movement caused by handling the patient and not caused by verbal instructions. Body segment adjustments, which are produced by the physical therapist, occur mainly in the trunk and neck, although the shoulder and pelvic girdles are also controlled. Both are involved with particular adjustments of the trunk.

Description of Technique

The unconscious patient is supported in either a sitting or a standing position. Specific patterns of body segment adjustment can then be produced.

Techniques Used in Sitting

In the sitting position, anteroposterior, lateral, and rotational adjustments can be produced by the physical therapist.

Sitting—Anteroposterior Adjustment. The patient is slowly moved between the positions of flexion and extension, and the physical therapist passively adjusts the head and trunk alignment as movement occurs. These adjustments are undertaken in the following manner. The body segment adjustments are controlled in the sitting position by supporting the patient's trunk from behind. In this position, the head and trunk can be supported and anteroposterior body segment adjustment is then performed. From the supported upright sitting position and with the head maintained in a normal alignment, the trunk is displaced backwards. During this movement posteriorly head and trunk are moved into an attitude of flexion (Fig. 2). From this position, the reverse movement is performed; the weight of the patient is brought forward and the neck and trunk adjusted into an extended position (Fig. 3).

Sitting—Lateral Adjustment. Before lateral adjustment is produced the physical therapist again supports head and trunk from behind. In addition the shoulder girdle is supported in the direction of the lateral adjustment (Fig. 4). From an upright starting position the trunk is moved to one side. At the same time as producing this lateral displacement of the trunk, the physical therapist adjusts the head towards the midline, and elongates the trunk on the side to which movement has occurred. The patient is then moved slowly back to the initial starting position and normal alignment is restored between the head and trunk. This lateral pattern of segmental adjustment and the return movement to the mid-line is repeated slowly a number of times.

Sitting—Rotational Adjustment. With the patient and physical therapist in the same starting position as for lateral adjustment, rotational adjustment can be produced. The head is rotated to one side, then this movement is continued with the result that the upper trunk is brought round in the same direction (Fig. 5). Trunk rotation in this form is controlled by moving the opposite shoulder girdle to the direction of the rotational movement. Initially, the shoulder girdle moves into protraction and, by continuing this movement, the upper trunk is brought round in the required direction. Throughout this rotational movement the physical therapist supports the patient and maintains a normal alignment of the head and trunk in the sitting position. This movement is repeated a number of times from the starting position. During the course of a treatment, this rotational movement should be performed in both directions. In addition, with the head and trunk rotated to one side, the patient can be supported and weight can be taken through each upper limb (Fig. 6).

The Basic Standing Position

To place the unconscious head-injured patient in a standing position with the intention of producing

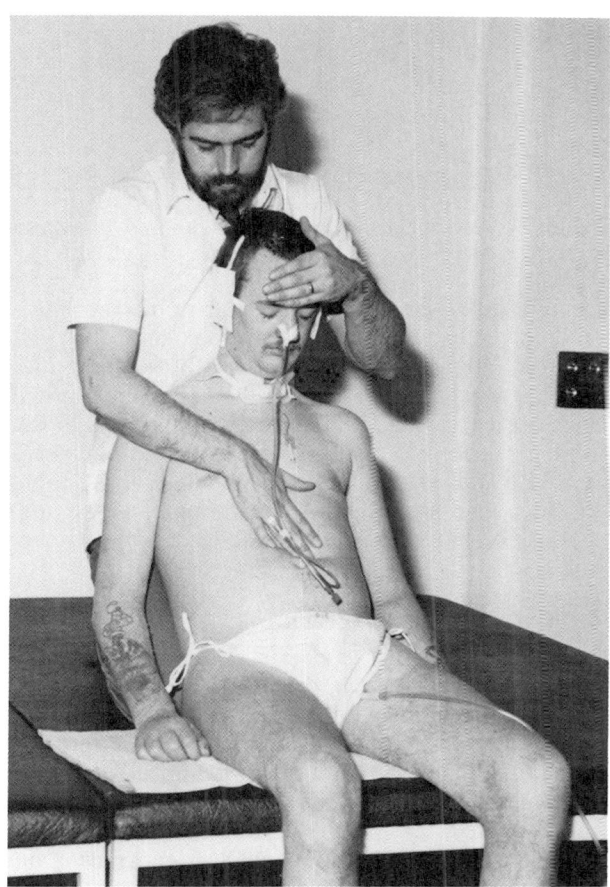

Figure 2 Posterior displacement of the trunk with adjustment into flexion.

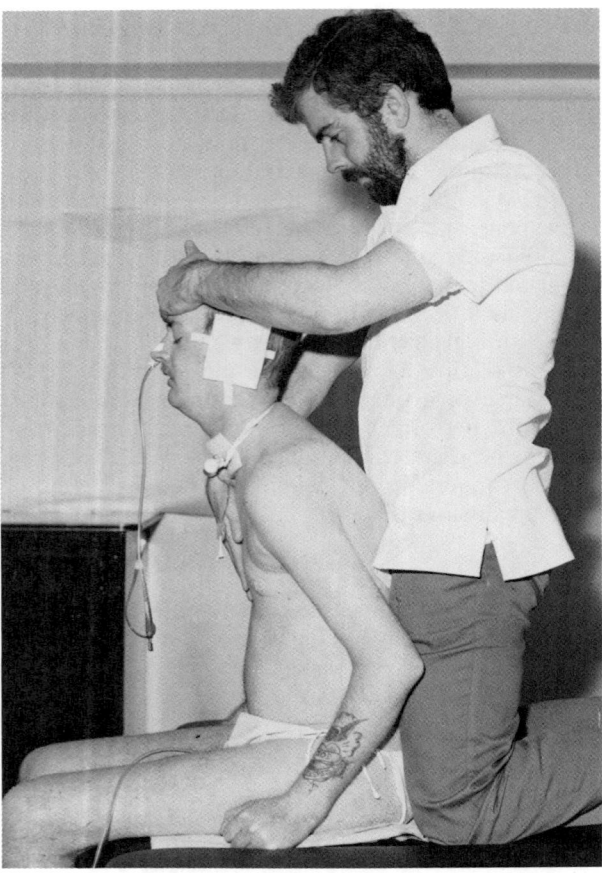

Figure 3   Anterior displacement of the trunk with adjustment into extension.

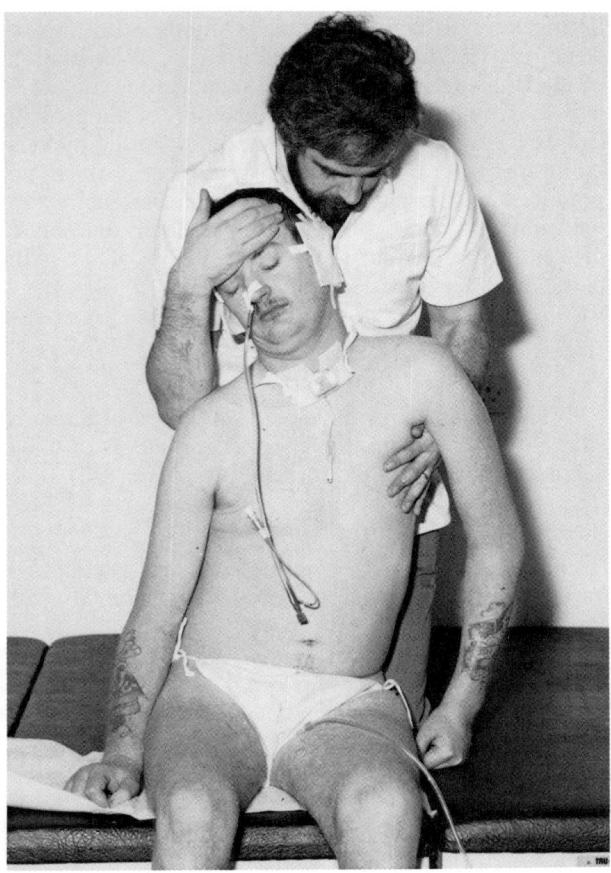

Figure 4   Lateral adjustment of the trunk in sitting.

specific body segment adjustments, requires the physical therapist to support the head, trunk and pelvic girdle in an alignment that is normal for standing. An assistant is required to support the knees in a normal degree of extension. An alternative solution is to use two leg gaiters, which maintain alignment of the knees in order that a standing position can be achieved. From this supported standing position the unconscious patient can be moved in order to produce body segment adjustment.

Techniques Used in Standing

With the patient supported and controlled in the standing position, the movements of anteroposterior, lateral, and rotational adjustment can be produced.

Standing—Anteroposterior Adjustment. From the starting position the physical therapist moves the pelvic girdle posteriorly. As this movement occurs the trunk and neck are passively moved into an attitude of flexion (Fig. 7). Throughout this movement the knees are maintained in an extended position. The patient is moved slowly back to the starting position and the sequence of adjustment is repeated.

The patient may present with established hypertonicity in the gastrocnemius and soleus muscles, which results in the ankle joints being maintained in a position of plantar-flexion. In this case, anterior adjustment of the pelvis can aggravate this increased tone. This appears to be caused by the transfer of body weight onto the fore-feet and the subsequent stimulation of an exaggerated positive supporting reaction. Where this problem does not exist, anterior movement of the pelvis can be produced and the trunk and neck can be adjusted into a position of extension. The movement involving posterior adjustment of the pelvis is most commonly used and has greater therapeutic value owing to the muscular responses that are invoked.

Standing—Lateral Adjustment. From the starting position, the pelvis is moved laterally (Fig. 8). This movement is controlled by supporting the head and trunk, then as lateral pelvic movement occurs, the head is encouraged to side-flex back to the mid-line. Simultaneously, the shoulder-girdle is elevated to cause elongation of the trunk on the side to which movement is taking place.

Standing—Rotational Adjustment. In standing, rotation is produced in the same manner as in

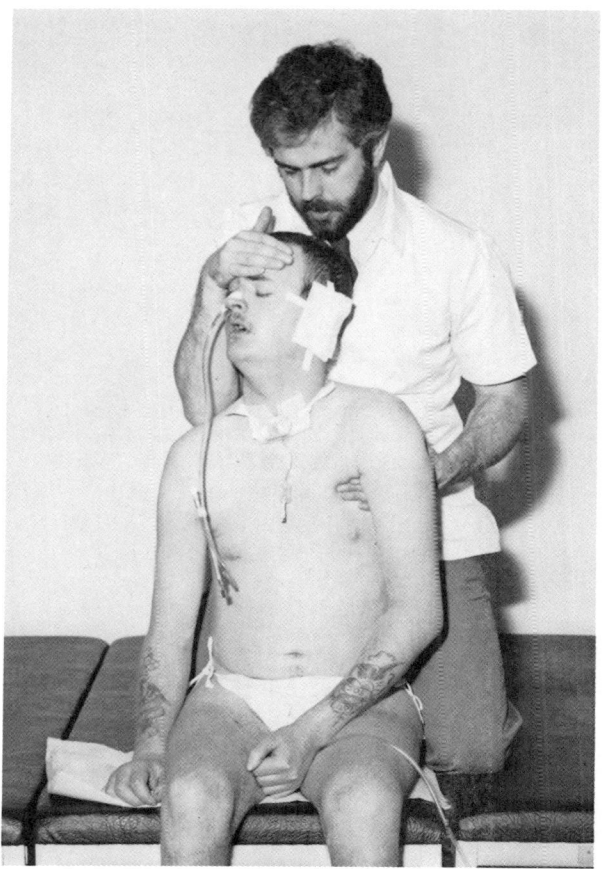

Figure 5 Rotational adjustment in a sitting position.

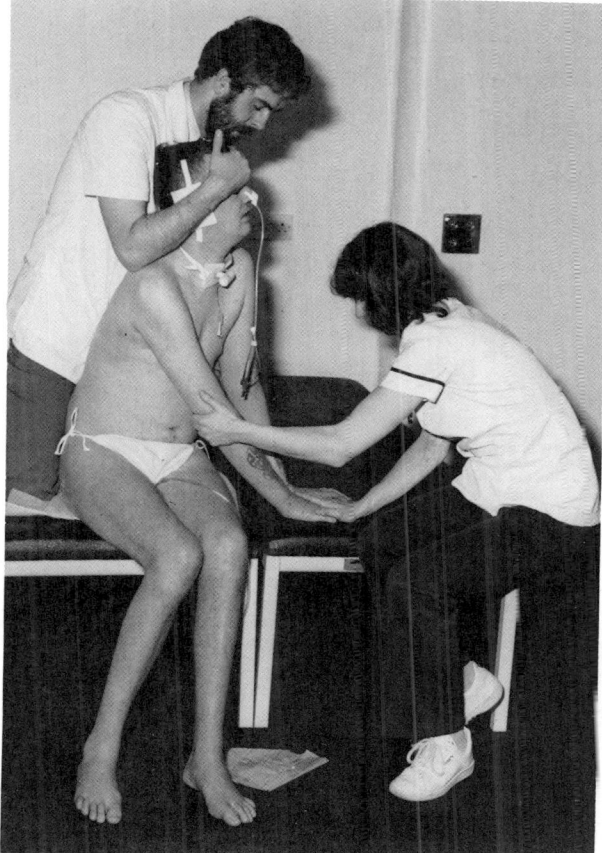

Figure 6 The arms taking weight in a rotated sitting position.

sitting. The head is rotated to one side and the opposite shoulder girdle is moved into protraction. By continuing this shoulder movement, the upper trunk is brought round into a rotated position. The physical therapist controls the distribution of weight through each foot and attempts to ensure that it is equal throughout the movement. During the return movement the alignment of the head and trunk is controlled as the patient is brought back to the starting position. As in sitting, this movement should be performed to either side (Fig. 9).

EFFECTS OF THE DYNAMIC APPROACH

The effects of this dynamic treatment approach are varied. Where the unconscious head-injured patient has reduced postural tone, the combined effects of movement and support in a normal weight-bearing position serve to stimulate an increase in postural tone to normal levels. With a return of consciousness, the stimulating effect of these two factors encourages an increased ability to sustain control of both the sitting and the standing postures. This then leads to an increased ability to perform functional tasks involving

the upper and lower limbs. The enhanced trunk and head control facilitates the relearning of functional tasks where balance is an important factor.

The patient with increased tone responds in a different manner to this type of treatment. In this type of patient, the effects of movement and weight bearing in an upright position serve to reduce the increased postural tone and, therefore, minimize the secondary soft-tissue problems that can develop in the presence of sustained hypertonicity. Where a patient has increased tone, which pulls the feet into plantarflexion and inversion, the effect of (a) being supported in a standing position and (b) the influence of body segment adjustment, combine to reduce the abnormal tone. As a result, during the course of a treatment the feet can adopt a plantigrade position. Once the patient has been placed in a standing position the effect of reduced postural tone is not instantly apparent. After a number of minutes in the standing position, during which the physical therapist has produced slow and rhythmical body segment adjustments, the plantar flexors and invertors of the ankle begin to show a reduction of tone and the feet an ability to adopt a

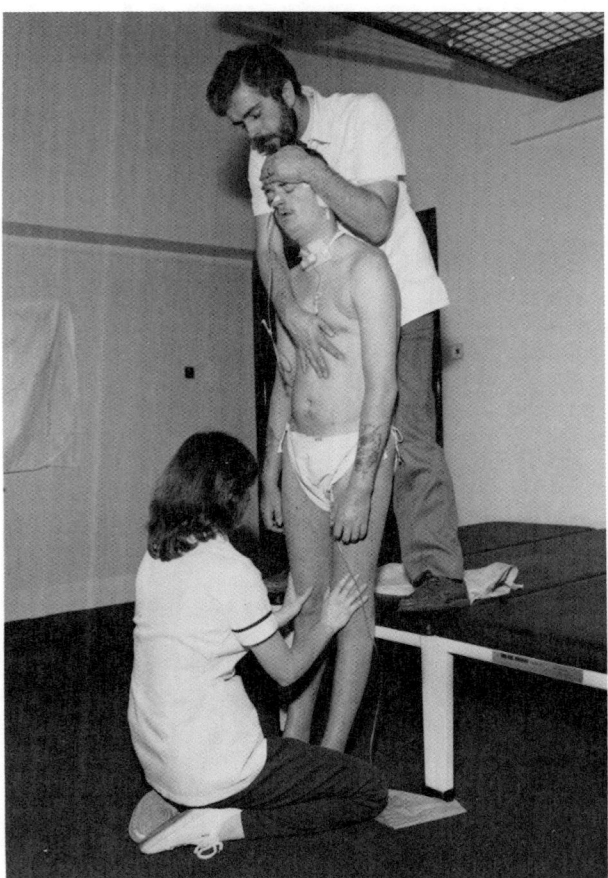

Figure 7   Posterior displacement of the trunk in standing.

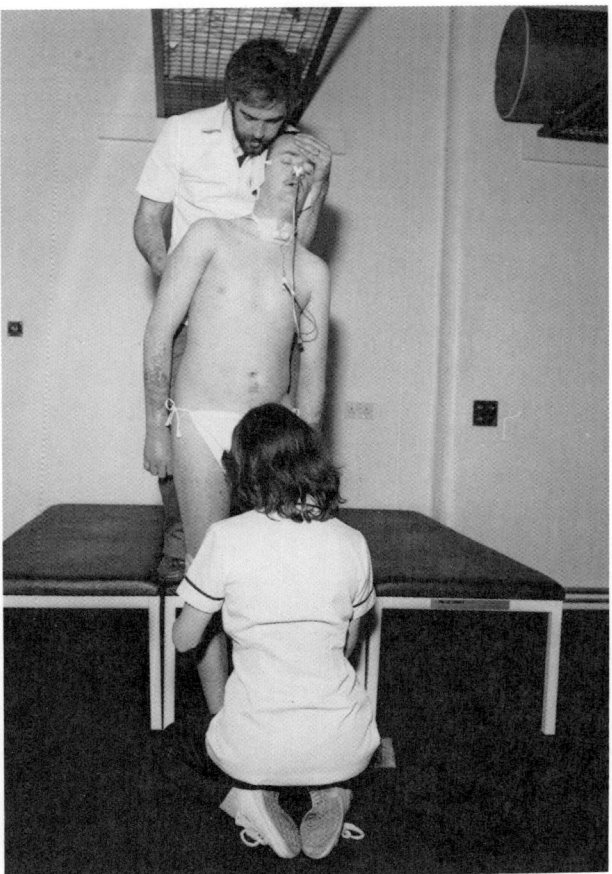

Figure 8   Lateral adjustment in a standing position.

plantigrade position. By repeating this particular standing technique the length of the achilles tendons and the posterior calf muscles can be preserved. A similar effect can be observed in the upper limbs where strong hypertonicity can produce flexion contractures of the elbow and glenohumeral joints. In this case, adjustments of body segments in either a sitting or standing position can reduce this tone and allow the physical therapist to extend the elbow and glenohumeral joints.

In addition to tonal and soft-tissue effects this dynamic approach to treatment serves to stimulate the unconscious head-injured patient in a general sense. During the course of a treatment the patient often opens his eyes, and there appears to be a slight rousing effect. The physical therapist speaks naturally to the patient during treatment using a quiet delivery; this may produce a stimulating effect. Movement itself can cause the patient to cough, and can cause both the rate and depth of respiration to increase. This can be an effective method for stimulating and reestablishing a normal cough reflex after the patient has been intubated over a prolonged period.

MECHANISM OF ACTION

The patterns of body segment adjustment which have been described are based upon the predictable changes in body alignment that occur during balance activities in the sitting and standing positions. The head and trunk adjustments, which occur during normal balance, are dependent upon the integration of optical, vestibular, tactile, and proprioceptive stimuli. Where normal integration occurs, these stimuli produce head righting and equilibrium reactions, which maintain balance against gravity. The intention in moving the unconscious patient is to reproduce the adjustments normally determined by the head-righting and equilibrium reactions. By externally initiating these reactions there should be a corresponding recruitment of normal levels of postural tone. The effect of movement itself has an influence on inhibiting increased postural tone. Sherrington described how reflex responses alter when the body position is altered. In the literature, differing rationales are given to explain this relationship between movement and inhibition of postural tone. Where there has been a cerebral lesion there

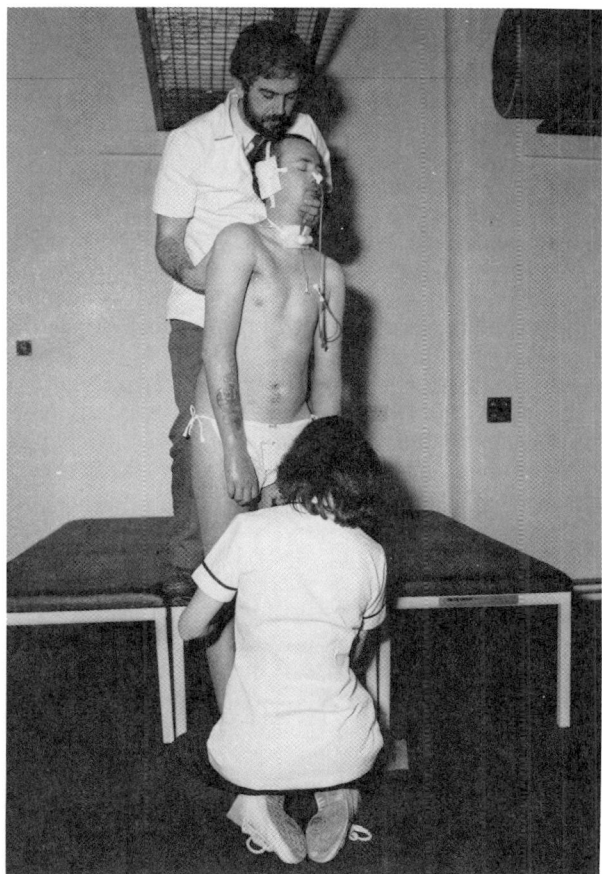

Figure 9 Rotational adjustment in a standing position.

are specific movement patterns that cause an inhibition of tone. Bobath has described these as reflex inhibitory movement patterns. These inhibitory patterns are movements that are in direct opposition to the abnormal patterns of spasticity. Where a head-injured patient presents with a decerebrate posture and the trunk is extended as a result of increased extensor tone, a reflex inhibitory movement involving trunk flexion is appropriate. By sitting the patient and producing a posterior displacement of the trunk, the abdominal muscles are stimulated and produce inhibition of the

extensor activity. These reflex inhibitory movements are most effective when they are concentrated on the trunk and head, and when they are combined with activities that stimulate balance.

The weight-bearing characteristics inherent in this treatment approach also contribute to the treatment effects. By supporting the unconscious patient in a weight-bearing position, the effect of gravity encourages the upper limbs to adopt an extended position. In the lower limbs, the body weight is transmitted through the feet, when the patient is in a standing position. This effect of weight bearing can assist to maintain the length of the achilles tendons if it is repeated a sufficient number of times.

THE PROBLEM-SOLVING APPROACH AND SELECTION OF TECHNIQUES

The selection of treatment techniques, which are appropriate for an individual head-injured patient, is made after careful assessment of the condition. Identification of specific released reflexes forms the most important element in assessment and determines the selection of particular treatment techniques. Techniques should be chosen in an attempt to oppose the abnormal reflex activity and to encourage the restoration of normal movement. A problem-solving process is inherent within this treatment approach. The patient's response to treatment should be continually evaluated; adjustments to treatment techniques can be made accordingly. In order to treat the unconscious patient effectively using this dynamic approach, it is important that this process of treatment evaluation be adopted.

SUGGESTED READING

Bobath B. Abnormal postural reflex activity caused by brain lesions. London: Heinemann, 1971

Carr JH, Shepherd R. Physiotherapy in disorders of the brain. London: Heinemann, 1985.

Carr JH, Shepherd R. A motor relearning programme for stroke. London: Heinemann, 1986.

Head injuries. Phys Ther (Special Issue) 1983; 63(12).

Jennet B, Galbraith S. An introduction to neurosurgery. 4th ed. London: Heinemann, 1983.

MANAGEMENT OF SPASTICITY

ANN L. McKEEMAN-MARCOTTE, M.Cl.Sc.(PT)
KEITH C. HAYES, Ph.D.

Spasticity is a familiar consequence of many different disorders of the central nervous system. These include disorders of genetic origin and those whose etiology derives from congenital defects or traumatic events. Readily identifiable in each case are the aberrations of voluntary movement and posture that characterize and define spasticity. These aberrations may include diminished strength and coordination of voluntary limb movement, appearance of involuntary and inappropriate movement patterns and the emergence of primitive reflexes.

The factors underlying the abnormalities of posture and movement are a reduction in the brain's capability to activate appropriate patterns of muscle contraction, and disruption of the brain's descending influence on the integrative properties of the spinal cord. The latter is evident in the common motor signs of spasticity namely, brisk tendon reflexes, clonus, and increased resistance to passive stretch. It is this hyperreflexia, together with later morphologic sequelae of immobilization (e.g., shortening of muscles and contractures), which compromise the ability of the patient to perform purposeful movement. It is also this hyperreflexia that provides the focus for much of the physiotherapeutic intervention aimed at controlling spasticity while the patient attempts to reestablish voluntary control over limb and axial musculature.

GENERAL CONSIDERATIONS IN PHYSIOTHERAPEUTIC MANAGEMENT

An important consideration in our management approach is the time course of development of the movement abnormalities. For example, in many patients with hemiplegia following a cerebrovascular accident, the movement deficit initially appears as flaccidity, and spasticity develops and increases in severity over a period of days, weeks, or even months. Early intervention, as soon as the patient is medically stable, almost certainly influences the extent of disability associated with the later stages, and in some cases may even prevent the development of spasticity. Therefore, physical therapy must be directed toward the prevention of spasticity and minimizing the associated dysfunction.

In a patient who already has spasticity, the focus is on managing the spasticity while enhancing residual function. Concurrently with management of the spasticity an attempt is made to prevent or to minimize the many complications that may develop from immobilization (e.g., pressure sores or contractures). Some of these complications are listed in Table 1.

Another important preliminary consideration in the management of spasticity involves the concept of total patient management. An attempt is made to coordinate carefully the physiotherapeutic management to complement treatment provided by other members of the rehabilitation team. The nature of the disability and its complications are such that the rehabilitation team may be called upon to follow a consistent 24-hour management approach that is incorporated into all aspects of patient care. It is important that patients, family members, and health care personnel recognize patterns of spasticity and be instructed on treatment strategies to compensate and minimize their effects on functional activities. This ensures that an adequate volume of therapeutic activity is undertaken, rather than limiting treatment activities to the time the patient is under direct supervision of the therapist.

Assessment of Spasticity

The direction of treatment depends heavily upon the findings from an assessment of the patient's capabilities and the extent of involvement of the primary and secondary complications of spasticity. Great care is given to the accurate assessment of the functional needs of each patient.

Traditionally, the clinical assessment of spasticity has been based upon subjective evaluations of motor signs such as clonus, deep tendon reflexes, resistance to passive movement, and abnormal primitive reflexes. Detailed assessments are usually conducted prior to therapeutic intervention and at scheduled intervals, in order to monitor progress. The variable nature of spasticity, and the extent to which it is influenced by both external and internal stimuli, may make such an assessment regime inadequate. It is preferable to undertake an ongoing daily evaluation that focuses on how the motor signs are disrupting functional capabilities. In turn, this evaluation is used to direct the treatment and to alter it, on an ongoing basis, according to the patient's needs. An attempt is also made to provide a quantitative assessment of various aspects of the muscular dysfunction and a torque motor

TABLE 1   Complications Related to Spasticity

Primary
    Stereotyped movement patterns
    Lack of coordination of movement
    Abnormal sensory input
    Loss of functional independence
    Abnormal gait
    Fatigue experienced in overcoming spasticity
    Sensations of muscle stiffness and heaviness of the limb

Secondary
    Joint contractures that lead to difficulties with self care and personal hygiene
    Pain
    Psychological consequences of disability
    Medical complications, i.e., pressure sores, urinary tract infections, which reinforce the effects of spasticity.

system is currently used to evaluate the resistive torque to a passive limb movement, i.e., limb hypertonia.

Physiotherapeutic Management of Spasticity

Treatment philosophy involves an eclectic approach that incorporates various physiotherapeutic management strategies, such as those advocated by Bobath, Rood, and Carr and Shepherd. The approach employs various techniques that activate sensory systems in order to selectively facilitate or inhibit motor output so that it more closely approximates normal function. Some of the therapeutic procedures are in fact designed to reduce the impediments to normal limb movement, whereas others are used to reinforce the patient's self-directed attempts to reestablish volitional control over limb and axial musculature. The ultimate goal is to improve functional status; therefore, all treatment is geared to achieving specific functional activities.

The specific physiotherapeutic treatment objectives are as follows:

1. Inhibition of spasticity;
2. Facilitation of normal movement;
3. Education or training of the patient and family to assume responsibility for spasticity management.

Spasticity interferes with and limits motor output and functional capabilities; therefore, it must be minimized in order to restore a normal functional movement repertoire. Once the spasticity has been inhibited, the patient must relearn various components of a movement and selective activation of the appropriate muscles for the movement. The complexity of the movement is gradually increased until complex motor patterns can be performed without the interference of spasticity. The third objective involves patient and family education and having the patient gradually assume responsibility for controlling his or her tone and treatment.

It is important to note that the first two objectives are not mutually exclusive, nor are they sequentially ordered. In fact, both are closely interrelated and attempts are made to attain objectives concurrently, in order to encourage normal purposeful movement. Likewise, for objective three, education of the patient and family about spasticity occurs concurrently with the attempt to meet objectives one and two.

In order to accomplish the objectives it is necessary to design an individualized treatment strategy that is born out of the assessment. Components are selected from the various sensorimotor approaches mentioned above and are administered according to the specific needs of the patient. Often it may be necessary to try a variety of different sequences or combinations of sensorimotor procedures in order to determine which are most effective for the individual. Tables 2 and 3 provide a brief—and by no means complete—list of procedures that can be used to inhibit spasticity and to facilitate normal movement. When using these various procedures, it is important to analyze carefully a response to a specific treatment and to ensure that the desired output is achieved; if it is not, additional sensory stimuli or different procedures may have to be added.

TABLE 2   Inhibition Techniques Aimed at Reducing Spasticity

Activity	*Comment*
Limb or trunk positioning	Reflex inhibiting
Passive and active limb movements	Reflex inhibiting patterns emphasizing rotation
Weight bearing	Joint approximation; greater than body weight
Maintained pressure	On tendinous insertions, abdomen or perioral
Light touch	Inhibitory cutaneous effects
Vibration	Low frequency <100 Hz to spastic muscle
	High frequency >100 Hz to antagonist
Maintained submaximal muscle stretch	
Slow repetitive rolling or rocking	
Inhibitive tone casting	
Biofeedback	Inhibition of spastic muscle
	Facilitation of antagonist muscle
Electrical stimulation	Facilitation of antagonist muscle

TABLE 3   Facilitation Techniques for Reinforcing Diminished Motor Output

Activity	Comment
Active movement	Trunk, proximal and distal limb control
Approximation	Of joint surfaces, less than body weight, to facilitate muscle cocontraction
Biofeedback	Facilitate appropriate action of the (spastic) muscle
Vibration	High frequency >100 Hz—facilitation of muscle action, e.g., dorsiflexion in hemiplegia
Electrical stimulation	Reinforce appropriate muscular control of limb movements
Tapping	Tendon, muscle belly
Developmental activities	Restoration of appropriate balance

Treatment should be an evolutionary process, which allows the patient progressively to assume responsibility for control of limb movements and spasticity, and especially to control spasticity within the context of daily living skills. All patients (regardless of their mental state or age) should be able to achieve gradual assumption of responsibility. Try to avoid having the patient become dependent on the therapist for relief from spasticity.

As the patient progresses, the complexity of the required task is increased by combining motor patterns and by introducing environmental influences. The amount of support or guidance offered by the therapist is gradually reduced, whereas the difficulty of the motor task is increased. The need to consider environmental influences is important because patients are often able to perform specific isolated components of an activity, e.g., gait, and even walk with minimal abnormalities, yet in the context of a stressful situation (crossing the street, walking on snow or ice) their gait pattern degenerates, and the disabling effects of spasticity return. Feedback to the patient—providing (a) reinforcement for success; (b) awareness of the need to extend capabilities; and (c) a reminder of the need for repetition in the practice of new skills—serves as necessary support and motivation.

A final point to reiterate is that, in order to influence spasticity, treatment must extend beyond the confines of the actual time spent within the physical therapy department and all patients should be given "homework" on tasks that they are to practice frequently throughout the day. For example, to inhibit extensor spasticity of the leg of a hemiplegic patient during sitting, the patient might be encouraged to practice pelvic movements such as sitting with the hips flexed and spine in extension.

SUGGESTED READING

Bishop B. Spasticity its physiology and management. Part 1–4. Physiotherapy 1977; 57:377–395.
Chapman CE, Wiesendanger M. Physiological and anatomical basis of spasticity: a review. Physiother Can 1982; 34:125–136.
Kandell E, Schwartz J. Principles of neuroscience. 2nd ed. New York: Elsevier, 1985.
Umphred D. Neurological rehabilitation. Toronto: CV Mosby, 1985.

BALANCE DISORDERS

KEITH C. HAYES, Ph.D.
ANN L. McKEEMAN-MARCOTTE, M.Cl.Sc.
(PT)

Our approach to the treatment of balance disorders in patients with nervous system pathology is based upon a theoretical framework derived from current neurophysiologic research. This framework views the maintenance of balance to be accomplished through the following two distinct control processes:

1. Anticipatory postural adjustments that are preparatory to an imminent and predictable loss of balance, and
2. Compensatory reactions that restore equilibrium after unexpected disturbance.

In the nomenclature of control systems these constitute a feedforward process and a feedback process respectively. The operations of both processes appear to be dependent upon each other, as patients often exhibit dysfunction in both systems. However, there are instances where patients show marked instability associated with impoverished preparatory adjustments, yet little or no instability in their feedback regulation of a maintained posture, or vice versa. The different types of instability that are identified by distinguishing between feedforward and feedback dysfunction provide direction for the prescription of treatment strategies that are specific to the needs of the individual.

Our treatment approach is thus predicated on a framework that differs from conventional theoretic bases. Nevertheless, we use assessments and treatment strategies that are not greatly different from existing programs. The differences that do exist are principally in the interpretation and rigor of the assessments and the relative importance ascribed to certain types of therapeutic activity. Indeed, the activities that we use often incorporate elements of neurodevelopmental sequencing, neuromuscular facilitation, and/or progressions in (biomechanical) stability. These are used to enhance performance on specified tasks. The activities thus become superficially indistinguishable from those used in conventional approaches.

Let us consider some hypothetical examples of patients with balance dysfunction, in order to clarify the distinction between the preparatory postural adjustments and the compensatory type of balance reaction.

Patient A, a young man, presents with a history of cerebellar ataxia resulting from a contrecoup injury sustained during a motor vehicle accident. When asked to stand with feet together and rapidly raise his arm, he loses his balance and uses an involuntary stepping reaction to regain balance. The basis of his instability is that he does not exhibit the preparatory activation of axial musculature to stabilize his trunk, and as a consequence of the dynamics of the arm movement, his center of gravity is displaced outside his base of support. The involuntary stepping reflex is brought into action as a final resort to prevent him falling.

Patient B is an elderly man who also presents with cerebellar ataxia; specifically, anterior lobe degeneration and polyneuritis consequent to chronic alcohol abuse. This patient rapidly raises his arm without loss of balance and exhibits all of the necessary preparatory postural adjustments in axial musculature. During quiet standing, however, this patient exhibits a marked postural tremor. The tremor characteristics (increased amplitude of sway at 1 Hz and 3 Hz) indicate abnormal proprioceptive input and/or processing of sensory feedback. In this case it is the feedback system that is deficient, rather than the feedforward control process.

Careful assessment of the *nature* of the instability constitutes an essential feature of our therapeutic approach. It is necessary to establish whether the dysfunction is present in his preparatory postural adjustment, or his feedback control, or both.

Assessment of the capability to generate the necessary preparatory adjustments includes consideration of postural adjustments in advance of both internal and external disturbances to equilibrium. By internal disturbances we mean the forces acting throughout the musculoskeletal system during a self initiated limb movement, such as in the arm raising examples given above. Impact from a heavy medicine ball that is thrown to the patient is an example of external disturbance that necessitates preparatory postural adjustments. Postural adjustments need to be made in advance of the impact rather than after the fact. Similarly, if forewarned of the timing and direction of the perturbation, a patient should be able to brace himself or herself in advance of being displaced by a therapist. Yet another example of the ability to generate appropriate preparatory postural adjustments is the weight shift to one leg that is necessary before raising the other leg.

In some of these examples the therapist can evaluate the appropriateness of the posture that the patient assumes, whereas in other cases palpation of the appropriate musculature is necessary. Table 1 provides

TABLE 1   Examples of Patient Generated Activities used for Assessment and Treatment of Feedforward Balance Dysfunction

*Hitting, kicking and throwing activities**	*Weight transfers†*
Hit a balloon (seated)	Look over L/R shoulder (seated/standing)
Throw a large ball (seated)	Reach to side (seated/standing)
Hit a balloon (standing)	Reach to front (seated/standing)
Throw a large ball (standing)	Reach behind (seated/standing)
Kick a ball—various sizes and weights (standing)	Cross one leg over the other (seated)
Play badminton (standing)	Shift to stand on one foot (not necessarily maintain)
	Weight shift and tapping with one foot
Catching	*Therapist interaction*
Catch various size balls	Prevent displacement when pushed or pulled by therapist (when patient knows direction and time of pull/push)
Catch medicine ball	Patient pushes therapist

* Note the progressive demand on stability required.
† These tasks should be possible with eyes closed or can be trained with eyes closed.

examples of other activities that may be used to verify the presence or absence of appropriate preparatory adjustments. These same activities, and others, may also be used for training feedforward postural control capabilities.

Evaluation of the status of feedback capabilities is done in both a global manner—identifying the presence or absence of appropriate balance responses to unpredictable disturbance—and in a more discriminating manner. In the former, standard tests such as unexpected pushes or pulls of the patient by the therapist can identify the appropriate functioning of the global sensory input associated with the loss of balance, i.e., vestibular, proprioceptive, visual. More refined assessments such as those indicated in Table 2 can identify which of the physiologic subsystems are dysfunctional.

Normally, there is some redundancy in the sensory information necessary to maintain balance, and failure of one source of sensation can be compensated by feedback from intact systems. Vision, which provides an important sensory reference for balance,

TABLE 2   Activities for the Assessment and Training of Feedback Balance Dysfunction

Global
  Large ball activities
  Four point kneeling
  Two point kneeling
  Half kneel-standing
  Seated position
  Standing
  Single leg standing
  Patient responds to a predictable total body displacement by therapist (seated/standing)

Specific subsystem tests
  Vestibular*
    Post rotary nystagmus
    Labyrinthine righting reactions
  Proprioceptive
    Tendon reflexes
  Visual
    Verticality test
    Eye closure effects on tasks
    Spontaneous nystagmus present?

Other reflex testing
  Asymmetric tonic neck
  Symmetric tonic neck
  Optical righting reflex
  Cortical righting reflex
  Protective reactions of abduction—extension of limb

* Vestibular stimulation therapy would be considered an approach for training feedback balance control. If the patient eventually learns to cue in advance of the stimulation, then preparatory adjustment training is taking place.

appears to be particularly effective at offsetting the deleterious effects of vestibular or proprioceptive dysfunction. Deprivation of vision can be ingeniously used to challenge the other sensory modalities and to reveal latent dysfunction.

When testing for feedback dysfunction (e.g., tests of righting reactions) it is important to recognize the need for the *unpredictable* nature of disturbances introduced to the patient. If the patient is aware of the direction and timing of an imminent push or pull, then feedforward protective strategies might be used. For example, the patient may cocontract and become rigid. The pseudostability introduced by such a strategy can mask the ineffective functioning of the feedback systems. It is also important for the patient not to *fear* the consequences of the disturbances that are introduced, for fear can similarly precipitate some patients into becoming rigid.

Once the nature and extent of balance dysfunction have been established, then the appropriate treatment strategies can be developed. The essence here is on focusing on the specific form of dysfunction, rather than providing a general catch-all of activities that may assist in the rehabilitation of balance. As with most therapeutic programs, it is appropriate to provide a sequence of activities and procedures to challenge progressively the dysfunctional balance mechanisms. As improvement is noted, so more demanding tasks are introduced. The sequence of activities we employ often follows a neurodevelopmental progression, with tasks performed in prone, four point kneeling, then two point kneeling, then half kneeling through to standing. Alternatively, a biomechanical progression is employed where the patient proceeds from positions of static equilibrium involving greater stability, to static position with less stability, and eventually to dynamic activities requiring balance. The neurodevelopmental and biomechanical progressions often complement each other.

Some of the activities and the sequences that we employ, specifically to enhance feedforward balance skills, may also be useful in specifically improving the feedback system. The difference exists in the way they are presented. Asking a patient to resist a push from the front, when the patient can clearly see the oncoming push, allows the patient to prepare in advance, i.e., a feedforward adjustment. The therapist can assess the effectiveness of the subtle preparatory adjustments that are made. Alternatively, if the patient's eyes are closed or if he or she is unaware of an impending push, then the response is one of feedback and should be assessed as such. It is important

to distinguish the predictability of the event to which the patient must respond.

It should also be recognized that the ability to perform preparatory adjustments depends upon the integrity of the senses. The physiologic mechanisms subserving the feedforward and feedback are by no means completely independent. Two distinctions need to be drawn: feedback control occurs *after the disturbance* and depends upon sensory consequences of the disturbance; whereas feedforward control depends upon anticipation, utilizing sensory information in *advance of the disturbance*. Often, feedforward control also reflects the learning that has taken place as a result of sensory feedback from previous experiences. With this is mind, it is appropriate to ensure the integrity of the sensory input that is necessary for the feedforward control process prior to identifying a dysfunctional preparatory control mechanism.

Many activities challenge both the feedforward and feedback systems. Activities such as use of wobble boards, walking on level ground, rough ground, or air mattresses, hopping, skipping, and running, fall into this category. We use these activities when patients exhibit dysfunction in both systems.

The therapeutic approach we take focuses on the nature of balance dysfunction rather than upon diagnosis per se. The diagnosis may assist in identifying and clarifying the nature of dysfunction. For example, if a diagnosis of polyneuritis is given, as in the case illustrated earlier, one might expect to find a balance dysfunction characterized by impaired feedback and compounded by deprivation of vision. The activities and techniques we use to assist in the rehabilitation process do not differ greatly from activities described by others. However, we feel that the specificity of their application and the response of the patient is enhanced by the focus provided by the theoretical framework.

SUGGESTED READING

Belenkii VY, Gurfinkel VS, Paltsev YI. Elements of control of voluntary movements. Biofizika 1967; 12:135–141.

Bouisset S, Zattara M. A sequence of postural movements precedes voluntary movement. Neurosci Lett 1981; 22:263–270.

Hayes KC. Biomechanics of postural control. In: Exercise and sport sciences reviews. Philadelphia: Franklin Institute, 1982:363–391.

Lucy SD, Hayes KC. Postural sway profiles: normal subjects and subjects with cerebellar ataxia. Physiother Can 1985; 37:140–148.

Nashner LM. Analysis of stance posture in humans. In: Towe AL, Luschei ES, eds. Handbook of behavioral neurobiology. Vol. 5. New York: Plenum Press, 1981:527.

FACILITATION TECHNIQUES

GEORGE I. TURNBULL, B.P.T., M.A., M.C.S.P., Dip. T.P.

The term "facilitation" is normally associated with the reeducation techniques referred to as proprioceptive neuromuscular facilitation (PNF). However, several additional procedures, which are also designed to elicit a predetermined motor response, are often included under the same generic heading. In common usage, the word facilitation is used to describe an action or process which makes something easier. However, the physiologic phenomenon of facilitation can briefly be described as the stimulation of action potentials, within a given neuron, in a manner which involves both spatial and temporal summation and which eventually causes that cell to exceed threshold levels resulting in discharge. These different but complimentary definitions of the same word may be the reason for the use of the term "facilitation" to describe therapeutic procedures beyond the PNF techniques and philosophy.

The purpose of this chapter is to describe selected factors that seem important in the effective application of the PNF therapeutic exercise paradigm.

PROPRIOCEPTIVE NEUROMUSCULAR FACILITATION (PNF)

The PNF approach was initially developed to deal more effectively with patients suffering from the disabilities that arise from poliomyelitis and multiple sclerosis. The basic aim of the technique is to influence the final common pathway by deliberate and controlled stimulation of factors known to excite or inhibit the alpha motor neuron pool supplying target muscles. Included amongst these factors is selective sensory stimulation, the volitional effort of the patient, and the stimulation of recruitment from complimentary alpha motor neuron pools, which includes the use of patterns of movement. Of utmost importance to the success of PNF is the skilled application of handling techniques and the coordination of all motor neuron pool influences by a physical therapist through the placing of optimum demand on the motor response throughout the range of movement and the application of verbal cueing.

The cornerstones of the PNF approach, in practical terms, are the patterns of movement. All patterns include movement in the sagittal plane, movement in the frontal plane and a specific rotatory component. The net result of this combination gives rise to the diagonal and spiral nature of the PNF movement patterns. In different terms, the target muscle group is placed in its fully elongated position at the commencement of the movement pattern. At the conclusion of the movement, the target muscle groups will have contracted throughout full range to terminate in the fully shortened position, thus causing movement about associated joints. In achieving this, MacConaill's laws of approximation and detorsion are observed with the origin and insertion of the target muscles moving closer together and rotating into the same plane. The concept of movement patterns is well known in the field of motor skills acquisition and refers, in that context, to generic movements of body components from which specific skills can be developed. The PNF patterns can be viewed in a similar manner in that the basic pattern will eventually be modified to achieve a desired therapeutic result. In other words, the patterns, though absolutely essential to the underlying concept of PNF, usually need to be modified in some way to emphasize the part of the pattern being treated. This goal is achieved through the techniques of emphasis, such as repeated contractions, reversals, and timing for emphasis—all of which serve to maximize the effect to the area that is the target of the therapy. Consistent with these concepts may be the demand for movement at a joint (the pivot) other than that which is most proximal, thus emphasizing muscle work about that joint. Therefore, in most therapeutic circumstances, the basic pattern of movement will be modified using these techniques of emphasis.

Another vital variable which requires identification is the role played by the operator. It is likely that the success of the clinical application of PNF is limited if applied by an operator who is not highly skilled. The reason for this is that in order to achieve spatial and temporal summation adequately at a given motor neuron pool, it would appear essential that all components of the technique be coordinated in terms of timing and intensity. In addition, the ability of the operator to detect, through their own sensorimotor mechanisms, discrete changes in the response of the patient and to adjust automatically the resistance being applied, is of paramount importance. These abilities require high levels of sensorimotor proficiency by the operator. In order to achieve a successful level of therapeutic performance, the physical therapist must become highly skilled in the application of the techniques, an objective that can only be achieved through adequate and consistent practice.

Clinical Usage of the PNF Techniques

Before discussing selected applications of PNF techniques, some myths should be addressed. PNF is but one therapeutic exercise approach, which has a number of advantages and disadvantages compared to other techniques. As such, it is probably inappropriate to consider PNF as a universal panacea for all conditions. Its application in the treatment of motor disorders characterized by hypertonicity of central origin, which can be regarded as over-excitation of the final common pathway, is highly questionable except perhaps in very limited situations. The overgeneralization of PNF to conditions for which it was not designed has perhaps led to a decline in the application of the technique. In addition, PNF is an operator-intensive technique. In days of over-crowded physical therapy departments, this technique is not an attractive option. Similarly, the high levels of operator skill required before the technique can be applied successfully is an additional disadvantage. However, no machine can reproduce the specificity and individualization of the exercise that is possible through the application of PNF in the hands of a highly skilled operator. As such, the PNF techniques can be used most successfully in the early care of certain conditions. Once the patient has reached a higher level of performance, the possibility of the treatment being progressed by the application of other techniques, which are less demanding of the therapist's time, might be seriously considered. In other words, it is probably redundant to continue applying PNF when the same effect could be achieved using another modality.

Application of the Technique

A certain process of decision-making logic appears to be undertaken relating to the application of PNF. I attempt to replicate this logic and to discuss the variables that appear important to the efficient application of the technique.

Decision to Use PNF

The condition being treated clearly influences a decision to apply PNF. Because the theoretic basis of the approach is directed towards influencing the final common pathway, conditions that affect the lower motor neuron seem well suited. Conditions characterized by muscle weakness, particularly where the weakness is disseminated throughout a body segment, appear to be the ideal circumstances under which to apply these methods. Included in this category are the cerebellar hypotonias whether or not in combination

with ataxia. In similar circumstances where instability around a joint is present, application of the technique of rhythmic stabilizations appears to be indicated. The same technique has been advocated to deal with problems of instability where the technique is applied proximally to enhance proximal fixation. Similarly, muscle spasm, of the type associated with pain and musculoskeletal disorders, seems to respond well to the relaxation technique known as hold-relax. Clinical presentations, where incoordination is a feature, may benefit from rhythmic repetitions of certain patterns (sometimes referred to as repeated movements through range) and the administration of reversals. However, it should be reiterated that application of techniques, which have the objective of increasing levels of central nervous system (CNS) excitation are likely to markedly increase the movement dysfunction in conditions characterized by spasticity of CNS origin.

Choice of a Pattern

Selection of the pattern of movement is based upon a knowledge of the function of the muscles that are the objective of the treatment. The pattern which most closely approximates the function of these target muscles is selected initially. For example, if the clinical condition being considered is a common peroneal nerve lesion, then the flexion-abduction-medial rotation pattern of the affected lower limb would be the pattern of choice. This is because the pattern includes dorsiflexion and eversion of the foot. Similarly, in the upper limb, if the radial wrist extensors were being treated, the pattern which would maximally work these muscles would be the flexion-abduction-lateral rotation pattern of the upper limb. If the trunk flexors are the target of treatment, then the response can be maximized by combining the trunk flexion pattern with a complimentary flexion pattern at the neck and perhaps the extension-adduction-medial rotation pattern of the upper limb. The purpose of these additional movement combinations is to induce recruitment from associated muscle groups to the weakened trunk flexors, thus maximizing the magnitude of the contraction in the target muscle group.

Teaching the Pattern to the Patient

There are four steps involved in thoroughly familiarizing the patient with the pattern, which is to be attempted. Initially, from a perceptual-motor learning viewpoint, the objectives of the procedure to be undertaken should be identified to the patient. Following this, the patient benefits from being shown, passively, the movement to be attempted. In terms of dialogue, a conceptual understanding of the nature of the movement pattern is the objective. Extensive, detailed dissertations are unlikely to be remembered once the instructions have been completed. Thus, the use of language that denotes the movement objective is mandatory (i.e., "I want you to lift your arm up and out to the side like this," or, "lift your arm up and out leading with your thumb") to identify the movement objective to the patient. These statements are made by the physical therapist while performing the movement passively. This procedure is undertaken more than once. The patient should then be asked to perform the movement in an active-assisted manner with the physical therapist providing guidance and correction for the most obvious errors. It would seem futile to attempt to achieve absolute perfection in the execution of the patient's pattern at this early stage. Finally, the patient is asked to undertake the pattern against resistance again with the therapist correcting the execution of the pattern. The precise movements of the fingers, wrist, elbow, and other components of the pattern is achieved as the treatment progresses through error correction conveyed in small but digestible amounts.

Verbal Commands

The purpose of verbal commands in PNF is to direct the voluntary effort of the patient maximally to the initiation and execution of the movement so that it coincides exactly with other facilitatory efforts carried out by the operator, such as stretch and traction. As such, verbal commands cue the patient. It seems logical that such commands must be short and must clearly imply the effort being demanded. Insipid and long, drawn-out commands do not achieve the desired facilitatory effect. Therefore, a command such as "lift!" or "pull!" seem the most appropriate. Perhaps more than one word may be used, such as "squeeze and lift!"; however, the more the patient has to process the information contained in the command, the more likely that the facilitation at the alpha motor neuron pool will be lost. As such, if the technique has been taught appropriately, extensive commands will be unnecessary and counterproductive.

In addition to the initial command, patient motivation can be influenced by the odd, well-timed instruction at strategic points throughout the range of movement. This may take the form of a correction of some component of the pattern or can simply be a further demand for maximal effort, which will be dictated by the response detected by the therapist. Again, the voice must imply, through intonation, that maximal effort is being demanded.

Feedback

As in the acquisition of all skilled movements, feedback from the operator is an essential ingredient in the appropriate application of PNF techniques. Corrective feedback should be used judiciously to achieve the correct execution of the pattern itself or

of any derivative of the pattern being used. It is, however, important to "get the pattern right" because that is when the facilitation of the target alpha motor neuron pool is at its greatest. In saying this, it must always be remembered that the object of the whole treatment is to initiate work in the target muscle group and to strengthen that response. For maximum effect, feedback should be specific rather than vague and should take into account the information processing capabilities of the patient. In most instances, attention to the correction of more than one factor at a time will likely be less than satisfactory.

Integration of Techniques of Emphasis

The techniques of emphasis, namely reversals, repeated contractions, timing for emphasis, rhythmic stabilizations and relaxation techniques, are the core of the practical application of PNF. Again, the skill by which these techniques are applied is of the utmost importance. As their name implies, these procedures further focus the demand towards the target alpha motor neurons and thus maximize the facilitation of the muscle groups being treated. In most instances, it is possible to utilize several of the techniques of emphasis in the same maneuver in order to maximize the motor response generated by the patient. For example, if the elbow flexors were to be facilitated, the operator could commence with a pattern which would include extension of the elbow. Reversal into the flexor pattern serves to facilitate the flexors through successive induction, whereupon the normal timing sequence could be altered by creating isometric holds at the shoulder and wrist components of the pattern. This timing for emphasis would result in recruitment from these components thus strengthening the response of the elbow flexors. This response could then be further enhanced by the establishment of an isometric hold within the elbow flexors followed by a well-timed stretch and a demand for a further isotonic contraction of the same muscle group.

The technique of emphasis referred to as rhythmic stabilizations is used in circumstances where instability around a given joint prevails. Such circumstances may include an unstable shoulder joint or a lack of proximal fixation due to cerebellar dysfunction. The aim of the technique is to facilitate cocontraction of all muscle groups around the joint, thus enhancing stability. If the technique were to be applied around the shoulder joint, the patient could be treated in supine with the shoulder joint flexed to 90 degrees and the elbow joint flexed to the same angle. The operator grasps the palmar aspect of the patient's hand with one hand while encircling the proximal part of the upper limb with the other hand. The patient's shoulder joint is then alternately internally and externally rotated. At the commencement of this manipulation, the patient is instructed "don't let me move your hand!". The procedure is judged as being successful when the operator can no longer detect movement taking place at the shoulder joint. Similar procedures can be applied at any other location but are particularly useful at the hip, knee, and around the body axis.

Hold-relax is a relaxation procedure that appears to be useful in conditions characterized by localized muscle spasm. It should be remembered that what is being considered here is the spasm associated with pain and not the spasticity of CNS origin. The rationale of this technique is that if a muscle is maximally contracted isometrically then this contraction will be followed by relaxation and an enhanced ability of the muscle to elongate. This elongation then tends to further the relaxation which has been achieved. The technique is useful in treating conditions characterized by limitation in range of movement either due to the muscle spasm or to adaptive shortening following a period of immobilization.

Frequency of Application of PNF

As in all other therapeutic exercise approaches, the techniques should be continued for as often as is necessary to obtain the objective of the treatment. In general terms, this is probably much more frequently than currently applied. A common criticism of PNF is that the effect is not lasting. In the acquisition of perceptual motor skills in normals, it is known that performance improves as a function of the amount of appropriate practice. Similarly, PNF is not designed

to produce instantaneous and lasting results. The desired motor behavior can be elicited by application of the technique; however, only repetition of this response will enable it to be produced by the patient on demand and at a level that is consistent with functional motor behavior.

It is beyond the scope of this chapter to include more specific detail pertaining to the PNF procedures. Continuing education courses and more extensive texts are available for this purpose. The points raised, however, are designed to provoke thought and to dispel some common misconceptions concerning this potentially useful but technically difficult series of procedures. Of particular concern is the urgent need for clinical research to demonstrate the value and limitations of these techniques. Such research, however, has to be conceived with great care and by those with adequate knowledge of the processes being tested. Regrettably, this has not always been the case in the past.

SUGGESTED READING

Eyzaguirre C, Fidone SJ. Physiology of the nervous system. 2nd ed. Chicago: Year Book, 1975:186–193.

Knott M, Voss DE. Proprioceptive neuromuscular facilitation patterns and techniques. 2nd ed. New York: Harper and Row, 1968.

Schmidt RA. Motor control and learning: a behavioural emphasis. Champaign, Illinois: Human Kinetic Publishers, 1982.

Sullivan PE, Portney LG. Electromyographic activity of shoulder muscles during unilateral upper extremity proprioceptive neuromuscular facilitation patterns. Phys Ther 1980; 60:283–288.

Voss DE. Proprioceptive neuromuscular facilitation. Am J Phys Med 1967; 46:838–898.

MUSCLE ENERGY: AN APPROACH TO THE EVALUATION AND TREATMENT OF SOMATIC DYSFUNCTION

ROBERT W. SYDENHAM, B.Sc., D.P.T., M.C.P.A., M.A.P.T.A., R.P.T.

The biomechanical approach to the treatment of musculoskeletal (somatic) dysfunction is becoming a prominent modality in the realm of physical therapy. Only a few years ago, expertise in the area consisted mainly of applying various forms of heat, cold, electricity, traction, and therapeutic exercise. Muscle energy is one technique within the realm of manual therapy that can be utilized in assessing and treating patients with somatic dysfunction.

Muscle energy techniques are primarily osteopathic in origin, but parallel the practice of proprioceptive neuromuscular facilitation (PNF). Many of the same principles, concepts, and theories apply to both; however, the main difference comes in the precise positioning of the joint and specific direction and intensity of an active contraction against a distinct counterforce. Fred Mitchell Sr. (1907–1974), an osteopathic physician, was the principal theorist and innovator of the muscle energy concept. Fred L. Mitchell Jr., also an osteopathic physician, organized his father's concepts and techniques with colleagues Moran and Pruzzo. They developed the *Evaluation and Treatment Manual of Osteopathic Muscle Energy Procedures,* which has served as the principal published resource of muscle energy techniques.

DEFINITIONS

The term somatic dysfunction, can be defined as impaired or altered function of related components of the somatic (body framework) system—skeletal, arthrodial, and myofascial structures, and related vascular lymphatic, and neural elements. In other words, it is a malfunction of a segment or segments of the spinal column, pelvis, or extremities, which may produce limited motion, muscle spasm, pain, tenderness, loss of strength, and even remote symptoms. In practice, it is common to see somatic dysfunction identified in terms such as myositis, fibrositis, sciatica, neuralgia, limited range of motion, and spasm, which are synonymous with and amplifications of the above concept.

Gross deviation from ideal or optimal body posture must be compensated for by altered joint position and increased muscle tension. In order for the body to maintain equilibrium, there must be some form of compensation for this altered state. As long as this compensation is within the body's tissue limits, it remains asymptomatic. However, if it exceeds these limits, the body's adaptive potential is also exceeded and symptoms arise. The onset of symptoms may be attributable to trauma or a gradual loss of the body's ability to compensate. Symptom characteristics are often indicative of the tissue in dysfunction; however, treatment techniques must aim to restore function to those tissues responsible for the body's compensatory or adaptive mechanisms. Failure of the above often results in a recurrence of symptoms or complaints. Thus, the therapist's approach to and management of dysfunction must include not only the common manual therapy techniques of mobilization and manipulation, but also a biomechanical analysis of movement and structure, specific instruction on exercise and posture, in addition to education.

ASSESSMENT

Palpation

Palpation is the principal skill for determining appropriate treatment using muscle energy techniques. With educated hands, qualities, such as softness, hardness, shape, texture, size, depth, thickness, position, temperature, and moisture can be detected and discriminated. Without much increase in pressure, the palpatory sense, which is a collection of many perceptual abilities, may be projected into the body, thereby allowing one to feel bones, fat, fascia, muscle, tendons, crepitus, and masses. These qualities are perceived by the examiner, and integrated with other information detected, such as motion, pulses, tissue tension, and reaction. Interpretation of this information is necessary to establish the possible relationships and techniques applicable to findings on assessment, and to determine appropriate treatment procedures. Although it is not the purpose of this chapter to go into detail on palpation, it is useful to be aware of a few subtleties that can enhance the perception of proprioceptive information. The pads of the fingers are most sensitive for fine tactile discrimination, such as tension, texture, and position. The dorsum of the fingers or hands are most sensitive to temperature. The palmar aspect of the metacarpophalangeal joints are seemingly more sensitive to vibration or movement, such as rib excursion. The center of the palm is most sensitive for gross shape recognition or stereognosis. Palpation is repeated many times a day in the clinic. However, what determines our treatment (to stretch, strengthen, mobilize, facilitate, or inhibit) is how the above information is interpreted and what significance is placed on the perceived proprioceptive information.

Observation

In addition to palpation, observation is an important part of evaluation of somatic dysfunction for it provides valuable information, such as gravitational adaptation, gross movement limitation, and observable compensation for injuries.

It is important to always position yourself so as to get a direct or true view of your subject. Failure to do so can lead to inaccurate impressions of displacement, depths, symmetry, and movement. Of equal importance, is use of the dominant eye, i.e., the one which is used predominantly for sighting. Often it is found that one eye is used for near sighting and the other for far sighting. Appropriate notation of the above often makes subtle differences much more apparent.

When assessing for symmetrical or bilateral movement, such as rib excursion, use peripheral vision. A common error is to look at one side then the other; however, a more effective method is to choose a midpoint and observe the movement of both sides simultaneously using peripheral vision, as it is more sensitive in some situations, and circumstances.

When assessing joint mobility, especially that of the spine, the resting position of the joint must be correlated to the mobility of that segment. A wide variety of resting joint positions can be consistent with normal joint function. However, if a decrease of range of movement is apparent, a restrictive lesion is present and warrants specific mobilization treatment. As well as motion restriction, these lesions also have visual and palpable signs of a facilitated segment. Naturally not only may vertebrae be altered in position or movement, but they may also be segmental or multisegmental. Multisegmental curves are generally adaptive to motion faults, or to movement restrictions above or below them. They may also be secondary to lower extremity dysfunction.

Segmental position faults are usually components of larger adaptive curves in the spine. They are often primary lesions, associated with facilitation, and become more apparent in either hyperflexion or hyperextension. This restrictive fault is ideally suited for the application of a specific muscle energy technique. Following the laws of spinal mechanics, the spinal segmental fault consistently demonstrates the following:

1. In hyperextension or hyperflexion, the segment is rotated and sidebent to the same side.
2. In hyperextension or hyperflexion, rotation and sidebending are restricted to the same side.

Thus, the restrictive fault can be named according to the position in which the joint is held. For example, when a segment is examined in hyperextension and it is found to be left rotated, it must also be left sidebent. Thus, the positional diagnosis would be flexion, rotation, and sidebending left (FRSL). In following, the mobility restriction or direction of treatment would be the opposite, i.e., extension, rotation, sidebending right (ERSR).

The use of specific but descriptive muscle energy language to describe position or movement faults, especially of the spine and pelvis, not only simplifies assessment and treatment recording, but also ensures accurate communication between colleagues.

PRINCIPLE OF TREATMENT

Basic to the muscle energy treatment approach is the understanding of the various systems within the body and the relationships that these systems form in both a state of health and in a pathologic state. It makes no sense to treat pain-producing hypermobility symptomatically, while leaving the non pain-producing hypomobility untreated. Equally, it makes no sense to treat an adaptive scoliotic curve without first treating an uneven sacral base.

Stress in many forms can influence the sympathetic nervous system and can manifest itself in somatic dysfunction. The somatic component of disease, the neurophysiologic, and the biomechanical and/or biochemical relationships of the body as a whole must be considered.

To understand the principles of muscle energy, one must be familiar with spinal reflexes and Korr's concepts of segmental facilitation.

Modern Manual Therapy of the Vertebral Column states:

According to Korr when the gamma motorneuron discharge to the muscle spindle is excessive, minimal external stretch or force is required to fire the annulospiral endings, which reflexively fire the extrafusal muscle fibers via the alpha motorneuron. The exaggerated spindle responses are activated by forces which tend to lengthen the facilitated muscle, and the increased muscle tension creates a restrictive spinal fault. The aim of muscle energy technique is to restore the normal neurophysiology of the segment.

These techniques are described as requiring active distinct controlled muscle contraction in a precisely controlled position, in a specific direction, against a distinct counterforce.

In the restoration of [segmental] joint mobility, accurate localization and specific muscle work are the key factors necessary if the technique is to be successful. According to Sherrington's Laws of reciprocal innervation, contraction of an agonist muscle [reflexively] inhibits its antagonist. The deep segmental muscles of the spine are essentially stabilizers, and their imbalance restricts joint mobility. The gamma discharge to the facilitated muscle can be reduced by specific contraction of its [agonists].

The stronger the contraction of the antagonist, the greater the relaxation of the agonist. However, too forceful a contraction increases synergist activity . . . and since the deep spinal muscles are stabilizers . . ., restoration of [normal] mobility is not achieved. [Segmental] palpation for appropriate muscle relaxation during application of the technique confirms the [amount] of counterforce necessary. . . . Contraction of the facilitated muscle in a lengthened position activates the golgi tendon organs causing reflex inhibition of both gamma and alpha [motorneurons] and subsequent muscle lengthening upon relaxation. Accurately localized, low intensity, *isometric contractions* of the agonist or antagonist segmental muscle are most effective in the treatment of segmental restrictive motion faults.

Whether autogenic or reciprocal inhibition is used is dependent upon which technique causes the best neurophysiologic change in the joint complex.

Faulty movement patterns become habitual, even at the segmental level, as a result of repeated excitation of the neural pathway in the central nervous system. The use of muscle energy techniques can result in the retraining of the stabilizing function of the intersegmental muscles.

In this instance, high intensity concentric isotonic contractions involving multiple segments achieve the best result. The counterforce applied by the therapist is less than the patient's force, thereby allowing muscle shortening and joint motion to occur. This technique is effective in restoring normal trunk motion patterns.

Muscle energy techniques can also be used to reduce localized tissue edema and to stretch intramuscular and fascial fibrosis. In this instance, high intensity eccentric isotonic contractions involving multiple segments give the best result. The counterforce applied by the therapist is greater than the patient's force, thereby lengthening the contracting muscle and stretching the intramuscular and overlying fascia. This is the most effective technique for treating multisegmental restrictive curves.

The muscle energy approach pays a great deal of attention to the quality of the motion restriction to determine what tissue or condition is restricting motion, whereas the mobilization approach tends to assume that joint restriction is the restrictive problem. Thus, the muscle energy approach may be more discriminating in determining the cause of a motion restriction (barrier), and by being more discriminating, the most appropriate technique can be employed to restore normal function or motion.

Since muscle energy techniques require patient participation and cooperation, they may not be appropriate for the acute patient since, during the evaluation process, often the only motion restriction or barrier is that of pain. Indepth mechanical evaluation often works better in the subacute conditions, where a differential of motion barriers may be detected (rather than just reflex guarding). Muscle energy techniques work well with chronic conditions, but often require emphasis on direct stretching techniques and home exercise programs, as many of these patients have actually undergone mechanical (histologic) shortening rather than neurophysiologic shortening, which is the basis of the muscle energy concept.

One of the major benefits of the muscle energy techniques, is that it requires active patient involvement. Not only is the patient participating, but on reassessment for motion restriction or barriers, following treatment, there should be an immediate improvement with respect to increased mobility and decreased pain. The techniques are such that they don't have to be done repeatedly to appreciate a positive change.

Precautions for the use of muscle energy techniques are few; the same ones apply as for other passive movement techniques. Occasionally dramatic emotional responses such as crying, depression, or euphoria may be experienced when pelvic and sacral dysfunctions are treated. Appropriate communication with patients, thereby preparing them for this possibility or explaining the potential emotional state usually alleviates any fear or concern they may experience.

No one approach to the treatment of somatic dysfunction can be used exclusive of all other. However, muscle energy as a concept and skill is a valuable treatment modality to the manual therapist. It has a sound clinical basis, is easily learned, and is a comfortable technique as patients control treatment through their own active movements. Most important, the treatment yields good results in the clinic with those patients whose main problem is subacute somatic dysfunction.

The author would like to acknowledge the contributions by the URSA Foundation and fellow colleagues for the implementation and acceptance of Muscle Energy in clinical practice.

SUGGESTED READING

Fowler C. Muscle energy techniques for pelvic dysfunction. In: Grieve GP, ed. Modern manual therapy of the vertebral column. Edinburgh: Churchill Livingstone, 1986:805.

Fryette HH. Principles of osteopathic techniques. Academy of Applied Osteopathy. Colorado Springs, CO. 1954.

Goodridge JP. Muscle energy technique: definition, explanation, methods of procedure. J Am Osteopath Assoc 1981; Dec:249–254.

Kabat H, Lichlt S, eds. Proprioceptive facilitation in therapeutic exercise. 2nd ed. Baltimore, MD: Waverly, 1969:327.

Korr IM. The collected papers of Irvin M. Korr. Presented by The American Academy of Osteopathy. Colorado Springs, CO, 1979.

Lee D. Principles and practices of muscle energy and functional techniques. In: Grieve GP, ed. Modern manual therapy of the vertebral column. Edinburgh: Churchill Livingstone, 1966:640.

Mitchell FL, Moran PS, Pruzzo NA. An evaluation and treatment manual of osteopathic muscle energy procedures. Valley Park, MO: Mitchell, Moran and Pruzzo, Valley Park, MO, 1979.

Sherrington C. The integrative action of the nervous system. New Haven, CT: Yale University Press, 1961.

POWER WHEELCHAIR TRAINING FOR HANDICAPPED CHILDREN

WILLIAM F. BOYCE, B.A., B.Sc. (PT), M.Sc.

Physical handicaps in children may include cerebral palsy, spina bifida, muscular dystrophy, arthrogryposis, head injuries, juvenile arthritis, and various syndromes. Physical mobility is of prime importance for the young (2 to 4 years) handicapped child since this is the most usual mode of interaction with the environment at this age. Limitations of physical mobility can impair the development of social, communicative, cognitive, fine motor, and adaptive skills. Traditional mobility training for handicapped children has emphasized independent walking for those with adequate lower extremity function, manual wheelchair skills for those with adequate upper extremity function, and expensive powered wheelchair mobility only for those with poor motor control, but near normal intelligence and behavior. The recent availability of public funding and techniques for assessment, prescription, and training have encouraged therapists to expand the use of powered mobility devices, which were previously considered unsuitable for many children.

ASSESSMENT

The usual reason for assessing the suitability of powered mobility for a child is a perceived need for independent, functional movement. It is the task of the therapist, in conjunction with a support team of medical, psychosocial, and technological specialists, along with the child and family, to determine (a) the importance of the mobility need, and (b) the likelihood of success in using powered mobility.

Need for Mobility

The need for mobility is demonstrated primarily through the desire of the child and the family for an alternate mode of movement. Of great importance are the potential levels of social and physical functioning that may be achieved if the child has control of his position in the environment. Anecdotal reports from teachers or therapists are also vital in determining the need for independent movement. Particular efforts at purposeful, directed physical movement, or interest in the movement capabilities of peers should be noted as they indicate a "readiness" for assisted movement. Children who are currently using manual wheelchairs may require the use of powered mobility if they have weakness or incoordination of the upper trunk and arms, which prevents them from being functionally independent in the community. Concomitant cardiovascular or respiratory disorders may also prevent the child from having the endurance to propel a wheelchair manually for any functional distance.

Likelihood of Success

Once a need for powered mobility has been established, it is then the task of the therapist to determine the likelihood of success of powered wheelchair use. Strengths and weaknesses of the child in many areas must be thoroughly evaluated in order to determine whether the provision of expensive equipment is justified.

Physical

In order to operate a power wheelchair successfully, a child must be able to perform a consistent physical movement. A complete neuromotor evaluation of muscle tone, gross motor level, active and passive range of motion, muscle strength, reflexes and reactions, and orthopaedic status is performed in order to determine movement capabilities. Proper positioning of the body with a seating insert is often required, in order to promote more normal muscle tone and isolated muscle control. Potential physical movements for mobility control have a wide range. One child may have the ability to move a standard joystick with the hand in all directions; another may be able to lean the head to one side to contact a switch; yet another may isometrically contract a single muscle that can be monitored by electromyography. The Single Input Control Assessment (SICA) developed by Hugh MacMillan Medical Centre, Toronto, Ontario, is a valuable tool for use in objectively determining the optimal movement pattern, site of interface, type of interface, and position of switch for power wheelchair control. The SICA software program is used with the Apple computer for assessment of response times, scanning skills, and hold and release capabilities. Complete computerized protocols for objective evaluation of power wheelchair control are also being developed currently.

Sensory

Recent assessments of vision, hearing, and sensation are vital, in order to determine how the child receives information about movement direction, speed, and obstacles while operating a power wheelchair. Visual acuity of 10 percent or greater in at least one eye is usually required for successful use of vision as the feedback mechanism. Nonetheless, a device is currently in development, which may be of value for the operation of power wheelchairs by completely blind persons. This device uses transmitters mounted to the wheelchair that transmit ultrasound signals ahead and to the side of the wheelchair. As the sound waves rebound off obstacles, doorways, or walls, receivers on the wheelchair transform the soundwaves to auditory or vibratory signals which the patient uses to determine position and speed. Use of this device is restricted to safe indoor settings where steps and overhanging obstacles do not pose a problem.

Satisfactory auditory skills are desirable in training situations where verbal feedback of performance skills is given. Safety in outdoor locations is also facilitated by the ability to hear noises that may indicate danger from vehicles.

If neither visual nor auditory skills are adequate for training in the operation of a power wheelchair, it may be possible to use sensation alone (e.g., vibratory awareness) to provide an environmental feedback mode. It should be noted that the lack of adequate visual or auditory skills often requires a corresponding increase in cognitive and communicative skills, in order to compensate during training in and use of power wheelchairs.

Communication

Adequate receptive language, but not necessarily verbalization, is required for training of power wheelchair skills. The ability to understand simple instructions—indicating start, stop, slow, fast, turn—is required. The age at which this level of receptive language is normally present ranges from 18 to 24 months. Use of a powered mobility cart for a child of 11 months has been reported in the literature, but it is doubtful whether this child responded consistently to instructions by caregivers. Sufficient expressive language skills should be present, thereby allowing the child to indicate the desire to move. This desire may be expressed verbally, or with gestures, pictures, or symbols.

Cognition

Certain cognitive skills are needed for successful implementation of powered mobility. A number of conceptual and perceptual processes are generally required for various degrees of independency in powered mobility. "Supervised" use of powered mobility requires at least an awareness of cause and effect relationships, movement awareness, enjoyment of movement, and self-initiation of activity. "Controlled" use in a safe environment requires additional visual and perceptual skills, such as spatial perception and discrimination of parts of the environment. The ability to separate from mother is also required. "Independent" use of powered mobility requires sustained attention by the child and knowledge of the need to avoid simple hazards such as steps and obstacles. In general, an 18 to 30 month cognitive range is required for the various stages of wheelchair independence. Severely and moderately intellectually handicapped children have successfully been trained to use powered mobility. However, in many of these cases, the element of behavior must be considered critical to success.

Behavior

Adverse or stereotypical behavior patterns may ultimately preclude use of the power wheelchair device by a child. Nonetheless, it should be remembered that behavior can often be altered and, thus, denial of a power wheelchair trial should never be based on behavior alone. Determination of appropriate reinforcers and behavioral contingencies can be undertaken in a trial situation. This procedure may require a significant trial period of 3 to 6 months to determine the feasibility of behavioral change. In particular, persistent aggressive behavior may prevent the successful use of a power wheelchair.

Environment

If it has been determined that a child has a desire for movement, and if the physical, communicative, cognitive, and behavioral skills necessary for successful use of a wheelchair are present, a number of other environmental factors must be considered. There must be a suitable location available for use of the wheelchair. A multilevel school, small living quarters, or unpaved outside areas are not conducive to power wheelchair usage. Accessibility to buildings, via ramps or lifts, must be available. Architectural changes to buildings may be required before a power wheelchair can be used. Transportation of the wheelchair by bus, van, or car must be available unless the device is to be used only in one location. In addition, parental motivation, supervision skills, and responsibility for wheelchair and battery maintenance should also be considered.

PRESCRIPTION

The process of prescription of a power mobility device for a handicapped child is essentially a process of patient-device matching. Having assessed the need for mobility, prerequisite skills, and environmental suitability, the therapist must then consider all available devices that match present and future needs and skills.

There are numerous devices available for power mobility, not all of which are wheelchairs. These devices may be classified by two main factors—body position and method of control.

Body Position

There are various body positions that allow both secure posture and an upright head position for sensory feedback from the environment, both of which are necessary for powered mobility. Sitting is the most common position, and most wheelchairs are designed to achieve a stable sitting posture with hips and knees flexed. Powered caster carts are also available for use in a long sitting position, which can be achieved closer to floor level. This is an important option for very young children whose peers are crawling or just beginning to walk.

A prone-on-elbows or supported kneeling position may be customized for those individuals whose respiratory or orthopaedic status does not allow an upright trunk position. The supported kneeling position may be an appropriate alternative for a child with severe scoliosis providing there is sufficient motor control to keep the head up. Powered bases such as the Everest and Jennings Muscular Dystrophy Base or the Fortress Scientific Power Base are readily adaptable for this posture.

Powered movement in a standing position can also be used as an alternative to a sitting position. This may be useful for a child with hip and knee extension contractures or sacral-coccygeal pressure sore problems. These upright mobility devices are used primarily indoors as their higher center of gravity makes them somewhat unstable on uneven or sloping surfaces.

Method of Control

Powered mobility devices may be controlled in a variety of ways. The most common method is through the use a proportional joystick with various handle shapes available, depending on fine motor control and grasp abilities. It is necessary to determine the optimal handle shape for hand access, maintenance of hand position, and ease of hand withdrawal. Handles such as a right-angled T-bar, dowel, toggle, small or large ball, or oblique-angled T-bar, may also be tried. A proportional joystick has two distinct advantages over other types of wheelchair controls. The proportional joystick allows a change in direction or speed without stopping the wheelchair. Proportional joysticks are available for use with the hand, upper extremity, foot, chin, lips, or tongue. It also allows simultaneous control over speed and direction.

Multiple switch controls such as the microswitch joystick, arm slot control, and tray touch plates are available for children with less accurate motor control. Multiple controls usually incorporate five switches (on/off, forward, reverse, left, right) and, thus, require five distinct repeatable movements. Children who learn wheelchair control with a microswitch joystick occasionally advance to use of a proportional joystick once they have learned basic skills and mobility.

Children with only one or two reliable effective movements may use single switch scanning systems for wheelchair control. Scanning systems present a visual representation of the five wheelchair functions, which are highlighted individually in a sequential fashion. As the desired function is displayed, the child contacts a single switch to activate that wheelchair movement. The movement then continues until contact with the switch is stopped. The visual scanning mode then repeats, and the child chooses the next desired function.

Occasionally if a commercially available device or control system is not suitable for the particular needs of the child, a therapist may obtain customized devices for trial purposes. The choice of a powered mobility device and control system is an individualized process, which uses all aspects of the assessment information previously gathered.

Consideration of possible growth and developmental changes during the prescription of a device ensures that the child will have use of the device for an appropriate length of time.

TRAINING

Training a disabled child to use a powered mobility device involves a number of areas of proficiency. These areas are interdependent and involve basic wheelchair operation, mobility skills, independence, safety, and maintenance. Different methods of instruction are also used for various children.

Basic wheelchair operating skills include turning the wheelchair on and off, and knowing the maneuvers necessary to go forward, to turn and to go backward. Knowledge of and access to optional devices, such as speed control, turn signals, and horn, are also basic skills. Basic skills may be taught without power being connected in the wheelchair.

Mobility skills include the ability to navigate straight hallways in forward or reverse, turning corners, and turning 180 degrees and 360 degrees. The ability to maneuver around obstacles and through doorways or over rough ground, ramps, and grass, are also necessary for mobility. These skills are usually learned within 6-months training. If the child does not achieve this skill level, a trial of different body positions or control methods may be appropriate.

Independence in powered mobility includes all skills required for the child to function as independently as possible within the environment. Independence skills include transfers or assistance with transfers by positioning the wheelchair and adjusting body position in the wheelchair. Also included is finding one's way around the home or school, i.e., to washroom, gym, kitchen, office, classroom, and outdoors. The child should also learn efficiently and accurately to approach a desk, dresser drawers, tables, cabinets, shelves, cafeteria counters, and coat racks. These skills involve knowing the physical space required for the task, approaching the object from the appropriate side for hand use, and reaching, securing, and placing objects on a tray or a lap. The child should also learn how to approach and maneuver on a wheelchair bus and van lifts or ramps as well as building elevators. Since this is a potentially dangerous activity, only those children with good motor control and judgment should be allowed to attempt independence in these situations. Partial independence may be possible for children with less than optimal skills. Detailed training instructions are available for many of these skills (Meeting Street School—Easter Seal Society of Rhode Island).

Independence in community mobility is of importance to the older child. Especially important is the ability to travel along sidewalks and to cross streets both at lights and at stop signs. Adequate visual perceptual skills are required for the child to be able to see oncoming traffic and to be able to discern the speed of vehicles. Judgment of the wheelchair speed required to cross streets is also vital for independence.

Safety skills are an essential component of powered mobility and independence. During the initial training stages, an attendant is usually present, but safety skills should still be introduced in order to emphasize their importance. The use of handbrakes for transfers, when stopped on slopes and when in vehicles, is the first safety skill learned. Power to the wheelchair must be turned off during transfers in order that inadvertent movement of the joystick does not cause the chair to move out of position. It may seem self evident but many young children need to be taught that they must release the joystick or switch in order to stop the wheelchair. Control of wheelchair speed in indoor versus outdoor settings is important, especially when other children are present. Knowledge of driving techniques and safety procedures should be taught if operating the wheelchairs on ramps or

lifts. Use of mirrors or looking over the shoulder when driving in reverse is also necessary. Stopping at corners to check traffic is vital, both indoors and outdoors. Basic knowledge of traffic safety rules is crucial for wheelchair users. Proper operation of a wheelchair in a parking lot is especially important since the wheelchair driver sits lower and is less visible than pedestrians. Many safety skills may be verbally tested and rehearsed in practice before attempting real-life situations.

Maintenance

Although all children might not be capable of actual maintenance of a wheelchair, they should be encouraged to become aware of the need for maintenance. If a child learns to pay attention to the normal sounds of motors and brakes, the normal smell of a charged battery, and the sensation of properly inflated tires, small problems can be corrected before major repairs are needed.

Proper battery care maintains the effective life of a wheelchair. Whereas only a very high-level child can physically manage this task, all children should be able to tell caregivers of the timing and location of the procedure to be followed. This is especially important in multiple caregiver situations and is usually well remembered after the child is "grounded" due to failure to charge a battery overnight.

Parents and caregivers must receive adequate training in power wheelchair maintenance. Use of sealed gel batteries may be indicated for parents who are reluctant to maintain regular acid batteries.

Instruction Format

The particular method of instruction in operation of a powered mobility device depends on the physical, cognitive, and communicative abilities of the child. Instruction may range from verbal cues to physical assistance or a combination of both. In general, young children require at least some physical assistance since their behavioral, perceptual, and judgmental skills may not be adequately developed. Direct verbal training instructions should be given, with consistent simple wording, once it has been established that the child knows the meanings of the cues. Visual signs should be kept to a minimum, especially for the hearing disabled, since vision should be focused on the environment. Tactile cues, such as hand-over-hand or tapping the person or chair on the side you want it to go, may be used. Allowing mistakes to be made is important in order for the child to learn the consequences of an action. Feedback should be immediate, direct, and should use cues that have been previously taught. Verbal and physical assistance should be decreased gradually until the child is as independent as possible.

Use of a plastic guide on the wheelchair control, with only forward and reverse directions, may help the child initially learn to operate a proportional or micro switch joystick device. "Free time" should be used at the end of each training session so that the child can practice new skills and learn true independence with the device. Behavioral limits should be outlined and strictly enforced. This is for the safety of the child and other individuals in the house or school environment. The child should occasionally be quizzed about operating rules (e.g., crossing the street) so that safety awareness can be determined before a child is placed in a potentially dangerous situation.

SUGGESTED READING

Butler C, Okamoto G, McKay T. Powered mobility for very young disabled children. Dev Med Child Neurol 1983; 25:472–474.

Lee K, Parnes P, Milner M. Single input control assessment. Toronto: Hugh MacMillan Medical Centre.

Lotto J, Milner M. Evaluations and development of powered mobility aids for two-to-five year olds with neuromuscular skeletal disorders. Toronto: Hugh MacMillan Medical Center.

Meeting Street School. Power wheelchair training program. Easter Seal Society of Rhode Island. East Providence, RI.

Zazula JL, Foulds RA. Mobility device for a child with phocomelia. Arch Phys Med Rehabil 1983; 64:137–139.

REHABILITATION IN SPINAL CORD INJURY

JENNIFER McEWEN-HILL, B.Sc. (PT)

The physical therapist's role in teaching the spinal cord injured patient to move again, lift paralysed limbs, transfer, walk, and maneuver in the environment has been clearly defined for some time. There have been some advances in equipment, such as improved electric wheelchairs and the development of lightweight sports chairs. Computer technology is assisting with environmental controls and is being combined with functional electrical stimulation to produce paraplegic and quadriplegic ambulation in a limited manner.

However, in spite of these changes patients who were previously unable to transfer are still unable to transfer. In a recent retrospective study over 10 years at University Hospital, London, Ontario, no change was found in independence achieved with specific level of injury. Quadriplegics injured at the sixth cervical level were the highest level of injury patients able to achieve an independent transfer. Few C6 quadriplegics were able to achieve independence.

This chapter focuses on dependent transfer techniques. The transfers described here are less well known and may be useful alternatives to those available in the literature. They may be used for both paraplegics and quadriplegics. They may be used on an ongoing basis or may help to solve the problem of an inaccessible home in the early stages of rehabilitation. This center does not wait for home modifications to be completed prior to the first leave of absence. Purchase of lifts and physical modifications may change once the patient has been home.

Some of the lifts may seem quite foreign when first tried, especially the one person towel transfer. Often people learning it express concern about injury because of the position from which the transfer is done; however, this has not been the case at this institution. There have been fewer injuries to both patients and staff.

TOWEL TRANSFER

This transfer may be used to transfer a light to medium weight patient (maximum 180 to 190 lbs) to a level surface. This may be done with one person, although in an institution with rotating staff two may be preferred for safety. The second person stands behind the wheelchair with one knee on the bed and assists by holding the patient's pants or buttocks. It may be used for a patient in a halo vest unless neck pain is experienced during the transfer. The transfer can also be used if the halo has been recently removed as this transfer causes less strain to the neck than a two-man lift. A patient with painful shoulders finds this transfer a relief, compared to a two-man lift or standing-pivot transfer, as no strain is placed on the shoulders. It may not be possible to transfer a patient with severe spasticity, contractures, or an inflexible spine using the towel transfer. Being unable to reach around the halo vest, a small lifter will have difficulties transferring a patient in a halo.

The transfer begins with the wheelchair positioned beside the bed with the casters pointing back. The patient's feet are removed from the foot rests and placed on the floor. The foot rests are swung out to the side. A towel is then slid under the thighs and positioned under the gluteal fold. Once the towel is positioned, the restraining belt and armrest may be removed—if they are removed before the towel is positioned, the patient is unsupported (Fig. 1A).

The person transferring the patient stands facing the patient, with feet on either side of the patient's feet. He or she then leans the patient forward, flexing him/her from the hips. The patient's head and shoulder rest on the lifter's hip opposite to the direction of the transfer. If the patient has enough upper extremity strength, he may reach around the lifter's hips. Alternately, the patient may rest his/her arms on his/her lap (Fig. 1B).

The lifter now grasps the ends of the towel, keeping both elbows straight. The motion used for this transfer is critical. It must not be viewed as a lift but as a transfer, where the lifter uses body weight to counter balance the patient's body weight. If done incorrectly, the lifter experiences discomfort in the thoracic or lumbar spine.

The motion used for the transfer is a rocking motion. To move the patient forward in the wheelchair, the lifter just leans back, keeping elbows straight and knees bent. Then, keeping elbows straight and knees bent the lifter rocks back three times to gain momentum for the transfer. On the third rock, the lifter swings the patient and pivots so that his or her buttocks come to rest on the bed. This movement is quite rapid. The lifter's elbow flexors must not be used (Figs. 1C, D, and E).

Rehabilitation staff have found this transfer to be much superior to a two-man lift as long as it is per-

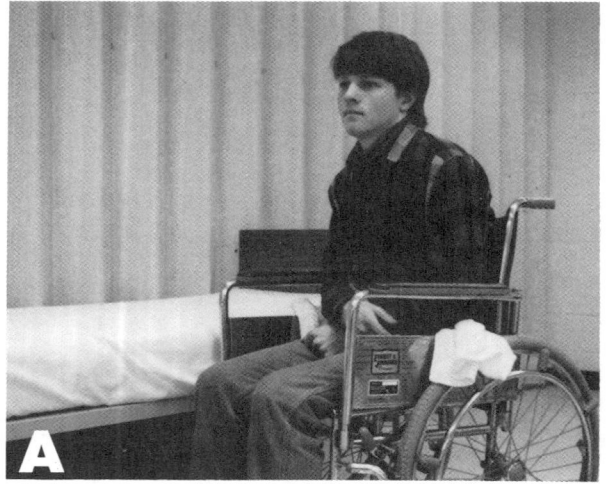

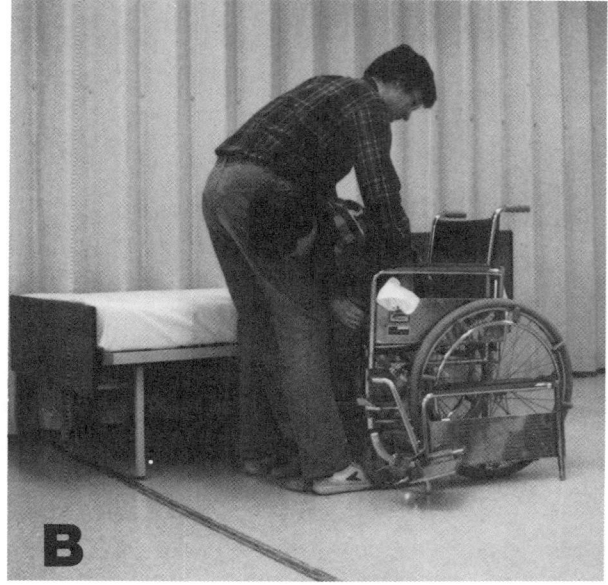

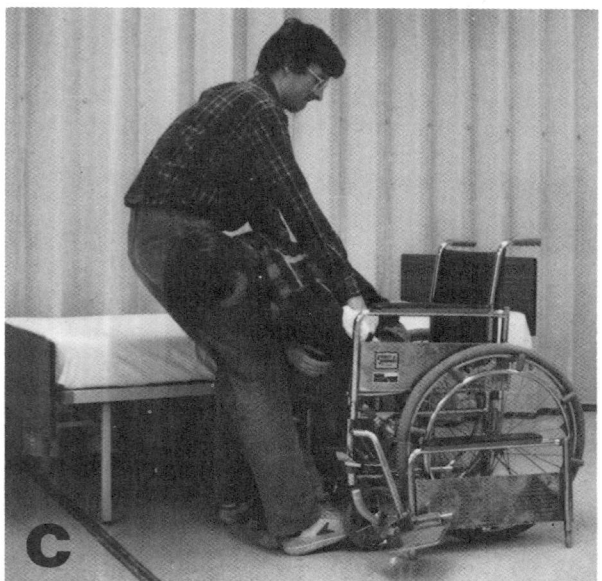

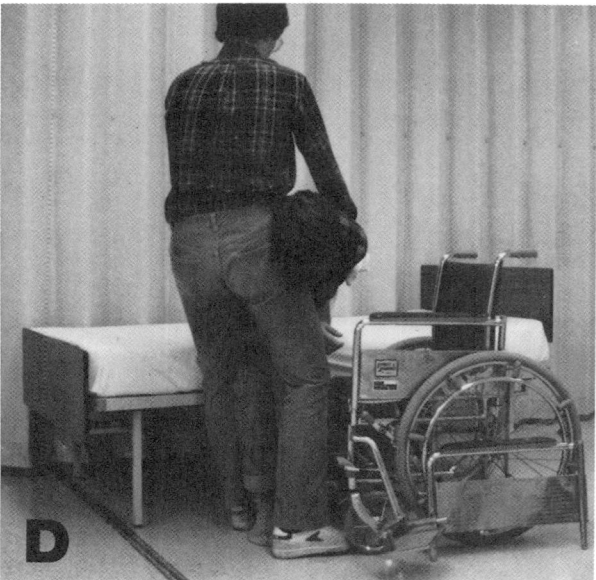

Figure 1 Towel transfer

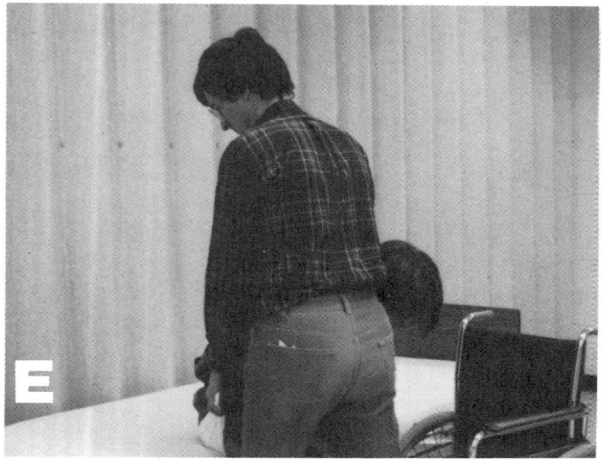

formed correctly. It may be done to a higher surface if a second person stands behind, one knee on the bed and grasps the patient's pants or buttocks to "boost" them up. A patient with a halo vest is transferred in the same manner although a flannel or towel may be needed on the hip to protect the lifter from bruising caused by the posts of the halo.

TWO-MAN TOWEL TRANSFER

This transfer may be used for lifting a patient to the floor or back to the wheelchair. It is an alternative

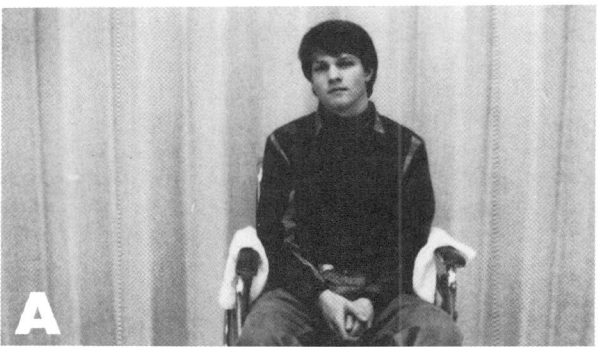

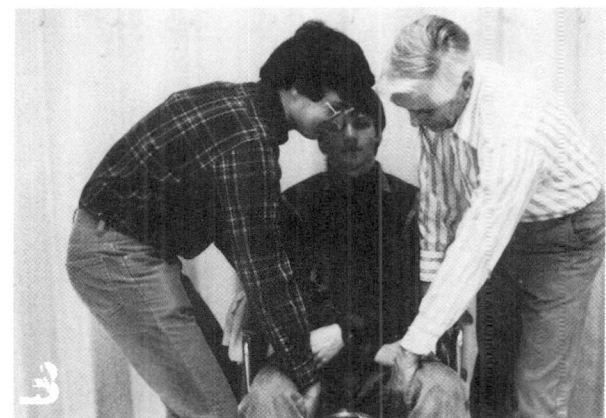

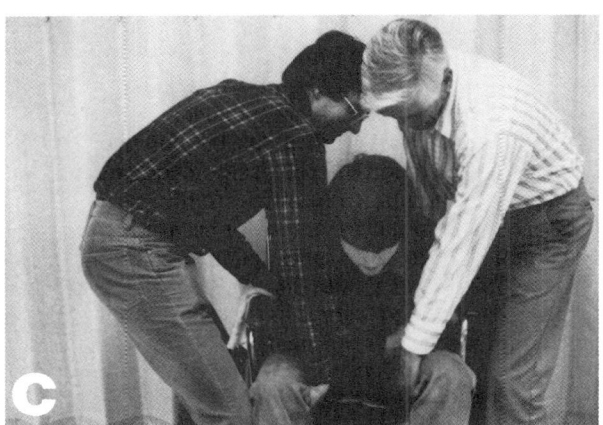

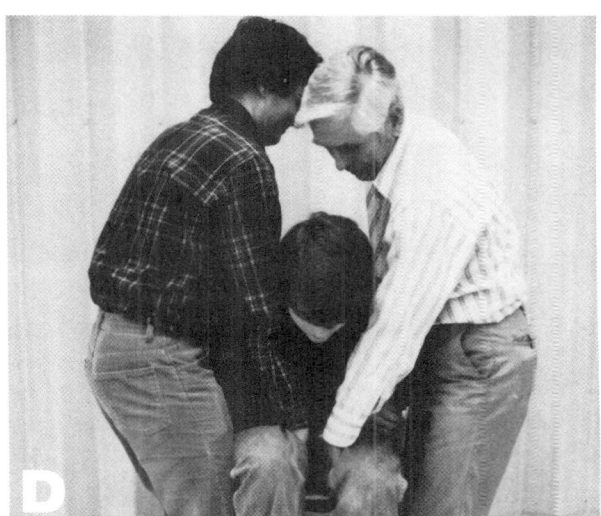

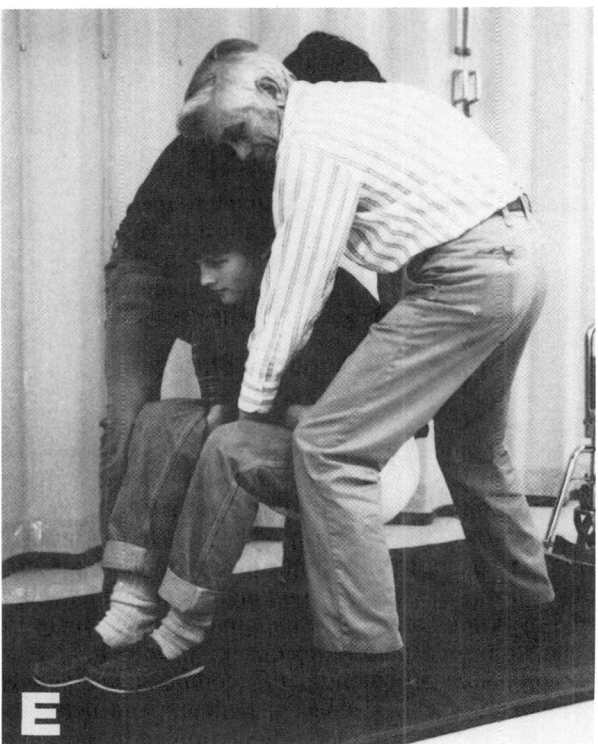

Figure 2 Two-man towel transfer

to a two-man lift or a Hoyer lift. It is especially useful for patients with painful shoulders or for those in wheelchairs or commodes with nonremovable arm-rests. The patient may be carried distances comfort-ably, making it useful for a wheelchair inaccessible room such as bathroom. It should not be used for a patient in halo traction.

The wheelchair is positioned facing the area where the patient will be placed. The armrests and footrests may remain in place. A towel is slid under the but-tocks so that one end hangs out from each side (Fig. 2A). The two lifters should face the wheelchair from opposite sides. Using the arm closest to the front of the wheelchair, each lifter grasps the patient around the inner thigh. The lifters' forearms are in a pronated position (Fig. 2B). The patient is then leaned forward to rest on the lifters' arms, which are supporting the thighs. The ends of the towel are grasped with the free hand (Fig. 2C).

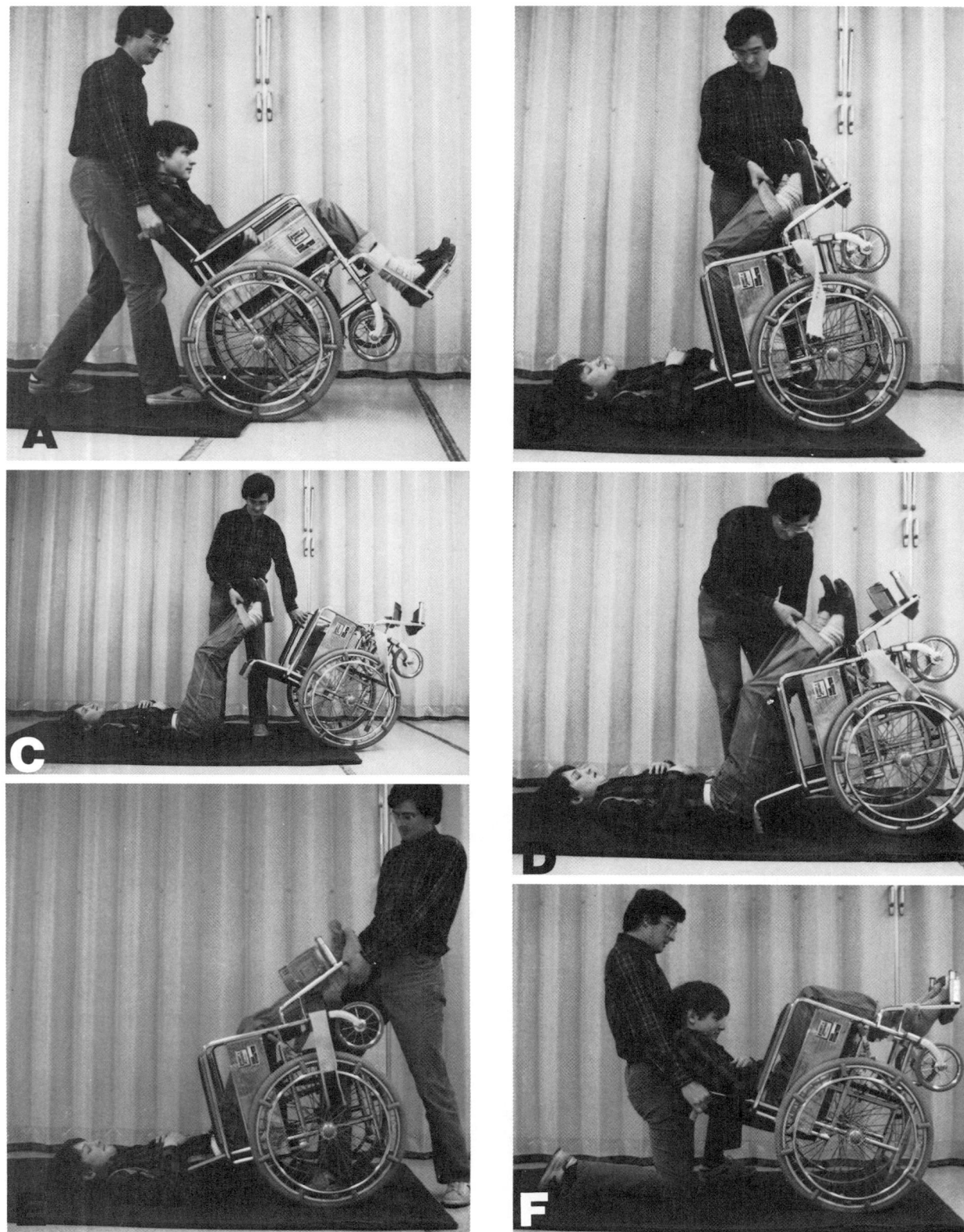

Figure 3   One-man transfer from wheelchair to floor

Before lifting, the lifters should widen their stance, bend their knees, tilt their pelvis and straighten their backs (Fig. 2D). The patient is lifted forward out of the chair and carried a little beyond where he is to lie or sit. Contact with the floor is made with feet first, followed by a smooth backward movement (Fig. 2E). The patient ends up in a long sitting position.

To get the patient back into the wheelchair it is easiest to position the towel with the patient in supine, by bending up his knees and sliding it in place. The remaining steps are then reversed.

ONE-MAN TRANSFER FROM WHEELCHAIR TO FLOOR

This transfer may be used to transfer a light to medium-weight patient to or from the floor by one person. It should be tried first with assistance available. A person with severe spasticity or very long trunk or some sports wheelchairs may make this transfer impossible. This transfer may be taught to a family member concerned about how they would get the patient back into the wheelchair if they were alone with the patient. It is not as easy to do as some other transfers and may not be possible for someone not in reasonable physical condition.

A belt is used to secure the patient's legs to the footrests. Next, the wheelchair is tipped backwards from behind until the handrips rest on the floor (Fig. 3A). The patient may experience some apprehension at this point because of the sensation that his legs will fall out of the wheelchair onto his face.

The lifter grasps the patient's pant legs with one hand and unties the belt with the other. If the patient is able he may now push with his elbows to slide off the wheelchair backwards onto the floor. Some patients may require assistance, but a patient injured up to the sixth cervical level should be able to manage this maneuver independently (Fig. 3B). As soon as the wheelchair back is free it is returned to the upright position (Fig. 3C).

To get the patient back into the wheelchair the lifter grasps the patient's pant legs with one hand, lifts the legs, and tips the wheelchair over backwards sliding the wheelchair back as close to the buttocks as possible (Fig. 3D). Then, the lifter, still holding the patient's legs, walks around so that he is facing the footrests. The footplates should be flipped up. The patient is grasped by both ankles and slid up the wheelchair back as far as possible (Fig. 3E). The foot plates are put down and the patient's feet tied to the foot rests. Now the lifter walks around to the patient on the floor. The lifter kneels and sits on his heels, raises the patient's shoulders and rests them on his thighs. This enables the lifter to reach the handgrips, support the patient's upper trunk and head, and have a better mechanical advantage. The wheelchair is now

tipped upright. The patient needs some support of the upper trunk while rising but slides down the back of the chair as an upright position is reached (Fig. 3F).

CAR TRANSFER WITH HALO TRACTION

Patients are arriving at rehabilitation centers much earlier than they used to. If no medical complications occur, they may arrive as early as 1 to 2 weeks post trauma. Quadriplegics in halo traction can only be involved in a limited and, therefore, frustrating rehabilitation program until the halo is removed. There is no reason why a medically stable patient in halo traction cannot go on a leave of absence in a regular car. With a shoulder harness in place, the neck is much better supported in halo traction than with a plastizote collar.

Certain cars do not accommodate the height of the halo. Four-door cars make the transfer more difficult because of the door post. A two man sliding board transfer is used. The patient must slide into the car hips first, sliding onto the seat and getting his halo past the car roof. The seat may have to be reclined. Not all patients fit in all cars, but families are remarkably resourceful in finding an appropriate car when given the opportunity of bringing a family member home.

The Quad Quip transfer board has been found to be useful when doing the transfer as it does not slide off the wheelchair cushion (Fig. 4). The post of the transfer board slides into the tube that normally accommodates the front post of the armrest. This cannot be used with a sports chair without modifications to the chair.

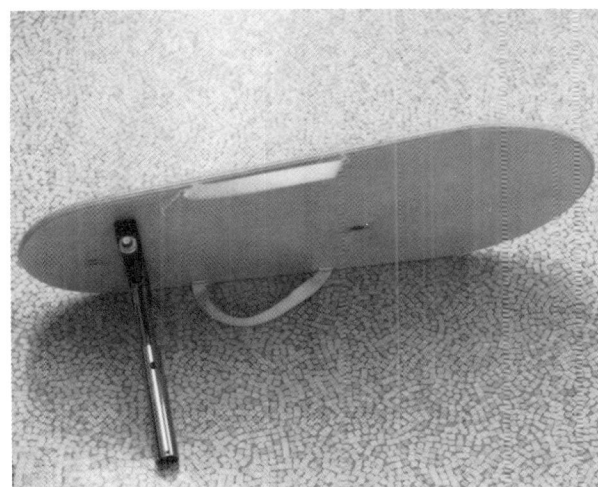

Figure 4 Quad Quip transfer board

The transfers described in this chapter may provide valuable alternatives to those described in the literature. They are easy to learn and, with the exception of the one-man transfer to the floor, may be performed by most people. They are very useful in the rehabilitation of spinal cord injured patients and can make home modifications and equipment purchases unnecessary.

FOUR-CHANNEL ELECTRIC STIMULATOR: AN AMBULATORY AID FOR SPINAL CORD INJURED PATIENTS

TADEJ BAJD, D.Sc., Dip. Eng.
ALOJZ KRALJ, D.Sc., Dip. Eng.

When several months or even years have passed after injury, the paraplegic patient has to undergo a program to strengthen disuse atrophied muscles. The strengthening program consists of daily application of cyclic electrical stimulation to the knee extensors, resulting in isotonic contractions. Stimulation periods of 4 seconds are followed by a pause of 4 seconds. Stimulation frequency of 20 Hz, pulse duration of 0.3 milliseconds and stimulation amplitude, such as enough to bring the legs to full extension, are used. The electrical stimuli are rectangular and monophasic. During training, patients are positioned supine—both lower extremities semiflexed—with a pillow under the knees. During the first week of the program the functional electrical stimulation (FES) session lasts for half an hour per day, while half an hour is added each following week. As a result of the FES training program, the muscle force is increased and the muscle fatigability is lessened. In this way, longer stimulation training sessions are made possible. The FES muscle strengthening is usually divided into two or three sessions, all together not exceeding 3 hours per day. The FES exercise can also prevent contractures, reduce spasticity, provide better blood flow within the stimulated extremity, and improve skin condition.

CRITERIA FOR SELECTION OF PATIENTS

The candidates for FES treatment are selected from patients with spastic paraplegia or tetraplegia resulting from complete or incomplete spinal cord lesion. The criteria for patient selection also include the following:

- upper motor neuron lesion
- well preserved skin
- intact joints and bones
- adequate balance
- good psychosocial condition
- motivation and good cooperation.

The following are the contraindications for FES application:

- peripheral lesions
- osteoporosis
- heterotropic ossifications
- contractures
- severe atrophy of muscles and no response to re-strengthening
- pressure sores
- obesity
- severe spasticity
- inadequate sitting balance
- lack of patient interest.

Standing-Up and Standing

When the maximal knee joint torque provided by FES exceeds 30 to 50 Nm (depending on patient's body weight) standing can be started. Continuous FES causes knee extensors to contract, maintaining the knee joints in extension, thus allowing standing. Through the use of two stimulation channels and arm support, the patients can stand from 5 to 10 minutes up to 1 hour or more, depending on posture, muscle fatigue, and exerted force. A pair of surface electrodes is held in place on both quadriceps femoris muscles by Velcro straps. The specific placement of the electrodes is not critical because of large quadriceps femoris muscles. The advantages of FES-assisted standing are manifold. It can help prevent decubitus, improve function of the bladder and other internal organs, and provide better blood flow in paralyzed parts of the body.

If standing is to be a useful functional activity (e.g., to get an object that is out of reach of the wheelchair), the person must be able to rise independently from a sitting to a standing position. The standing-up procedure can be accomplished by stimulating both knee extensor muscle groups. The patient assists FES by lifting with the arms. If a patient is not obese or extremely weak in the arms, rising from sitting to standing can be easily accomplished.

Stimulation parameters are the same as in the training program. During the motion of standing-up, stimulation voltage up to 100 V is to be applied. It is then lessened (for each leg separately) to the minimal value, allowing full knee extension during standing.

Standing at any location is facilitated by a special wheelchair equipped with a collapsible supporting frame. The supporting frame is lightweight and designed to slip into the arm support holders (of a regular wheelchair). The height of the handles can be adjusted according to the patient's needs. When the frame is collapsed it does not interfere with the normal use of the wheelchair. The wheelchair, together with the supporting frame, can be stored in a car.

Walking and Stair Climbing

When patients are able to stand safely for at least 20 minutes, FES-assisted walking is commenced. It can be performed in parallel bars or with the help of a special frame on wheels, designed for initial walking trials. For safety reasons, the patient can be attached to the frame with leather belts.

During reciprocal walking, the stimulator must be controlled through three different phases of walking: double stance, right swing, and left swing. The stimulator is controlled by two hand switches. When neither of the switches is pressed, both knee extensors are stimulated. On pressing the switch in the right hand, the right leg is stimulated to flex; the same is true for the left switch and the left leg. In the very first experiments, both switches are held and controlled by the physical therapist. Later, the switches are built into the handles of the walker or crutches, and the patient controls them. The duration of the swing phase is equal to the time of pressing the switch. A special electronic circuit takes care of possible erroneous simultaneous pressing of both switches. In this case, no change occurs in the stimulator output.

Surface electrical stimulation of knee extensors is delivered to the muscles through large (6 × 4 cm) electrodes made of sheet metal from stainless steel covered with several water-soaked layers of gauze. Flexion of the swinging lower extremity is elicited through two small (2.5 cm diameter) round electrodes made of sheet metal and covered with water-saturated gauze.

Stairs represent a major obstacle in the transportation of wheelchair-confined patients. Therefore, stair climbing is the most important advantage of FES-assisted rehabilitation of complete paraplegic patients. The reciprocal gait pattern is used also in walking up stairs. The synergistic flexion response is strong enough to lift the leg to the next stair. The switch control must be in one hand only as the patient is holding the handrail with the other hand. Swing-to gait with continuously stimulated knee extensors is the most appropriate for walking down stairs.

USE OF FES IN INCOMPLETE SPINAL CORD INJURY (SCI) PATIENTS

In the last decades, different traffic preventive measures, improved vehicle engineering, more effi-cient first aid, improved transport to the hospital, and advanced treatment in an emergency center, have resulted in a reduction in the number of complete paraplegic and tetraplegic patients. Consequently, many more incomplete cases are arriving in spinal units. According to statistical observations, there is a greater number of incomplete patients among tetraplegics than among paraplegics. On the basis of these findings, it can be concluded that incomplete tetraplegic patients represent an interesting group of paralyzed patients suitable for FES treatment.

Because of the complex neurophysiologic state of incomplete SCI patients it is impossible to predict the outcome of the FES rehabilitation process when the patients are admitted to the spinal unit immediately after the accident. Similarly, it is not possible to decide what rehabilitation aid the patient will need after recovering from the spinal cord injury. Therefore, the first step in the FES program is the application of therapeutic electrical stimulation.

Therapeutic electrical stimulation is applied daily and consists of cyclic stimulation of partially paralyzed knee extensor muscles where 4 seconds of stimulation alternate with 4-second pauses. The training program lasts for about 2 months.

After the training program, three different groups of incomplete SCI patients are encountered as follows: (1) in the first group, both voluntary and electrically stimulated muscle strength is improved; (2) in the second group, only the stimulated muscle strength is increased; and (3) in the third group, neither voluntary nor stimulated response is augmented.

The final goal of an electrical stimulation training program is restoration of ambulation, in incomplete SCI patients, with the help of functional electrical stimulation. In many incomplete paraplegic and tetraplegic patients, exaggerated extensor tone can be observed in the lower extremities, thereby providing more or less safe standing for some patients. Many are unable to break this exaggerated extensor tone during standing and, hence, are unable to achieve adequate flexion for gait. It has been shown that in thoracic and cervical incomplete patients electrical stimulation of an afferent nerve augments dorsiflexion, knee, and hip flexion in a total lower limb flexion reflex pattern. In this way, peroneal stimulation can be used efficiently to initiate a step from an incomplete SCI patient.

Four different groups of patients are encountered with respect to their needs for application of different orthoses based on FES. (1) Incomplete SCI patients who are able to stand, but require unilateral peroneal stimulation to elicit the flexion response and initiate a step. (2) Patients where bilateral peroneal stimulation is found helpful. (3) In a great number of incomplete tetraplegic patients one leg is almost completely paralyzed, whereas the other leg is under voluntary control and is sufficiently strong to provide safe standing—with crutches—for short periods. Unilateral stimulation of knee extensors and an afferent nerve is helpful in these patients. (4) In the last group there are patients for whom a minimum of four channels of FES is required for synthesis of a simple reciprocal gait pattern, such as in complete thoracic patients.

ADVANTAGES AND DISADVANTAGES OF TREATMENT

When introducing FES to complete or incomplete SCI patients, it is necessary to be aware of the benefits and problems of the new rehabilitation approach. The following are the advantages of FES:

- patient's own muscles and metabolic energy are used
- patient's bone support and joints are functionally used
- no external bracing is required
- preserved neuromuscular reflexes can be functionally used
- muscle atrophy and ossifications are prevented
- blood flow and muscle strength are improved
- skin condition is improved
- spasticity may be reduced
- the patient may be rehabilitated to a higher functional level
- therapy is promoted
- electrodes are easily applied to the extremity
- appearance is not undesirable
- no attachments are present to cause pressure spots or decubiti
- cost is less than, or the same as, orthoses
- need not be custom made, thus eliminating production problems

- does not depend upon extremity size for fit, thereby eliminating problems caused by change in girth.

Some disadvantages of surface FES application in spinal cord injured patients are as follows:

- electrode placement is time consuming
- stimulated muscle fatigue and hence functioning time is limited
- muscle force is lower (in comparison to normal muscle)
- selectivity is inadequate
- time of use of surface electrodes is limited
- stimulators are bulky
- control of stimulator by patient is inadequate
- multisite application possible when restoring complex movements
- skin irritations are possible with improperly used stimulator.

SUGGESTED READING

Bajd T, Kralj A, Turk R. Standing-up of a healthy subject and a paraplegic patient. J Biomechanics 1982; 15:1–10.

Benton LA, Baker LL, Bowman BR, Waters RL. Functional electrical stimulation: a practical clinical guide. 2nd ed Downey, CA: Rancho Los Amigos Hospital, 1981.

Cybulski GR, Penn RD, Jaeger RJ. Lower extremity functional neuromuscular stimulation in cases of spinal cord injury. Neurosurgery 1984; 15:132–146.

Kralj A, Bajd T, Turk R, Krajnik J, Benko H. Gait restoration in paraplegic patients: a feasibility demonstration using multichannel surface electrode FES. J Rehabil Res Develop 1983; 20:3–20.

Marsolais EB, Kobetic R. Functional walking in paralyzed patients by means of electrical stimulation. Clin Orthop 1983; 175:30–36.

Vodovnik L, Bajd T, Gračanin F, Kralj A, Strojnik P. Functional electrical stimulation for control of locomotor systems. CRC Crit Rev Bioeng 1981; 6:63–131.

PRINCIPLES OF ELECTROMYOGRAPHIC FEEDBACK AND ITS CLINICAL APPLICATION IN STROKE REHABILITATION

G. ELIZABETH TATA, B.P.T., M.Cl.Sc.

BASIC PRINCIPLES

Biofeedback is a methodology that uses instruments to detect physiologic processes of which the subject is not normally aware and then teaches the subject to modify the physiologic activity by using external representation of that activity in the form of an auditory or visual signal.

Biofeedback has been termed a "behavioral medicine" technique because its objective is to train a certain behavior such as the control of heart rate, skin temperature, or, in the case of electromyographic (EMG) biofeedback, muscle activity. As such, the basic principles of learning are adhered to. It is well established that learning is maximized if knowledge of results is given immediately. Biofeedback techniques make this possible. The clinical physical therapist should be aware of the terminology used to describe learning principles. "Shaping" is the modification of a behavior (e.g., muscle activity) by defining a desired response and reinforcing closer and closer approximations to this response. "Reinforcement" is given in the form of an auditory or visual display, which is a reward for successful approximations. The desired response or goal should be set at a level that the subject can attain on at least 75 percent of attempts in order that motivation be maintained. "Weaning" involves withdrawal of the feedback display in stages as the subject learns control of muscle activity independently of the artificial feedback. Follow-up reinforcement may be required at intervals to maintain the learned control.

SELECTION OF PATIENTS

Appropriate conditions for the use of EMG biofeedback are those in which motor control is impaired due to problems of proprioceptive deficit or motor output of the central nervous system. Vision and hearing must be intact in order that the patient can perceive the feedback, and there must be an intact motor pathway to the muscle. Because the biofeedback is instantaneous the patient learns very quickly that the visual or auditory signal can be turned on by production of the required movement. Patients must be motivated to try to improve the selected motor response and repeatedly to activate the feedback display. The ability to understand and follow instructions is essential, and success will therefore be limited in those patients with receptive aphasia. Patients with hemiplegia following stroke probably comprise the largest population for whom biofeedback is used. Age, sex, side of lesion, previous rehabilitation, and length of time since stroke are not good indicators of a patient's ability to benefit from biofeedback training. Significant improvement may still be possible several years after a stroke. Success might be limited in those patients with left hemiplegia and an associated neglect of the left side of the body.

EMG Biofeedback Equipment

EMG biofeedback equipment uses surface electrodes to detect motor unit action potentials. It amplifies and processes the resulting electrical signal and displays it to the patient in the form of an auditory or visual signal, which is proportional to the state of tension or relaxation of the muscle. EMG equipment is able to detect single motor unit activity, thus providing evidence to the patient and therapist of extremely low levels of muscle activity at a stage before movement can be observed or felt. This permits an earlier start to training than would otherwise be possible.

Surface electrodes are available in a variety of both reusable and disposable types. A saline electrode gel is applied to the electrode for electrical conduction between the skin and electrode. The electrode is then fixed to the skin by an adhesive collar. Self-adhesive disposable electrodes are available, which may have a sponge surface to which gel is applied or may be already impregnated with gel. These electrodes are quick and easy to apply and may be left in place for several days with the advantage of assuring consistent electrode positioning from one training session to another. This is important for accurate documentation of progress and especially if the patient is using numerical or meter readings as feedback. A change to a less optimal electrode position may result in lower recorded levels for the same effort by the patient that previously gave a higher reading: this could be discouraging.

174

Surface electrodes have a wide area of pick-up and will detect activity of surrounding as well as target muscles. This can be minimized by close spacing of the two active electrodes over the center of the muscle belly. Spacing up to 2.5 cm apart, depending on electrode size, and along the longitudinal axis of the muscle is optimal for maximum signal detection where minimal muscle activity is present. It may be necessary to try different positions to find the strongest signal in a muscle with very low activity. Wider spacing over a single muscle or muscle group may be used where the goal is reduction of excessive amounts of muscle activity. A ground electrode is also necessary and is placed at a nearby point. Disposable electrode strips may have the ground as the center of the three electrodes.

Reduction of skin impedance is usually required to allow adequate conduction of the EMG signal. This involves cleaning with alcohol, shaving if necessary, and abrasing with pumice or light sandpaper. EMG units are now available with a high input impedance making skin preparation minimal or unnecessary.

The amplitude of the EMG signal is very small, ranging from 0.2 to 0.5 microvolts (μv) at resting level to around 500 μv on maximum contraction of a large muscle. Amplification is required before the signal can be processed and recorded.

For ease of interpretation in the clinical setting the biofeedback unit processes the raw EMG signal by rectifying and then averaging the total amount of electrical activity over a set period of time. Examples of time constants used are 0.3 seconds, 1 second or 3 seconds. Some units give a choice of time constant, whereas others are fixed. A short time constant causes the feedback display to be more sensitive to changes in muscle activity levels, which may be frustrating initially for a patient with poor control who is trying to maintain a constant level of activity.

More sophisticated equipment gives a choice of average or peak microvolt level for a specified time constant. There may also be a band width choice for the selection of lower or higher frequencies of the signal. The higher frequency band width setting ensures more selective pick-up of motor unit action potentials close to the electrodes since higher frequencies become attenuated as distance from the electrodes increases.

Feedback Modes

Various types of feedback display are available. Meter readings indicate rise and fall of microvolt levels by deflections of a needle. Sensitivity of the instrument is usually adjustable to more than one range, e.g., 0.1–10 μv, 1–100 μv, 10–1000 μv. The ranges vary on different makes of machine. Some units provide light-emitting diodes or light bars, which light

up proportionately to the amount of muscle activity. Alternatively a single light may be triggered to go on or off at a preset microvolt or threshold level. Some units give a digital read-out of microvolt levels.

Auditory feedback may be given as a series of clicks or a tone. Firing of larger numbers of motor units causes a progressively higher rate of clicking or higher frequency tone. Some units have only an on/off tone triggered at a preset threshold microvolt level. Head-phones allow the patient to work independently so that the sound does not disturb others in the area and also eliminates environmental noise, which may be distracting. Connection may be provided for external "environmental control" of tape recorders, television, or electrically operated toys, which can be used to help motivate the patient. Recent developments of equipment are providing features previously available only for research purposes, such as connection to an oscilloscope for display of the raw or processed signal and automatic print-out of the signal. The more advanced features are not essential for clinical purposes but are useful for keeping precise records for assessment of progress and for research and publication purposes.

PROBLEMS OF MOTOR CONTROL IN HEMIPLEGIA

In hemiplegia there has been damage to inhibitory and excitatory pathways, which influence motor output. This results initially in flaccidity or hypotonia followed by the development of varying degrees of spasticity or hypertonia with the loss of inhibitory and modulating influences of the supraspinal centers on alpha and gamma motor neurons. Impaired gamma motor neuron and muscle spindle function produces abnormal proprioceptive feedback. There is also abnormal coordination of agonist and antagonist muscle groups with lack of isolated joint control and the problem of abnormal total movement synergies.

Functional deficits resulting from this abnormal motor control include upper extremity impairment of reach, grasp and manipulation. Lower extremity dysfunction during gait causes loss of stable support, reduced stride length and inability to dorsiflex the ankle during swing-through and heel-strike.

Training strategies for the hemiplegic patient are aimed at producing more normal levels of muscle tone, improving agonist-antagonist interaction, and thereby gaining coordinated movement. Clinical EMG biofeedback equipment can be useful in the assessment of muscle tone as well as for training in raising or lowering of muscle activity levels.

Hypertonic muscles may have abnormally high resting levels and during passive movement are much more sensitive to stretch, reacting more quickly than normal to produce higher bursts of activity. The relaxation time to return to resting level takes longer. On active contraction the time to reach peak activity and the relaxation time may be abnormally prolonged. A hypertonic muscle is usually weak and maximum voluntary contraction may attain peak EMG levels considerably lower than normal. Deficits in contraction and relaxation timing result in loss of efficient phasic activity.

Hypotonic muscles may have normal or below normal resting levels and low levels on both slow and rapid passive movement demonstrating unresponsiveness to stretch. The patient may have great difficulty in generating higher microvolt levels. Prior to beginning biofeedback training, baseline microvolt levels should be recorded as part of the initial assessment (Table 1).

In addition to EMG levels, passive and active range of motion should be noted as these are useful outcome measures for assessing the ability to relax and to isolate movement.

Defining Goals

From the initial assessment and baseline measures training goals are developed. In behavioral medicine terminology this is termed response selection. In the upper extremity raising the EMG level of hypotonic finger and wrist extensors may be an initial selected response progressing to active wrist and finger extension, with the ultimate functional goal being development of prehension. As recovery proceeds, varying degrees of spasticity develop and reduction of EMG levels of finger and wrist flexors are a selected response at rest, on passive, and then with active wrist and finger extension. Simultaneous increase in extensor activity with flexor inhibition can be achieved using a two-channel biofeedback unit.

At the shoulder movement problems include lack of isolated glenohumeral abduction and hypotonia or hypertonia of the scapular musculature causing abnormal scapulohumeral movement. If spasticity of retractors and downward rotators of the scapula is the identified problem, the responses selected would be reduced activity in these to allow normal orientation of the scapula. Target muscles might be the rhomboids, teres major and latissimus dorsi. A progression from this would be to increased activity of deltoid to achieve shoulder abduction.

In the lower extremity, hypotonicity is an initial problem, which causes instability of the hip and knee on weight bearing and drop-foot during swing and early stance phases of gait. Initial responses would be raised EMG levels of target muscles—hip abductors, quadriceps femoris, tibialis anterior, and toe extensors. As spasticity develops biofeedback is directed towards inhibition of hypertonic hip adductors and plantarflexors at rest, on passive movement, and on active movement of agonist muscle groups.

Selection of target muscles is based on careful assessment of their levels of tone and how this is affecting movement. Working with one muscle group in an abnormal synergy may help in normalizing tone of other muscles contributing to the synergy.

Training Procedures

Introduction of biofeedback training to the patient involves a simple explanation of the procedure and demonstration on an unaffected limb of how muscle contraction and relaxation result in auditory and visual feedback. This is usually quickly realized by the patient and fine levels of control can be obtained in normal muscle in a few minutes of practice. Care should be taken not to give too high expectations. It

TABLE I   Baseline Measurement of EMG Levels

	Initial date	Follow-up date
Resting level (μv)		
Peak during slow passive movement (μv)		
Peak during rapid passive movement (μv)		
Relaxation time following passive movement (secs)		
Peak EMG on maximum isotonic contraction (μv)		
Time to reach peak EMG (secs)		
Relaxation time following peak EMG (secs)		
Peak EMG of antagonist during agonist contraction (μv)		

is explained that biofeedback is a part of the total rehabilitation process to help gain improved motor control.

After demonstration on the corresponding muscle of the unaffected limb electrodes are applied to the target muscle and, if able, the patient can try moving to observe changes in the feedback display. Baseline measurements as suggested in Table I are recorded at this and future sessions for evaluation of progress.

Procedure to Increase Activity of a Hypotonic Muscle

There may be little or no evidence on observation or palpation of activity in a severely weak or hypotonic muscle. In order to detect maximum microvolt levels, meticulous skin preparation is needed and electrodes are placed close together in the center of the muscle to avoid pick-up of activity from surrounding muscles. Experimentation with different sites may be necessary to find optimal pick-up. Skin preparation and electrode site must be consistent from one session to another so that meter readings give valid indication of progress, and the patient is not discouraged by lower levels due to poor and inconsistent electrode placement. If there is doubt as to whether activity is from the target muscle or a nearby muscle a second feedback channel could be used to distinguish between the two.

The lower microvolt scale is used initially. The threshold level is set at the peak microvolt level attainable on active contraction (e.g., 10 μv on a 1 to 30 μv scale). Feedback is usually given continuously with additional feedback such as the turning on of a light or sound when threshold microvolt level is reached. The threshold level is set so that the patient is successful on at least 75 percent of repetitions. As strength of contraction improves the threshold for triggering of feedback is progressively raised and the scale is switched to the next microvolt range when the maximum level on the lower scale is reached.

Facilitation of activity in a hypotonic muscle is achieved using any of the usual techniques. Gravity free positioning, compression, quick stretch, proprioceptive neuromuscular facilitation techniques, passive or assisted movement through range to give the patient the feel of the movement, and mechanical vibration of the hypotonic muscle may all be tried in an attempt to elicit activity. Once a successful technique has been found it is repeated as much as possible before fatigue to help the patient to become aware of the "feel" of the movement so that it can be remembered at a later session. Fatigue may occur rapidly if high levels of concentration and effort are required to produce the required response. This will determine the length of the session and number and length of rest periods. Thirty minutes, with appropriate rest periods, is probably the maximum time for efficient concentration on a single task before fatigue.

The patient must be given time to build up to a peak contraction and maintain it for as long as possible. Verbal encouragement and manual stimulation can be given, but the patient should also be allowed quiet time with the biofeedback alone to develop an internal awareness of the movement.

If maximum effort is used, there will probably be excessive activity in antagonistic and synergic muscles, thus producing abnormal patterns of total limb movement. Though this can be permitted initially and may be necessary to facilitate contraction of the target muscle, the ultimate goal will be to activate the agonist muscle, together with active inhibition of the antagonist, and to achieve isolated control of the target muscle. Appropriate progression of positioning will help to achieve this. For example, dorsiflexion may be allowed as part of a total flexor synergy at first and progression made to dorsiflexion with the knee extended as is required for normal gait. Relaxation of hypertonic muscles first and the use of dual channel feedback will help to reduce excessive antagonist activity.

Functional electrical stimulation of a hypotonic muscle is useful to demonstrate movement to the patient and to find optimal electrode sites. Newer biofeedback units are available with EMG-triggered electrical stimulation, which allows a minimal EMG signal from a weak muscle to trigger the electrical stimulation with the goals of increasing strength and range of motion.

Joint stiffness, especially of the hand, is a frequent problem in hemiplegia. Passive movement prior to beginning the biofeedback session helps to reduce joint stiffness as well as increasing the patient's awareness of the movement to be executed.

Procedure to Reduce Activity in a Hypertonic Muscle

Fluctuations in the feedback signal can again be demonstrated on a muscle with normal tone before placing the electrodes over the target muscle or muscle group when inhibition of activity in a hyperactive muscle is the goal. If general body relaxation is required frontalis is the chosen target muscle.

Resting microvolt levels are recorded initially. The patient should attempt to raise and lower the feedback signal levels and to thoroughly understand the relationship between muscle activity and feedback changes. If resting levels are high, training is directed toward reducing microvolt levels with the help of general relaxation techniques or tone inhibiting postures.

Training strategies can include passively stretching the muscle to a new length. If the passive stretch has raised the microvolt level the patient will try to reduce the level before stretching to a further position. Slow, smooth repetitions can be made while the patient concentrates on keeping microvolt levels below a set threshold. The threshold will initially be high and is lowered as ability to relax and to inhibit unwanted muscle activity improves. Progression is made towards voluntary contraction of the agonist whilst inhibiting antagonist activity using feedback from either one or both target muscles. Increasing the speed of passive and active movement will further challenge the ability to inhibit excessive activity.

As time to reach peak activity and relaxation time of spastic muscles is usually prolonged, the biofeedback can be used to train more efficient on/off timing of the target muscles. Both hypotonic and hypertonic muscles are usually weak, and training to maintain 5-second sustained maximum contractions helps to increase strength.

Number, Frequency, and Length of Training Sessions

The optimal parameters of training must be judged for each patient individually and depend on such things as severity of the dysfunction and fatigue factors. Simple movements such as dorsiflexion required for gait may be more quickly and easily learned than the control of more complex movements of the shoulder or arm as required for manipulation.

Reported studies on hemiplegic subjects give times varying from 10- to 40-minute sessions, daily or two to three times weekly for up to 3 months.

Practice and Repetition

Development of motor skill is accompanied by decreasing levels of coactivation, decreased effort and energy expenditure, and more efficient timing. The key to achieving this is practice and repetition into the millions. In the normal nervous system practice facilitates excitatory neuronal pathways and is accompanied by progressive inhibition of antagonist and synergistic groups. The damaged nervous system probably requires as many or more repetitions to achieve this.

Insufficient repetitions may be the reason why patients who show good initial learning of a movement cannot maintain it and are unable to incorporate it into a functional pattern. There must also be minimal failure in repetitions as only successful repetitions lead to learning. The patient should be successful in reaching the set goal or threshold on at least 75 percent of repetitions.

Precision of practice is also essential for optimal learning. Each repetition should be identical with consistent electrode placement and limb positioning. This requires that the movement chosen be initially a sim-

ple, one joint movement that can be integrated later into a more complex pattern.

Functional movements are multijoint, compound movements and highly automatic. Patients who demonstrate success in learning simple movements under controlled conditions may not be able to incorporate them into functional activity. Use of biofeedback during gait training or manipulation can help in achieving functional carryover. Repetition should occur until movement can be performed without conscious monitoring of component parts and without excessive effort.

Weaning

As the patient acquires better control a weaning process can begin by giving feedback only intermittently during a session to encourage increased awareness of internal physiologic feedback and the sense of effort required to produce the movement. Also the frequency of sessions can be reduced. Once improved control is established, biofeedback should be withdrawn as continued use may not be helpful and may actually interfere with development of the patient's own sensory-motor integration.

The degree to which the learned movement is maintained after withdrawal of the biofeedback depends on recovery of proprioceptive feedback. If this does not occur to a sufficient degree a new motor program will not be established, and although the patient may be able to perform the movement on a conscious level it will not become automatic, will not therefore be functional, and will not be used.

Outcome Measures

The ultimate outcome of rehabilitation incorporating biofeedback varies depending on the severity of dysfunction and degree of recovery of the nervous system. Lower extremity training seems to have better outcome success than upper extremity training. Movements are less complex and the patient must use the leg for gait which is a highly repeatable pattern from stride to stride, whereas upper extremity movement is more complex and less stereotyped. It is also easier to compensate by use of the unaffected arm. Aphasia and proprioceptive impairment may have a greater impact on negative outcome in the upper extremity.

Outcome measures, which may be used to determine treatment effectiveness, include EMG levels as used for baseline assessment (see Table 1), passive and active range of movement, and muscle strength measurements. A broad grading scale might be used, such as: 0=relief from spasticity, 1=assistive capacity, 2=prehension, 3=normal function. Functional outcome measures include manipulative abilities and gait parameters, such as velocity, stride length, or ability to dorsiflex during swing-phase and heel-strike.

EMG biofeedback training is used to help compensate for proprioceptive deficits in patients with hemiplegia and allows precise training of motor control to begin early in the rehabilitation process. It can be of benefit to patients with recent or long-standing hemiplegia and is used with other neuromuscular training techniques to help the patient relearn more normal movement patterns.

SUGGESTED READING

Basmajian JV, ed. Biofeedback—principles and practice for clinicians. Baltimore: Williams & Wilkins, 1979.

Basmajian JV, Blumenstein R. Electrode placement in EMG biofeedback. Baltimore: Williams & Wilkins, 1980.

Hurrel M. Electromyographic feedback in rehabilitation. Physiother 1980; 66:293–298.

Kottke FJ, Halpern D, Eaton JKM, Ozel AT, Burril CA. The training of coordination. Arch Phys Med Rehabil 1978; 59:567–572.

Wolf SL, Baker MP, Kelly JL. EMG biofeedback in stroke: effect of patient characteristics. Arch Phys Med Rehabil 1979; 60:96–102.

Wolf SL, Binder-Macleod SA. Electromyographic biofeedback applications to the hemiplegic patient. Changes in upper extremity neuromuscular and functional status. Phys Ther 1983; 63:1393–1402.

Wolf SL, Binder-Macleod SA. Electromyographic biofeedback applications to the hemiplegic patient. Changes in lower extremity neuromuscular and functional status. Phys Ther 1983; 63:1404–1413.

Wolf SL, Edwards DI, Shutter LA. Concurrent assessment of muscle activity (CAMA). A procedural approach to assess treatment goals. Phys Ther 1986; 66:218–224.

ELECTROPHYSIOLOGIC AGENTS

FUNCTIONAL ELECTRICAL STIMULATION IN SPINAL CORD INJURY

ANNE L. McDERMOTT, B.S., L.P.T.

Treatment of spinal cord injury or disease continues to be one of the greatest challenges facing rehabilitation medicine today. Research in the area of spinal cord repair and regeneration continues to progress but, as yet a cure has not been realized. Until a cure is found, those of us working in rehabilitation must take full advantage of the technological advances going on around us. Functional electrical stimulation represents one such advancing clinical modality.

Electrical stimulation has been used widely in various forms for many years and has seen physical medicine applications to peripheral nerve injuries, phrenic pacing, and management of spasticity and bladder control. However, functional electrical stimulation (FES), as differentially defined by Rancho Los Amigos, refers to the external control of nondenervated, but paretic or paralytic muscles by electrical stimulation to achieve functional and purposeful movement.

Paralysis may be due, in part, to lower motor neuron involvement that can occur at or around the level of the spinal cord injury (SCI) or in low level injuries of the cauda equina and conus medullaris. However, in the majority of traumatic spinal cord injuries, the peripheral nervous system remains essentially intact. Loss of voluntary control may result in rapid and extensive atrophy below the level of the lesion, but in most instances, the reflex arcs (consisting of upper motor neuron, afferent, and efferent nerves, and skeletal muscle) remain viable as functional units. Clinical access through FES to intact but weakened or paralyzed motor units involves the application of electrical current to initiate muscle contraction.

The effectiveness of FES in muscle strengthening has been widely demonstrated both in this country and abroad. This work has been done primarily with hemiplegics and SCI patients and encompasses a full spectrum from surface to implanted electrodes and from simple, single muscle stimulation to sophisticated, multichannel, computer-controlled systems of stimulation.

Much of the recent work with FES focuses on its utilization with chronically paralyzed limbs for the purpose of computer-controlled ambulation or exercise. Although this discussion incorporates many of the same treatment principles, it has a different focus—that of facilitation of *voluntary* movement with an emphasis on early intervention. Thus, the purpose of this chapter is to (1) highlight some factors affecting patient response to FES and to (2) outline an effective treatment protocol for enhancing return of voluntary motor control after SCI.

EVALUATION AND PATIENT SELECTION

One of the primary goals in any SCI rehabilitation program is to improve functional status. An increase in strength is an inherent objective in that process. Traditional means of strengthening include neuromuscular facilitation techniques and modalities such as vibration and biofeedback in addition to conventional progressive resistive exercises. We have found the combination of FES with any or all of these techniques to be particularly effective in many cases.

However, not every SCI patient is an appropriate candidate for FES treatment. Although there are no rigid criteria for patient selection, certain factors, such as time since injury and completeness of injury, have been recognized as reliable prognostic indicators. In general, it appears that those more recently injured and those with incomplete injuries demonstrate greater increases in strength with FES. This is not to say that patients who do not fall into these categories do not benefit to some degree, but rather that the outcome for them cannot be predicted as reliably.

Any prospective FES candidate must first be evaluated to rule out evidence of obvious lower motor neuron involvement. This can be qualitatively done through clinical evaluation of the contractile response that can be achieved with FES or quantitatively through specific diagnostic electroneuromyography (EMG). A clinical evaluation suffices when a strong positive response is noted. The picture becomes less clear, however, when an obvious contraction cannot be elicited, and it is not possible to ascertain conclusively whether the poor response is due to (1) the loss of contractility that accompanies disuse atrophy or (2) the loss of a viable reflex arc secondary to lower motor neuron involvement. When presented with a poor contractile response, the therapist may proceed with a low level FES conditioning program to see if contractility improves over time. However, the optimum course of action is to obtain more definitive EMG studies in order to establish a clearer picture.

Furthermore, the clinical FES evaluation is an important procedural step in that it enables the therapist to identify optimum sites for electrode placement. Motor points can often be located through a quick trial and error procedure that evaluates various electrode placements. A more objective and often more efficient identification of sites can be made with a motor point finder or "tap key" type direct current probe. Appropriate sites should then be documented photographically or with an indelible skin marker for subsequent treatments.

TREATMENT PRINCIPLES

When initiating a clinical program for strengthening with FES, there are several basic principles that should be considered. One such principle is early intervention, which may optimize the benefits of FES. In most cases, our patients begin FES less than 3 months postinjury, although we have also treated patients who are chronically injured, some longer than 8 years. With shorter acute stays and earlier rehabilitation admissions, we are often able to begin FES treatments as early as 2 to 3 weeks post injury. Whenever possible, this early intervention appears optimal in minimizing atrophy, maintaining muscle health, and promoting muscle reeducation as soon as possible.

Additionally, it must be stressed that FES is not a passive modality. Volition is a critical element in maximizing facilitation and neural retraining. For this reason, the patient is instructed to contract actively with the stimulus.

Patients whose injuries are diagnosed as neurologically motor complete receive stimulation to muscle groups one level below the clinical site of their lesion. These guidelines are further delineated in Table 1. Patients with neurologically incomplete injuries receive stimulation to any muscle group demonstrating a reasonable potential for return. When muscles to be stimulated are being identified, priority should generally be directed in a proximal to distal fashion following the progression of natural neurologic recovery. Attention must also be given to maintaining balance between agonist and antagonist muscle groups, especially in the spastic incomplete SCI patient. For example, strengthening the triceps of an incomplete

TABLE 1 Stimulation Site by Neurological Level

Functional Level	Muscles to be Stimulated
C4	Deltoids
	Biceps
C5	Wrist extensors
C6	Triceps
	Wrist flexors
C7	Intrinsic hand muscles
T12	Hip flexors
L2/L3	Knee extensors
L4/L5	Dorsiflexors and evertors
	Hamstrings
	Hip abductors
L5	Gluteals
S1	Plantar flexors

quadriplegic with increased extensor tone may interfere with biceps function.

FES is intended to augment the strengthening program and should be used in conjunction with general principles of progressive resistive exercise using positioning and resistance as indicated. A standard triceps strengthening program might progress as follows:

1. *Gravity eliminated* with powder board and (a) skate—to minimize friction, progressing to exercise with (b) towel—adding weight of hand and arm as resistance until patient can manage additional (c) resistance—adding weights at wrist until able to work
2. *Against gravity* using only inherent weight of arm and hand, progressing to
3. *Against gravity with resistance.*

Lower extremity strengthening progresses in the same manner.

TREATMENT PARAMETERS

Experience has shown that with a treatment of moderate intensity and length (15 to 20 minutes per muscle group) acutely injured individuals benefit optimally from a daily FES program. It should be understood that a daily reevaluation of active movement in the stimulated muscle is also required to minimize the danger of overfatigue of very weak muscle fibers. Ongoing evaluation of the contractile response should also be done during the treatment session to ensure that adequate muscle endurance is present to complete the session. An inability to produce consistent muscle contractions throughout a 15-minute treatment session warrants discontinuing the treatment and maintaining or decreasing "dosage" of subsequent treatments until a full session can be achieved. Progression is indicated only with increased endurance and resistance to fatigue.

Frequency and length of the treatment sessions are two of a number of parameters that can be varied in an effort to individualize an FES program and to optimize patient response. For instance, various wave forms are available within and between different stimulators. Clinical trial of various wave forms is the most effective way of ascertaining which one will elicit the best response in a particular patient.

After an appropriate wave form has been selected, several parameters can be varied to alter the shape and the effectiveness of the stimulus (Fig. 1). One of these variations is the rise time or ramp, which refers to the manner in which the stimulus reaches the set intensity level. Clinically, it is important to use a rise time that is comfortable for the patient, but still quick enough to minimize accommodation. Generally, a 2-second rise time is effective, although a shorter rise time may be more effective with a hypotonic muscle, and a longer rise time may be more appropriate in the presence of marked spasticity.

Pulse width and amplitude can be discussed together since it is their product that determines the total amount of stimulation received at any one time. In a useable range of 40 to 300 microseconds, pulse widths of 250 to 300 microseconds have been found to be clinically most effective and comfortable. With surface FES, the fibers closest to the electrodes are excited first. Increasing the intensity and amplitude excites additional fibers, but the increase must be limited by patient tolerance. In treatment, the goal is to adjust the intensity so as to obtain the strongest consistent contraction within the sensory tolerance. The degree of sensory sparing is therefore an important consideration as it may limit the amount of current that can be applied and subsequently the strength of the contraction that will be elicited. This consideration is compounded in individuals with significant adipose tissue overlying the stimulated muscle since fat markedly increases electrical resistance, but unfortunately

does not shield the cutaneous pain receptors from the increased intensity required to elicit a contraction.

In addition to sensation, fatigue may be a complicating factor that is differentially affected by treatment parameters. The therapist must remember that although FES contractions may look normal, electrically induced contractions differ from voluntary muscle activity. Normally, an energy efficient system prevails where smaller fatigue resistant fibers are selectively recruited before larger, faster fatiguing fibers. Motor units are also fired asynchronously to further minimize fatigue of the muscle as a whole. With surface applied FES, the larger, more superficial and faster fatiguing fibers are stimulated first and then repeatedly. This obviously leads to a quicker depletion of muscle energy stores and subsequently, to faster fatigue. In light of this inherent characteristic of FES, parameters should be adjusted to minimize fatigue as much as possible.

The frequency (i.e., pulses per second [pps]) used must be high enough to obtain muscle tetany in order to realize strengthening benefits. This may occur anywhere within a range of 30 to 100 pps. Clinically a pulse rate of 50 to 100 pps may be perceived as more comfortable, but also results in rapid neuromuscular fatigue. Thus, a frequency in a lower range of 40 to 50 pps is generally indicated.

The duty or "on-off" cycle also influences the rate of fatigue. A 1-second on-1-second off cycle will result in rapid fatigue as compared to a cycle of 1-second on-5-seconds off. The required off or rest time is also dependent on the level at which the muscle is working. Dr. I. M. Kots, recognized for his work with Russian athletes, felt that a 50-second rest period was required for recovery after a 10-second maximal contraction. However, if working at a submaximal training level with an emphasis on endurance, then a shorter rest period may be sufficient. With the SCI population, both strength and endurance need to be incor-

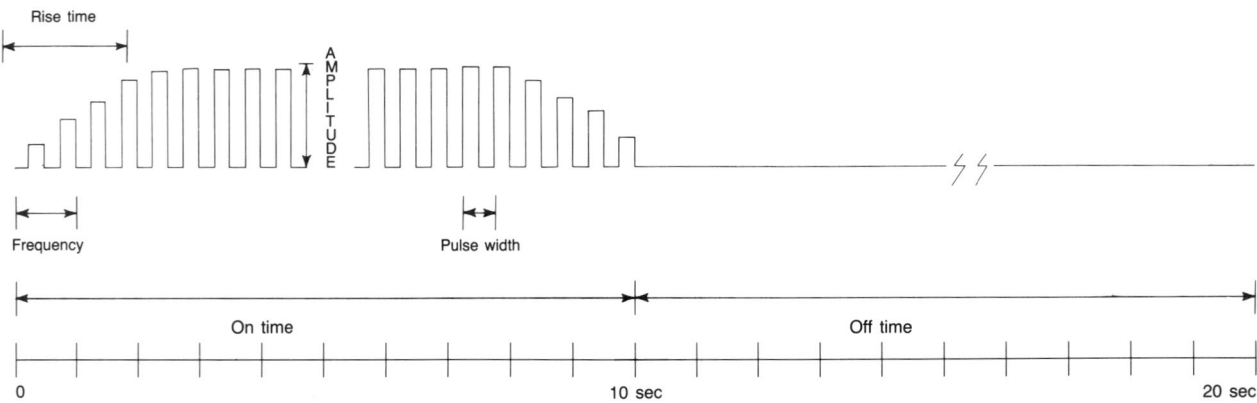

Figure 1   Treatment Parameters for FES.

porated into the training regimen. An FES program designed for this purpose and utilizing a submaximal training level is generally effective with a duty cycle of 10-seconds on-10-seconds off. It may, however, be necessary to begin with a longer rest period that is reduced gradually over a period of several days or weeks as fatigue resistance is built up.

ASSESSMENT

All of the aforementioned parameters are selected in an effort to optimize the return of active range of motion, gross strength, muscle endurance and subsequent function. This is readily evaluated with conventional goniometry, manual muscle testing, and functional assessment. Experience has demonstrated that if response to FES is favorable, benefit from treatment may continue for weeks or months until maximal functional level is reached. At the very least, early FES should deter atrophy and improve the health and contractility of the muscle, thereby maintaining the muscle in a state of readiness in the event that any further neurologic recovery occurs. Intervention affords the therapist an element of control over what has previously been considered a "wait and see" situation.

DISCUSSION

Let us briefly review the most pertinent arguments both for and against the clinical use of FES as a strengthening tool in SCI. There remains some unresolved controversy over the mechanism and potential harm caused by overfatigue of a weakened muscle. As this fatigue could certainly be brought on by electrically-induced contractions, it is always best to proceed cautiously and to monitor muscle endurance closely.

Another issue is our limited ability to quantify the effect that FES plays in recovery of function in the acutely injured SCI patient. With a chronically in-jured, neurologically stable patient, any obvious improvement in strength following initiation of FES treatment could validly be considered a result of FES. In the acutely injured individual, however, this correlation cannot be clearly drawn because of the unpredictable nature of neurologic recovery and the greater possibility of spontaneous return. Therefore, it may be more difficult to justify the time, energy, and perhaps cost involved in providing a full-scale clinical FES program.

On the other hand, FES has clearly been shown to deter muscle atrophy and to maintain the health of muscle tissue, thereby reducing complications of immobility—skin breakdown, osteoporosis, contractures, and circulatory changes. For these reasons alone, FES may be indicated even without guaranteed improvements in strength. However, more important is the knowledge that the risk-benefit issue is on the side of the patient. The benefits just mentioned certainly outweigh the minimal known risks such as temporary reddening of the skin and possible sensory discomfort. For this reason, the investment in a clinical FES program may be worth the peace of mind that comes from knowing that the SCI patient, who stands to benefit with even the smallest improvement in his now limited function, has been given the best chance to do so.

SUGGESTED READING

Benton LA, Baker LL, Bowman BR, Waters RL. Functional electrical stimulation—a practical guide. Downey, CA: Rancho Los Amigos Rehab Eng Ctr, 1981.

Cummings G. Physiological basis of electrical stimulation in skeletal muscle. Certified Athletic Trainers Association Journal 1980; March.

Hambrecht FT, Reswick JB, eds. Functional electrical stimulation—applications in neural prostheses. New York: Marcel Dekker, 1977.

Mortimer JT. Motor Prostheses. In: Brooks VB, ed. Handbook of physiology, section I—the nervous system. Vol. II. Bethesda, MD: American Physiological Society, 1981:155.

Peckham PH, Mortimer JT, Marsolais EB. Upper and lower motor neuron lesions in the upper extremity muscles of tetraplegics. Paraplegia 1976; 14:115–121.

CLINICAL APPLICATIONS OF POSTOPERATIVE TRANSCUTANEOUS ELECTRICAL NERVE STIMULATION

KATHERINE TRIST RICHARDSON, B.Sc., P.T.
LINDA S. MOORE, B.Sc., P.T.

Pain is a sensory phenomenon that can interfere with or inhibit many aspects of postoperative rehabilitation. Using only narcotics to relieve pain can result in unwanted side effects, such as respiratory depression, nausea, and mental clouding. This delays the exercise or ambulation phase. Transcutaneous electrical nerve stimulation (TENS) is being extensively evaluated as an adjunct to medication for pain control in an effort to reduce the need for narcotics. At the same time, researchers report that the use of TENS results in decreased incidence of postoperative complications such as deep vein thrombosis, atelectasis, ileus, and muscle spasm. Patients with fewer complications and decreased pain can be mobilized without delay. This mobilization may result in decreased length of stay in hospital. Effective postoperative pain control without high doses of narcotics is desirable.

Experience suggests that conventional high frequency TENS provides the best control of postoperative pain. This is readily tolerated by patients in acute stages of recovery. Experimentation has demonstrated that the mode of action of low-rate high intensity TENS is through release of endogenous opiates (endorphins). This response is not found with conventional TENS. The exact mechanism by which analgesia is produced from high frequency TENS stimulation is not fully understood. Melzack and Wall suggested the gate control theory to account for pain modulation with TENS. This theory may, in part, explain why TENS diminishes the sensation of pain. Investigators continue to expand on and propose modifications to this theory.

TENS EQUIPMENT FOR POSTOPERATIVE APPLICATION

The TENS Unit and Parameters

The frequency and pulse width can be preset and adjustments made only if the pain cannot be effectively managed by adjusting the amplitude setting. Frequency settings with the range of 70 to 150 pulses per second (pps) and pulse width settings between 60 and 250 microseconds (μsec) are suggested. It has been found that 150 pps and 150 μsec are effective in the management of pain for postoperative orthopaedic patients and these settings have been used as a starting point. The newer model TENS units provide therapists with an accurate readout of the frequency and pulse width settings. Older and less sophisticated TENS units have dials indicating an output ranging from 0 to 10. It is not possible to determine accurately the frequency of a particular setting on the dial. If the range of the TENS unit used is from 10 to 200 pps, it can be assumed that the 0 setting corresponds to 10 pps and that the 10 setting corresponds to 200 pps. It cannot be assumed that a 5 dial setting is equal to 100 pps. This would depend on the output distribution of the machine. Manufacturers can supply a reference chart correlating dial settings with internal output ranges of the unit. For clinical application, it is not essential for frequency or pulse width to be exact. It is more important that output remain within the high frequency range as outlined above. The latest TENS units now offer the option of modulation of frequency and pulse width. The machine automatically varies the output between 50 and 100 percent of the set value. Patients experience a continual fluctuation of the pulse parameters. This added feature may prove to be an effective alternative for postoperative patients.

If possible, the TENS unit chosen for postoperative use should have recessed dials or a protective cover to avoid accidental changes in dial settings. If patients experience a "jolt," they stop using the machine.

Batteries versus Rechargeable Packs

The choice between alkaline or rechargeable batteries is a matter of preference. If a new set of alkaline batteries is provided with each unit, this decreases the frequency of call-backs to check nonoperating machines. Alkaline batteries generally last 4 days with continuous use and longer when used intermittently. It is advisable to leave extra new batteries with patients for periods when therapy services are unavailable.

Electrode Selection

Sterile electrodes have been designed and manufactured specifically for application close to the surgical site. These electrodes do not require the use of gel. They are self-adhering and conform easily to body contours. A variety of sizes are available, but electrodes can also be cut to the appropriate lengths (consult the manufacturer for the minimum effective length before cutting). As the area of analgesia produced is primarily under the electrode, it is desirable to choose large electrodes. When they are to be placed outside the dressing, nonsterile electrodes may be used.

Skin Care

Before applying the electrodes, the skin must be thoroughly rinsed with water or saline solution to remove all traces of the iodine-based surgical skin preparation. This is necessary to achieve optimal electrical interface and avoid chemical or allergic reaction. Normal skin function is compromised during prolonged application of electrodes. Improved contact is achieved if the area is free of body hair.

Ideally, the electrode site should be checked daily for skin irritation; however, the presence of dressings often does not permit this. At dressing changes, lift a corner of the electrode and examine the skin beneath. If skin reaction is evident (slight redness is normal), the electrodes should be reapplied in an alternate location or removed. 3M Tenzcare postoperative sterile electrodes have been used and left in place for up to 4 days without any adverse skin reactions in a population of 75 patients. If there is a history of sensitivity to tape or adhesive, a sample electrode may be applied to similar skin in another location and checked regularly as a control. Patients with marked skin sensitivity should be excluded from TENS treatment.

If patients describe a "burning" or "prickling" sensation, this indicates that the contact at the electrode-skin interface is inadequate and a change of electrodes is required. Stimulation should be discontinued until this can be done.

Electrode Placement

Postoperative pain is not only caused by the incision but by surgical trauma to the other structures in the region. Postoperative TENS electrodes must be placed to provide stimulation to the entire painful area. In abdominal or thoracic surgery, it is desirable to place electrodes parallel to and 5 to 7 cm from the incision. This separation increases the depth of penetration of the stimulation. A second set of electrodes (with a dual channel model) may be placed paravertebrally at the corresponding spinal segments. Electrodes should not be placed over the carotid sinus.

When treating peripheral joints postsurgically, electrodes may be placed parallel to the incision, but medial-lateral or anterior-posterior to the joint. Electrodes should be at least 2 to 3 cm from the incision. Avoid contact with steristrips, if these are being used.

An alternate method is to place the electrodes proximal and distal to the joint. The exact placement may require modification to suit a specific surgery. When a long incision is used, as in anterior cruciate ligament reconstruction or total knee arthroplasty, the trauma to the superficial nerves often results in an area of paresthesia. Electrodes placed over an area of paresthesia are ineffective. The use of long electrodes (i.e., 15 cm) generally ensures that at least part of the electrode is on skin with intact sensation. The general area of paresthesia can be determined by performing sensory testing on a sample of postoperative patients who have had the same surgical procedure. Where the electrodes cannot be placed near the surgical site as in hand or foot reconstruction, modification is required. Adequate treatment can be provided with stimulation along the peripheral nerves that supply the surgical site using electrodes that have been trimmed to conform to the contours of the area.

The positioning of electrodes may be influenced by practicality. Electrode lead wires must extend beyond the dressing so they are accessible in the recovery room and can be connected to the TENS unit leads. If range of motion of the joint is required immediately postoperatively, the electrodes must not interfere with motion or loosen as a result of the movement.

ESTABLISHING A TENS PROTOCOL

Preoperative Patient Information

Patients participating in a TENS program require detailed preoperative instructions. Most patients have fears and anxieties about surgery; the anticipation of pain following surgery is probably the greatest. Therefore, a preoperative interview with each patient is extremely important. This interview should be performed by a qualified health care professional who is familiar with the TENS program.

It is helpful if patients receive written information sheets that outline the purpose of TENS and the operating instructions for the machines. The interview allows the opportunity to review the written material, to assess the patient's level of anxiety about TENS, and to observe initial reactions to the machine. Patients must understand that the health care team is concerned about comfort and safety. It should be stressed that the postoperative treatment is the same with or without the use of TENS. Patients should be aware that some pain from surgery is expected and that appropriate analgesic medication will be prescribed by their physicians and is available upon request. TENS alone, or a combination of TENS and medication, may not relieve all of the pain and this should be discussed. The use of TENS allows patients another pain management tool.

Participants should be allowed to experience the

sensation of TENS preoperatively and to practice adjusting the controls to familiarize themselves with the machine. Electrodes are applied to an area close to the proposed surgery site. The pulse rate and width may be preset and locked.

Patients adjust the amplitude to produce a strong but comfortable "tingling" sensation. They should perceive a deep sensory paresthesia, but should not experience muscle contraction or fasciculation. It is important that patients handle the machine confidently. The amplitude settings they choose should be recorded and used postoperatively as the initial intensity levels. Patients should understand that they may adjust the amplitude and that a higher setting may be required after surgery to provide the necessary analgesic effect. Without this reassurance, many choose to leave the dial at the immediate postoperative setting. Ample time for discussion and questions must be allowed. Patients should be informed that they are free to discontinue the use of TENS at any time.

Postoperative Procedure

The TENS unit is connected to the electrodes in the recovery room and the amplitude adjusted to the setting determined preoperatively. In cases where the surgical area has been locally anaesthetized, or an epidural anaesthetic has been used, initiation of TENS should be postponed until sensation returns. Patients require follow-up when they are alert to readjust the amplitude settings. Slight increases in the pulse width may be necessary if the stimulation is not felt throughout the area of pain. Accommodation to the current within the first 5 to 10 minutes of stimulation necessitates increases in the amplitude. The activity level of the patient also determines the intensity necessary to be effective. Damage to the machine and the leads can be minimized by attaching the unit to patients.

Continuous stimulation is suggested for the first 12 to 24 hours postoperatively. After this time, most patients are alert enough to start an intermittent program. Each session may last up to 1 hour with patients commencing stimulation when a moderate level of pain is perceived. A pain scale (visual analogue or numerical rating) illustrates to patients the meaning of moderate pain. There is often a latent period of approximately 20 minutes before an analgesic effect is experienced. Generally, TENS is continued for 3 to 4 days postsurgery. Postoperative complications may necessitate the discontinuation of TENS.

Implementation of a TENS Program

To establish an effective postoperative TENS program in a hospital, education of all personnel involved is essential. Manufacturers of TENS equipment can be helpful in supplying the information and audio visual aids for staff education. A team leader should be designated to coordinate the program and offer support to staff.

Contraindications

The following contraindicate TENS treatment: (1) presence of cardiac pacemaker; (2) pregnancy; (3) senility; (4) application of electrodes over carotid sinus; and (5) marked sensitivity to adhesive tape.

Indications for the Use of TENS

Postoperative Patients

Success with TENS has been reported on patients after the following surgical procedures:

1. Thoracic and abdominal surgeries: thoracotomy; abdominal aortic repair; gastrectomy; cholecystectomy; colectomy; bilateral nephrectomy and splenectomy; and gynecological laparotomies.
2. Spinal surgery: spinal fusion; laminectomy; discotomy; and chemonucleolysis.
3. Peripheral orthopaedics: arthroplasties of the hip, knee, shoulder, and elbow; podiatric procedures; arthrotomy with menisectomy; anterior and posterior cruciate reconstruction; and rotator cuff repair.
4. During stages of labor and post caesarean section.

To Augment Physiotherapy Treatment

Postoperatively, TENS is effective to decrease pain and to permit early treatment following cast or dressing removal. If TENS is used prior to or during treatment, patients tolerate joint mobilization and contract-relax stretching.

Special Considerations

Patients may meet the surgical requirements for inclusion in a TENS program, but still not be appropriate for this mode of treatment. Other factors that must also be taken into consideration include the following:

1. Patients who, in the preoperative interview, demonstrate a high level of anxiety about the surgery or the use of TENS may not benefit. Without close supervision, these patients have been found to set the TENS units at ineffective intensities or to discontinue its use. However, there is indication that these patients may benefit from the placebo effect of TENS.
2. Patients must be able to understand the pre-

operative instructions and be comfortable with and physically capable of operating the machine independently.

3. Patients whose history includes long-term narcotic use generally report no benefit from TENS.

4. Caution should be used when placing electrodes under a cast. Stimulation should not exceed 4 days, although, in the absence of any history of skin irritation, the electrodes may be left in place for up to 2 to 3 weeks. If stimulation is necessary beyond the fourth day, it is advisable to cut a window in the cast so the electrode site can be checked daily.

EXPECTED OUTCOMES

1. The concept of TENS is generally well received by patients. When offered this tool for pain control, most people agree to participate in a TENS program.

2. Patients usually operate the machine effectively. Compliance is higher when staff offer follow-up support during the postoperative period.

3. Patients like to use TENS. Most state they would use it again for pain control.

4. A decrease in medication requirements may not be evident. Trends indicate that patients use TENS to make the time between medications more tolerable. Some patients extend the length of time between analgesics. The delivery of narcotics is often determined by the health care personnel rather than by the patients' needs. It must be reinforced that not all patients require medication for comfort.

5. The subjective reduction in pain permits earlier mobilization and introduction of other therapeutic techniques.

6. The length of stay in intensive care may be shortened. Overall length of stay in hospital may not be affected. This variable can be influenced by doctors' philosophies of treatment, hospital policy, protocol, and other factors.

7. A decrease in the occurrence of postoperative pulmonary complications and ileus has been documented.

8. The use of TENS may be particularly important in those patients undergoing surgery for the first time as they appear to experience more pain and to request more medication than those with previous surgical experience.

9. TENS is a safe method of treatment with minimal adverse effects.

10. In some cases, patients using TENS at in-effective intensity levels subjectively report decreased pain. This suggests a placebo effect.

In the initial stage of establishing a postoperative TENS program, the coordinator finds this is a time-consuming project. Frustration is encountered when introducing this concept of pain management, but the use of TENS gradually becomes routine. Personnel in direct patient care begin to recognize the effectiveness of TENS. Once all staff are comfortable with TENS, they are able to oversee the patient's use of the machine and, therefore, the coordinator's responsibilities are decreased.

Most surgical patients would benefit from the use of TENS, but the expense in time and machinery may be prohibitive. Few hospitals can afford the luxury of a TENS unit for every surgical patient, and each institution must establish its own guidelines for patient inclusion in these programs. The benefits to patients participating in a well-established postoperative TENS program outweigh the initial expense of the machines and staff time involved in education and coordination.

SUGGESTED READING

Ali J, Yaffe CS, Serrette C. The effect of transcutaneous electric nerve stimulation on postoperative pain and pulmonary function. Surgery 1981; 89:507–512.

Alm WA, Gold ML, Weil LS. Evaluation of transcutaneous electrical nerve stimulation (TENS) in podiatric surgery. J Am Podiatry Assoc 1979; 69:537–541.

Cooperman AM, Hall B, Mikalacki K, Hardy R, Sadar E. Use of transcutaneous electrical stimulation in the control of postoperative pain. Am J Surg 1977; 133:185–187.

Harvie KW. A major advance in the control of postoperative knee pain. Orthopedics 1979; 2:26–27.

Hymes AC, Yonehiro EG, Raab DE, Nelson GD, Printy AL. Electrical surface stimulation for treatment and prevention of ileus and atelectasis. Surgical Forum 1974; 25.

Mannheimer JS, Lampe GN. Clinical transcutaneous electrical nerve stimulation. Philadelphia: FA Davis Company, 1984.

Moore LS, Richardson K. The use of transcutaneous electrical nerve stimulation for the relief of pain following repair of the anterior or posterior cruciate ligament of the knee. 1987; (Unpublished).

Melzack R, Wall PD. Pain mechanisms: a new theory. Science 1965; 150:971–979.

Rooney S, Jain S, Goldiner PL. Effect of transcutaneous nerve stimulation on postoperative pain after thoracotomy. Anesth Analg 1983; 62:1010–1012.

Smith MJ, Hutchins RC, Henenberger D. Transcutaneous neural stimulation use in postoperative knee rehabilitation. Am J Sports Med 1983; 11:75–82.

Solomon RA, Viernstein MC, Long DM. Reduction of postoperative pain and narcotic use by transcutaneous electrical nerve stimulation. Surgery 1980; 87:142–146.

VanderArk GD, McGrath KA. Transcutaneous electrical simulation in treatment of postoperative pain. Am J Surg 1975; 130:338–340.

LOW FREQUENCY CURRENTS: ELECTRICAL STIMULATION OF MUSCLE

KATHERINE A. JOHNSON, B.M.R. (PT)

Electrical muscle stimulation (EMS) is a physical therapy modality used to facilitate muscle strengthening. There are many reported uses of EMS including the treatment of central nervous system muscle weakness; however, this discussion focuses on the utilization of EMS in musculoskeletal conditions.

There is little evidence to support the belief that EMS enhances a strengthening program for normal muscle. Interest in this area arose in the late 1970s when Kots claimed a technique of EMS (commonly referred to as the Russian technique), which utilizes a medium frequency current with a 10-second contraction followed by a 50-second rest repeated ten times per session, could significantly increase muscle strength in athletes. His results remain unsubstantiated. In fact, studies on normal muscle demonstrate that strength gains with exercise alone versus exercise plus EMS are comparable. Therefore, there is no advantage in using EMS to obtain strength gains in normal muscle. Ample evidence is available to demonstrate strength gains when EMS is used as an adjunct to exercise in abnormal or atrophied muscle. Though exercise alone can strengthen muscle in certain abnormal physical conditions, the addition of EMS enhances strength gains. Therefore, the following approaches are based on these premises.

The major criteria for selection for this treatment is muscle weakness; the aim of treatment is to facilitate strengthening of muscle. Acute conditions would be expected to respond more favorably initially due in part to the short length of time of muscle disuse. Examples of such acute conditions include postoperative knee conditions where EMS could be initiated immediately postoperatively providing there is an area for electrode placement (such as windows cut in the cast). Treatment that is frequent and of short duration is desirable since EMS can be used, in conjunction with voluntary isometric contractions, for a joint still in the nonweight-bearing phase of rehabilitation. Such treatment is appropriate for use following upper extremity surgery. There is an emphasis in the literature on strengthening muscle of weight-bearing joints, whereas little information on upper extremity strengthening programs is available. When using the type of low frequency EMS described here, a major criteria in patient selection is that the muscle receiving stimulation must have an intact nerve. Depending on its stage of growth, a regenerating nerve may respond to stimulation. The pulse widths of most commercial units are not long enough to stimulate denervated muscle, and a special machine is required for this function.

Weakness following peripheral nerve disorder, especially when the muscle is unable to move the joint through full range of motion (ROM), is reduced with EMS. In such a circumstance, EMS initially aids in reeducating muscle movement. However, progression of strength gains remains a function of nerve regeneration. Acute muscle weakness, such as occurs post surgery, is usually treated with EMS; however, chronic orthopaedic conditions (such as residual weakness following an old fracture or ligament injury) are suitable. The extent of differences in strength gains that can be achieved in acute versus chronic muscle weakness in orthopaedic conditions is not known.

Any condition that results in muscle disuse or atrophy is suitable for strengthening using EMS, that is with the exception of contraindications. Age is no barrier; however, muscle strength is expected to decrease as a normal part of the aging process—a consideration to be made when treating the elderly. Obesity may present problems since fat acts as an insulator to electrical currents. A higher current amplitude is necessary to achieve contraction, and since this may result in greater discomfort to the patient, the goals of treatment must be well delineated before using EMS.

Stimulation following muscle transplant is most suitable for reeducation provided the appropriate postoperative rest period is followed as outlined by specific technique or surgeon; this can be especially appropriate following hand surgery. The skin over the area of electrode placement must be intact and healthy. Any cuts or abrasions cause discomfort to the patient as these areas have lowered skin resistance.

EMS should be used with discretion when treating children and the therapist must ensure they have a good understanding of what to expect. EMS should not be considered as a priority adjunct treatment in children. If a patient is unable to understand the use of EMS, it may not be of benefit since adequate voluntary effort is required. Patient motivation should be considered a criteria for selection. Since effective EMS requires voluntary effort, the patient must be willing to contract the muscle with the stimulation in order to gain optimal results and time utilization.

Contraindications for the use of EMS are usually relative and not absolute, depending on the area of application. In patients with cardiac pacemakers, treatment should not occur in the thoracic region or, as an extra precaution, in the shoulder region. Areas distant from the chest (i.e., lower extremities) could be treated once the clinician is familiar with the nature of the pacemaker, though if in doubt do not use EMS. Patients with cardiac conditions should receive the same consideration as those with pacemakers. EMS is contraindicated in the area of the abdomen during pregnancy, but can be used on the extremities. EMS should not be used over the carotid sinus in order to avoid effects on blood pressure, and great caution should be used when stimulating anterior neck muscles to avoid muscle spasm and resultant breathing difficulty. Dermatologic conditions may be exacerbated by electrode irritation; therefore, if there is uncertainty, the clinician should reassess alternative treatment methods. Undiagnosed muscle weakness must be considered a contraindication since the clinician cannot develop treatment plans involving EMS in this case, and the weakness may indicate a more serious diagnosis.

There are no definitive treatment techniques for EMS; however, many guidelines are necessary in developing treatment protocols. There are many different types of machines and currents used in treatment, including interferential, high voltage, galvanic, and high frequency; however, evidence suggests that low frequency currents are one of the most appropriate in facilitating muscle strength gains.

Traditional machines for EMS consist of low frequency, low voltage currents. Current intensity ranges from 0 to 100 milliamperes; frequency is usually adjustable at 1 to 100 pulses per second (pps); and width has a range of 50 to 300 microseconds. Current generators are either constant voltage or constant current. The former causes increases in current if impedance is decreased and vice versa while voltage does not change. If impedance is decreased the patient may feel surges of current. The latter type of generator causes voltage increases if impedance is increased and vice versa while current remains constant. Current intensity does not change with changes in impedance, thus avoiding current surges, if a voltage limitation is built in. Most commercial machines are constant-current generators, and use of this type of current generator is recommended.

EMS machines offer either spike or square waves or both. The important aspect of pulse shape is a quick rate of rise. There is no evidence to suggest the superiority of either wave form, and clinically this may be an individual preference depending on the patient's response. Both spike and square waves should be biphasic to allow ion flow in both directions and to prevent unnecessary skin irritation. Most commercial machines do have ion flow in both directions with a large pulse in one direction and a smaller postpulse recovery in the opposite direction. Square waves may be either symmetrical, which delineates an equal shape curve in the positive and negative direction, or asymmetrical. Either form is suitable and neither has been shown to be more effective in producing strength gains. Sinusoidal currents are rarely used for muscle stimulation.

There are no definitive values for pulse frequency, width, or amplitude from studies to date; however, a range of values for clinical use exists. A frequency range of 20 to 50 pps provides a high enough rate to produce muscle tetany, yet not so high as to cause muscle fatigue. Though a muscle contracts at much higher frequencies (some machines up to 100 or 200 pps) this is not the most efficacious method of achieving strength gains. An average frequency at which to commence treatment is 30 pps though this may be adjusted slightly higher or lower in order to achieve muscle tetany.

Pulse width and amplitude are related by the strength-duration curve; a shorter pulse duration requires a greater amplitude (up to a point) to produce a contraction. A pulse width range of 50 to 500 microseconds may be available clinically, but an average width of 300 microseconds is recommended. Generally, a shorter pulse width is more comfortable providing the amplitude necessary for stimulation is not so high as to cause discomfort. Constant current EMS machines have an amplitude range usually of 0 to 100 milliamperes and, depending on patient impedance, the current amplitude (or intensity) will differ. All machines should be examined by electronics personnel prior to clinical use to establish the accuracy of the manufacturers reported parameters and to examine waveforms if not demonstrated elsewhere. An oscilloscope test is necessary as a result of variations in machine output. Once pulse width and frequency are set, amplitude is turned up, and the patient produces a synchronous voluntary contraction when the level of maximum tolerance is reached.

After the above parameters are appropriately set, the therapist must consider duty cycle (current on and off times) and rise and fall times of the current. The pulse rise time, which must be shorter than the on time, provides a gradual rise to peak intensity and is necessary for patient comfort. A 2 to 3 second rise time is sufficient for the purposes of muscle strengthening in orthopaedic conditions, and a current fall time is not necessary. The duty cycle is a 1:2 or 1:3 ratio, for example, an on time of 10 seconds, off time of 20 seconds (1:2) or an on time of 10 seconds, off time of 30 seconds. In the very early stages of rehabilitation, a larger ratio may be necessary to reduce fatigue, especially if the muscle is unable to move the joint throughout its range. As rehabilitation progresses, so does the duty cycle ratio, and though a

1:1 ratio may be used, earlier fatigue may occur as a result.

Though many types and sizes of electrodes are available, carbon impregnated with silicone is now the most common electrode for clinical use. The smaller the electrode, the larger the current density (or concentration of current), therefore care is necessary with very small electrodes to avoid skin burns. If a larger muscle group (e.g., the quadriceps) is the target stimulation area, larger electrodes, in the area of 5 cm × 10 cm, are desired. The standard smaller size electrode, in the area of 5 cm × 5 cm, is more appropriate for shoulder or forearm muscles. These sizes are reduced further for smaller muscles such as those in the hand.

If different size electrodes are used, the concept of current density must be remembered—where more current, and therefore more stimulation, will occur under the smaller electrode. The advantage of using a smaller stimulating electrode is gained when attempting to isolate a smaller muscle with the large electrode acting as the indifferent electrode. The exact electrode size varies considerably depending on both patient and muscle group, therefore an element of trial and error is necessary to achieve the best muscle facilitation.

Machines are single channel or multi-channel with each channel housing a positive and negative electrode. Choice of machine depends on patient use, but a multi-channel machine is more versatile. The small portable EMS machines usually consist of dual channels with one channel used per muscle stimulated. The second channel may be used to facilitate antagonist muscles in conjunction with agonist facilitation or two patients could be treated on two different channels; however, all machine parameters would be identical since most machines do not allow independent control for each channel except amplitude. Two channels can be combined when treating larger muscle groups such as quadriceps. In this case both positive leads are placed in one electrode, whereas each negative lead is attached to a separate electrode. Some EMS machines have built-in timers, others may have a patient-activated switch. The choice depends on assessment of the patient's level of comprehension and motivation.

Two broad categories of electrode placement are unipolar and bipolar. In a unipolar technique one larger electrode is placed over the nerve trunk, whereas the smaller electrode, usually the cathode is over the muscle to be stimulated, however, this may vary in some individuals. A bipolar technique consists of placement of both electrodes over the muscle to be stimulated. Both placements are suitable as evidence does not indicate a greater advantage of either. Each of these requires the use of one channel.

Electrodes in close proximity tend to stimulate only the surface of the skin and as distance is increased between electrodes, the current penetrates deeper. Larger muscle groups such as the quadriceps may respond better to a unipolar technique since longer distance between electrodes allows a deeper current penetration, thus facilitating greater muscle area. The clinician should try both approaches before choosing the most appropriate; choice will be based on subjective response. A minimal distance of 3 to 6 cm is recommended for this purpose.

Before applying electrodes, the skin must be cleansed and if necessary shaved to reduce impedance. Clean carbon electrodes are used only with an electroconductive gel. This obtains the best conductivity and reduces electrode-skin impedance, which minimizes skin irritation. There are many forms of gel including pre-gelled electrodes, karaya, tac gel, and standard gel some of which require tape for fixation. Choice depends on the clinical setting and therapist preference, however, standard gel and tape is most cost effective in a busy clinical practice.

The mechanism of providing muscle stimulation through low frequency EMS is by stimulation of peripheral nerves, provided the amplitude of the current is sufficient to stimulate the nerve. Nerve stimulation produces muscle contraction, and because of the "all or none" principle, increasing stimulation intensity will cause a greater number of fibers to contract.

There are a number of factors contributing towards the results of EMS use including motivation, treatment duration, and frequency. Patient motivation, specifically the exertion of a maximal voluntary muscle contraction during current application, is necessary. Isolated EMS in the absence of voluntary effort does not produce strength gains.

The duration of each EMS treatment session is usually an average of 20 minutes. Muscle weakness resulting from nerve pathology where contraction is present but very weak would best receive EMS for short periods frequently through the day. A patient receiving EMS towards the end of a rehabilitation program may have stimulation of 30 minutes or longer, however, 20 minutes is often a feasible clinical time.

Recommended training frequency is a minimum of three times per week. Since different diagnoses and machine parameters are described in the literature it is often difficult to compare training frequencies directly. Training results are also a function of the amount of resistance applied to the contracting muscle. Once a muscle is able to move a joint fully against gravity, the therapist must consider the application of resistance, either isometric, isotonic, or isokinetic, concurrent with use of EMS. At this stage, progressive resistance supplemented by EMS is necessary for achieving strength gains.

The therapeutic response is assessed at time of application to determine that proper machine parameters and electrode placement have been utilized. As current amplitude is increased a tetanic muscle contraction is apparent. If the muscle only twitches, an increase in frequency may be necessary. As the contraction increases, the patient is instructed to indicate when the sensation is maximally tolerable. Once this point is reached, resistance, if indicated, is added, and treatment is initiated.

Long-term therapeutic response involves assessment of muscle strength since the function of EMS is to enhance this response. Ideally, an objective measure of muscle strength such as a myometer or isokinetic dynamometer should be used. This type of measure contributes to the decision of when to discontinue EMS since it may not be practical to continue use of EMS until full strength is obtained.

The side effects of EMS are minimized through an understanding of proper technique. Skin irritation or burn is prevented by proper skin preparation, the use of electroconductive gel, nonallergic adhesive tape, proper electrode size and frequent change of electrode site. Muscle ache from fatigue is prevented through proper frequency range and treatment duration. Current surges are avoidable with a constant-current stimulator and avoidance of changing electrode-skin contact while the EMS machine is operational.

The major advantage of EMS as an adjunct to strengthening is that it can be used at any phase of muscle rehabilitation—from early postsurgery to minimize muscle atrophy while the limb is immobilized, until the patient has almost full strength gains. Low frequency EMS machines are portable and simple to use, thereby facilitating patient home use when appropriate. The most important advantage of EMS is the ability to strengthen weak or atrophied muscles effectively when used as an adjunct to voluntary movement.

SUGGESTED READING

Benton LA, Baker LL, Bodman BR, Waters RL. Functional electrical stimulation: a practical guide. 2nd ed. Downey, CA: Rancho Los Amigos Hospital, 1981.

Kottke FJ, Stillwell AK, Lehmann JF. Krusen's handbook of physical medicine and rehabilitation. 3rd ed. WB Saunders, 1982.

Kramer JF, Mendryk SW. Electrical stimulation as a strength improvement technique: a review. J Orthop Sports Phys Ther 1982; 2(4):91–98.

Lloyd T, DeDomenico G, Strauss GR, Singer K. A review of the use of electro-motor stimulation in human muscles. Aust J Physio 1986; 32(1):18–30.

Wolf SL, ed. Electrotherapy: clinics in physical therapy. Vol. 2. New York: Churchill Livingstone, 1981.

CURRENT APPLICATION OF ULTRAVIOLET LIGHT

JOYCE L. MacKINNON, Ed.D., M.P.T.

Ultraviolet light has long been used as a therapeutic modality. Initially, patients were exposed to sunlight to obtain the desired effects and, even today in some underdeveloped countries, sunlight is still used as an ultraviolet modality. This method of using the sun's rays for their beneficial effects is referred to as heliotherapy.

Direct sunlight is a mixture of infrared and ultraviolet radiation, with approximately 60 percent of the radiation in the infrared range and the remainder in the visible and ultraviolet range. Only approximately 0.1 percent of the latter are ultraviolet wavelengths in the therapeutic range. The intensity of the radiation is variable and is affected by the distance between the earth and the sun, the amount of dust and other particles in the atmosphere, the time of day, and the altitude.

When heliotherapy is used as a therapeutic modality, the main risk to a patient is that of overexposure. A patient should be monitored for an increase in oral temperature above 98.6° F and an increased pulse rate. Complaints of headache, nausea, or fatigue may be signs of overexposure. However, due to the difficulty of determining accurate absorption of the sun's ultraviolet rays and the many variables that can impact on the use of heliotherapy as a therapeutic modality, artificial sources of ultraviolet light are now usually used to provide ultraviolet therapy.

Artificial light therapy was first introduced in 1893 by Neils Finsen. He was able to demonstrate that certain stimulating and bactericidal effects were produced with ultraviolet rays from artificial sources. Examples of these artificial light sources that are in use today include the full-body, quartz mercury arc ultraviolet lamp and the spot quartz ultraviolet lamp.

PHYSICAL PRINCIPLES

Ultraviolet light is produced in the range of 136 to 3,900 A. This range is divided into two segments, a far range of 136 to 2,900 A and a near range of 2,900 to 3,900 A. Since various wavelengths have different effects, a physical therapist must know the wavelength that a particular lamp emits. For example,

germicidal effects can best be obtained with a wavelength of approximately 2,535 A, whereas erythema is produced between 2,500 and 3,000 A. To aid in the formation of vitamin D, the wavelength should be shorter than 3,150 A; a feeling of well-being appears to be generated by wavelengths between 2,800 and 3,200 A. The therapeutic effects of general ultraviolet light exposure are as follows: (1) aids in the formation of vitamin D; (2) improves resistance to infection; (3) increases skin pigmentation and condition; and (4) provides a general tonic effect. The therapeutic effects of local ultraviolet light exposure are as follows: (1) provides counter-irritation for the reduction of pain; (2) encourages desquamation, which is useful in treating skin conditions such as acne; (3) increases blood supply and nutrients; (4) stimulates the growth of epidermis; (5) destroys bacteria and increases the production of white blood cells; (6) increases the resistance of the skin to infection; and (7) destroys tissue.

Two physics laws should be kept in mind when treating a patient with ultraviolet light. The Grotthus law states that rays must be absorbed in order for their effects to be produced. The effects are produced at the point of absorption, and maximum absorption occurs when the rays are at a 90 degree angle to the treatment surface. Therefore, a therapist needs to ensure that the ultraviolet rays being emitted from the source are striking the skin surface at a 90 degree angle. The second physics law of importance to therapists using ultraviolet radiation is the inverse square law. This law states that the intensity of the ray varies inversely with the square of the distances from the source. For example, if a lamp is held 2 in from a patient's skin and is then moved closer to the skin surface by 1 in, the intensity of the rays is increased by a factor of four.

PRECAUTIONS

Some dangers are associated with the use of ultraviolet light therapy, and some precautions should be taken for the safety of both patient and therapist. Ultraviolet light can damage the eye; the condition that occurs is usually conjunctivitis, which manifests itself by a gritty feeling and by tearing. The possibility of eye damage can be eliminated if the patient's eyes are covered with moistened cotton pads and if the therapist wears goggles when treatment is being administered. There are certain agents that increase sensitivity to ultraviolet radiation, such as recent exposure to infrared treatment, certain foods such as eggs and lobster, recent multiple radiographic exposure, and drugs such as tetracycline, insulin, thyroid hormone, and gold therapy. There are individuals who are inherently sensitive to ultraviolet radiation. Prior to treatment, patients should be questioned to ascertain possible ultraviolet radiation sensitivity. If predisposition to sensitivity is suspected, another treatment may be chosen or a reduced dosage of ultraviolet radiation with careful patient monitoring may be considered.

There are several general facts about ultraviolet lamps that therapists should know. The burners in the lamps deteriorate with use, and therefore the amount of radiation being emitted needs to be monitored periodically. One method of monitoring involves obtaining a minimal erythemal dose (MED) level for each lamp. The way in which an MED is obtained for a lamp or for a patient is explained later in the chapter. Another fact concerning lamps is that the lamp's burner lights up as soon as the current is turned on, but a warmup period of several minutes is required before the lamp emits maximum radiation. When the lamp is turned off, the burner must cool before the lamp lights again. Approximately 10 minutes is required for this cooldown. Therefore, sequential patients are to be treated, the therapist may want to leave the lamp on between treatments, with the ultraviolet source covered by shutters or a hood. Quartz is sensitive to skin surface oils; therefore, the burner should not be touched with fingers as the lamp is being cleaned, since this impairs the lamp's efficiency.

TREATMENT

Before starting ultraviolet treatment on a patient, an MED should be obtained. This should be done for each patient, but some clinicians calculate an MED for a particular ultraviolet lamp and then use that calculation to determine a patient's initial ultraviolet exposure. If a lamp MED is calculated in lieu of an individual patient's MED, the procedure should be performed using an individual who is light-skinned. It is better to err on the side of caution rather than expose a patient to too much ultraviolet radiation.

There are several methods that may be used to determine a patient's MED, (that is, the time of exposure required to produce a minimal visible erythema that disappears in 12 to 48 hours). Small areas of skin surface are exposed to ultraviolet light for 15, 30, 45, or 60 seconds, respectively. The patient is then asked to return to the clinic the following day, and the site that appears faintly red is considered the MED.

Depending on the purpose of the ultraviolet light treatment, a physical therapist may want a patient to receive a first, second, third, or fourth degree erythema. The erythema obtained is visible 1 to 8 hours after exposure rather than immediately after; this fact is important to remember so that a therapist does not overexpose a patient in an attempt to obtain the desired effect immediately.

A first degree exposure, chosen for its tonic effect, appears as a faint reddening, which fades in 12 to 48 hours. A second degree exposure, chosen for its stimulative effect, is equivalent to a mild sunburn. The skin reddening is plainly visible. There is usually some slight desquamation and pigmentation. Sometimes the patient notices a slight itching. The reddening subsides in 3 to 4 days. A third degree exposure, chosen for its counterirritant effects, resembles a severe sunburn. There is intense reddening, slight edema, desquamation, and pigmentation. The reddening subsides in about a week. A fourth degree exposure, chosen for its destructive and bactericidal effects, results in severe reddening of the skin. There is usually exudation and blistering. The visible effects persist for several days, and the exposure leaves a deep pigmentation. Ultraviolet rays only penetrate 1 to 2 cm; thus, the bactericidal effect is limited by the shallowness of penetration.

When treating a patient using a full-body, quartz mercury arc ultraviolet lamp, the principle factors affecting dosage are the distance of the lamp from the skin surface and the length of exposure. The lamp is usually positioned 76 cm (30 in) from the most elevated body part to be exposed; areas not to be treated are covered. The lamp should be at a right angle to the skin surface to be treated. After obtaining a patient's MED (or using the lamp's MED), dosage is usually increased 15 seconds per treatment, although patients can be progressed more rapidly than this, depending on tolerance to ultraviolet light and desired treatment outcome. A suggested frequency of treatment is as follows: (1) for first degree erythema, treat daily or every other day; (2) for second degree erythema, treat every second or third day; (3) for third degree erythema, treat once a week and (4) for fourth degree erythema, treat every 10 days to 2 weeks. If a treatment is missed, do not increase the dosage at the next treatment, but use the same dosage as was last administered. When skin is inflamed or if eruptions are present, the surface is more resistant to ultraviolet radiation and can therefore tolerate a higher dosage than can surrounding skin. Consequently, the therapist must make sure that the surrounding skin surfaces, which are not to receive treatment, are well covered.

In general, ultraviolet light promotes healing, improves skin condition, and improves general health and resistance. It may be used for a number of dermatologic conditions, such as psoriasis, acne, and pityriasis when improvement in skin condition is desired. Ultraviolet light can be used on open wounds and ulcerations to promote healing and to markedly reduce the presence of bacteria. It can be used in the presence of calcium deficiency to activate vitamin D.

Treatment protocol starts with knowing the diagnosis and the reason for choosing ultraviolet light treatment. At the initial appointment, using the method outlined earlier in the chapter, the patient is exposed to varying dosages of ultraviolet light so as to determine the MED. The patient should be instructed to return to the clinic within 24 hours so that the MED may be noted. If the patient cannot return the next day, the therapist may describe the skin reaction to be noted, and ask the patient to do so. However, some patients seem to belong to the "more is better" school of thought and report a longer exposure time than was needed to obtain the MED.

During the first and subsequent treatments, exposure time, distance of ultraviolet source from the skin surface, and treatment date should be recorded. Since the ultraviolet lamp needs to warm up before actual treatment can begin, it usually makes sense to get the patient into position, move the lamp into position and measure 76 cm (30 in) from the closest point of skin surface to be exposed to the lamp, and then move the lamp out of the way and turn it on to allow the burner to warm up. If the lamp remains situated over the patient as treatment preparations proceed, there is the possibility of ultraviolet leakage due to improperly closed shutters, and particular danger to the eyes of the patient, especially if the patient is positioned supine and is looking up at the lamp. In addition, sometimes a therapist has a tendency to glance up frequently at the lamp to see if it is on, and this exposes the therapist's eyes to danger. Finally, if the lamp is positioned over the patient as treatment preparations proceed, it hampers movement and might become a hazard.

Treatment should be explained to the patient. The area to be treated should be inspected for any unusual coloration or features and should be cleaned if necessary. For instance, a patient may have applied body lotion or moisturizer earlier in the day. These substances reduce ultraviolet light penetration and therefore need to be removed.

Only the area to be treated should be exposed to the ultraviolet light. Surrounding areas should be draped. This is of particular importance when the area to be treated is more resistant to ultraviolet radiation than the surrounding skin surfaces. The patient's eyes should be covered with moist cotton pads. Once the patient is positioned, he or she should be cautioned not to move once treatment has started.

After the therapist has put on protective goggles, the lamp should be moved into place for treatment. The distance from lamp to skin surface should again be measured. It is important that the lamp be positioned so that the ultraviolet rays strike the skin surface at a right angle. When the equipment and patient are in the proper position, the shutters of the lamp should be opened and treatment timing should begin.

When the shutters are being opened, care should be taken not to tilt the lamp.

Treatment should be terminated when the appropriate amount of time has elapsed. At that time, the shutters should be closed immediately. If the lamp is to be used for a subsequent patient treatment, it may be left on and pushed out of the way. If the lamp is not needed within the next 15 minutes, then it should be turned off.

With subsequent patient treatments, ask about any unusual reactions that may have been noticed following ultraviolet light exposure. Observe the skin surface to be treated in addition to the surrounding area, noting any adverse reaction. For example, some skin surfaces may appear more reddened than others, thus indicating that, for some reason, they are either receiving a larger dose of ultraviolet radiation as compared to the surrounding skin, or the area perhaps is more sensitive to the effects of the radiation. Often, these areas are slightly raised bony prominences, such as the patella or coccyx region, and may need to be covered during all or part of the next treatment.

LOCAL APPLICATION

When only a small body surface area is to be treated with ultraviolet radiation, it may be more efficient to use a spot quartz ultraviolet lamp rather than a full-body lamp. Since it is portable, the spot quartz lamp is especially convenient when treating patients at home or in the hospital. The lamp is usually used when a bactericidal effect is desired, such as when treating open wounds or skin ulcerations. Also, when treating patients with ulcerations the ultraviolet radiation increases the blood supply and nutrients to the area, thereby aiding the healing process. Rather than positioning the spot quartz lamp at some distance from the patients's skin, the lamp may actually touch the skin or be positioned $2^1/_2$ cm (1 in) from the surface to be treated. At contact, a first degree erythema is produced in 6 seconds; with the lamp held $2^1/_2$ cm (1 in) from the body surface, a first degree erythema is produced in 12 seconds. As when using the full body ultraviolet lamp, care must be taken to cover the surrounding body surfaces that would otherwise be exposed to the light, but are not in need of treatment. Other precautions previously mentioned also apply; the lamp operator should not look directly at the ultraviolet light being emitted and should wear goggles during treatment, the patient's eyes should be protected, and questions should be asked to determine ultraviolet radiation sensitivity, whether inherent or as a result of contact or ingestion of certain substances. Remember to clean the skin surface to be treated, and to remove any dressings, including transparent ones. Allow several minutes for the lamp to stabilize before beginning treatment. Record date of treatment, exposure time, and any adverse reactions. When using ultraviolet treatment for its bactericidal effects, the patient can be treated every other day, increasing the dosage one MED per treatment, and continuing treatment until the wound closes or until the area is free of infection. With patients who are on long-term ultraviolet light treatment, such as those with large ulcerations, the treatment dose is stabilized at 3 minutes once that dosage is reached. Having cultures taken from the wound makes the decision of when to discontinue treatment more objective than if only visual or olfactory cues are relied upon.

Ultraviolet light therapy is of value in the treatment of ulcerations, open wounds and with certain dermatologic conditions. The ulcerations and open wounds respond well to therapy. Usually complete closure is obtained, or, in the case of deep ulcerations, infection is reduced to the point where surgical closure can occur with good results. Patients with lo-

calized dermatologic conditions respond well to therapy in a relatively short time period (2 to 3 weeks).

Ultraviolet light is an effective treatment modality when used for appropriate conditions. Care must be taken to provide a therapeutic patient dosage: although the patient should not be exposed to too much ultraviolet radiation, enough radiation must be received for treatment to be effective. Precautions should be remembered and taken into account when providing treatment.

SUGGESTED READING

Griffin JE, Karselis TC. Physical agents for physical therapists. Springfield, IL: Charles C. Thomas, 1978.

Light S, ed. Therapeutic electricity and ultraviolet radiation. Baltimore: Wavery Press, 1967.

MacKinnon JL. Ultraviolet light treatment of a patient with Pityriasis Lichenoides et Varioliformis Acuta (Mucha-Habermann disease). Phys Ther 1986; 66(10):1542–1543.

INTERFERENTIAL CURRENT THERAPY

SANDY RENNIE, M.Sc., B.P.T.

PHYSICS

Interferential current therapy was originally developed in Vienna, Austria in the mid 1950s by Dr. Hans Nemec. The name interferential stems from the concept of two currents "interfering" with each other. The two currents that interfere with each other are medium frequency currents (3,000 to 6,000 Hz), and the result of their interference is a low frequency (1 to 200 Hz) current that is produced in the subcutaneous tissues. Medium frequency currents are introduced in the tissues via low frequency current in order to overcome the naturally high impedance of the skin. When the frequency of an alternating current is increased, the capacitive reactance (high impedance) of the body tissues falls. Thus, at 4,000 Hz, the effective skin impedance may be as low as 40 ohms per 100 cm^2, as opposed to a 3,000 ohm resistance per 100 cm^2 for a 50 Hz current. Such a low skin impedance with a medium frequency current means the voltage required to produce stimulation of the tissues is considerably less than with low frequency currents. The patient experiences less cutaneous sensation and the current feels more comfortable.

Current Format

Figure 1 shows two medium frequency currents, one at 4,000 Hz and one at 4,100 Hz. When these two currents are superimposed on one another (A), the two positive half cycles of the current are added together to produce an increased positive amplitude of the resultant wave. In the next half cycle (B), the two negative half cycles again summate, giving an increased amplitude in the opposite direction.

Owing to the slight difference in frequency, there comes a point (C) where one half cycle is positive in direction, and the other equal and opposite in a negative direction. At this point, the resultant current is zero. The result of the blending or interfering of these two medium frequency currents is a low frequency current where there is a variable increase and decrease in amplitude (intensity) occurring in rhythmic manner. This is described as the "beating" of the two cur-

rents. The beat frequency is the number of times in each second that the current rises in intensity to its maximum and falls away to minimum value. The beat frequency in Hertz is simply the difference in frequency between the two medium frequency currents (i.e., 4,100 Hz − 4,100 Hz = 100 Hz).

The "envelope" effect (dotted line) shows the shape of the beat frequency cycle. The number of these envelopes per second represents the beat frequency of the current. Each envelope has only one cycle of peak intensity—an intensity strong enough to cause stimulation of the tissues. The probable "effective" stimulus characteristics are found in Figure 2. The rectangular area represents the effective stimulus—in the sense that the amplitude of the signal on either side of this area is likely to be insufficient to produce effective stimulation of the tissues. At a frequency of 4,000 Hz, the pulse duration of each half cycle is about 125 μsec. The first half cycle is probably the effective stimulus since the second phase occurs at a time when the neurons cannot respond because of their refractory period.

The beat frequency can be delivered in a constant or variable mode. In the constant mode, there is a constant difference between the two medium frequency currents, and this results in a constant beat frequency. Almost all commercially available interferential machines allow the physical therapist to choose any constant frequency between 1 and 100 Hz or higher.

In the variable mode, the difference between the two circuits is always changing, and in this way, there is a rhythmic change in beat frequency. In most interferential machines, this rhythmic change in beat frequency can be controlled throughout a number of ranges, usually a low range (1 to 10 Hz and back to 1 Hz), full range (1 to 100 Hz and back to 1 Hz), and a high range (80 to 100 Hz and back to 80 Hz). At present, there is little evidence to favor the use of either constant or variable mode of operation. However, there is likely less accommodation of the sensory nerves to a variable beat frequency, and thus it may be more effective than the constant beat frequency.

Localization with Interferential Currents

Interferential currents are normally applied with two pairs of electrodes. This has one principal advantage over a 50 Hz sinusoidal waveform, that being the depth of the stimulation produced. Maximum stimulation is not produced near the electrodes, but in an area near the geometric center of the four-elec-

196

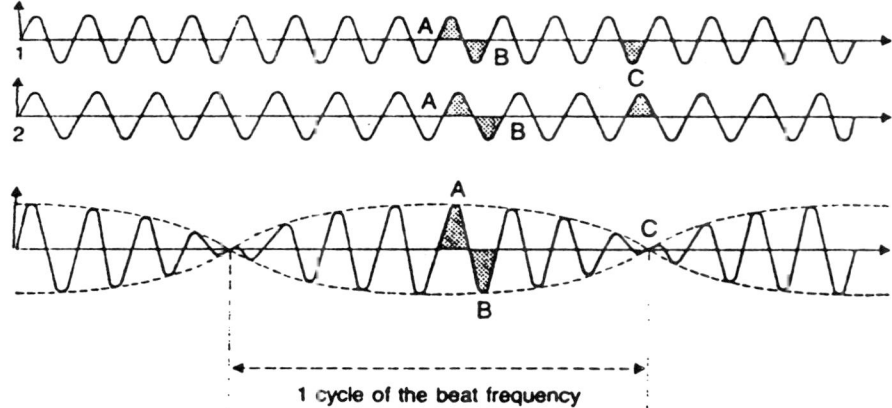

Figure 1 Diagrammatic representation of interferential current. (From De Domenico G. Basic guidelines for interferential therapy. Ryde, Australia: Theramed Books, 1981:6.)

trode arrangement. Figure 3 (A, B, and C) demonstrates the difference in depth penetration of three current formats.

The main interference effect occurs in those areas bounded by the "clover-leaf" shaded middle portion as shown in Figure 4. Current flow is not uniform over the area treated since the tissues of the body are not homogeneous. The maximum interference effect is felt in the directions shown by the arrows (see Figure 4).

Certain manufacturers provide their interferential machines with a method of increasing the area of maximum stimulation. This is often called the "vector

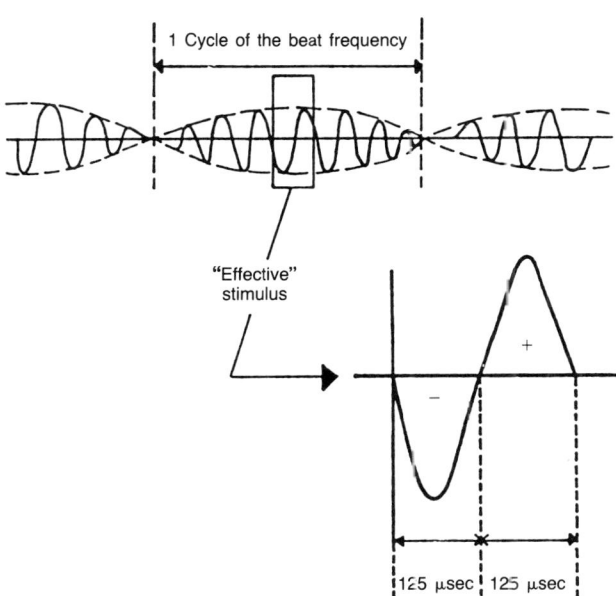

Figure 2 Probable "effective" stimulus characteristics. (From De Domenico G. Pain relief with interferential therapy. Aust J Physio 1982; 28(3):17.)

sweep." By alternately modulating the intensity of each interferential channel, the current pattern in the tissues is "moved" 45 degrees, thus providing a more uniform total distribution of the interferential current in the tissues.

PHYSIOLOGIC AND THERAPEUTIC EFFECTS

The physiologic and therapeutic effects of interferential current therapy originally were based on manufacturer's information brochures, and although there is now published information regarding these effects, more clinical and experimental research is required to determine the mechanism of these effects.

The factors affecting the physiologic and therapeutic effects include the following:

1. Frequency range selected
2. Use of constant or variable frequency
3. Intensity of current
4. Circuit intensity equalization
5. Accuracy of electrode placement
6. Patency of circulation
7. Intact cutaneous neurologic sensation
8. Knowledge of underlying pathophysiology in relation to the desired effect.

Physiologic Effects

The physiologic effects of interferential current are summarized as follows:

1. Depression of action of the sympathetic nervous system
2. Stimulation of large diameter sensory (mechanoreceptor) nerve fibers
3. Stimulation of intact motor nerves
4. Increased vasodilatation (decrease in sympathetic tone of vessels)

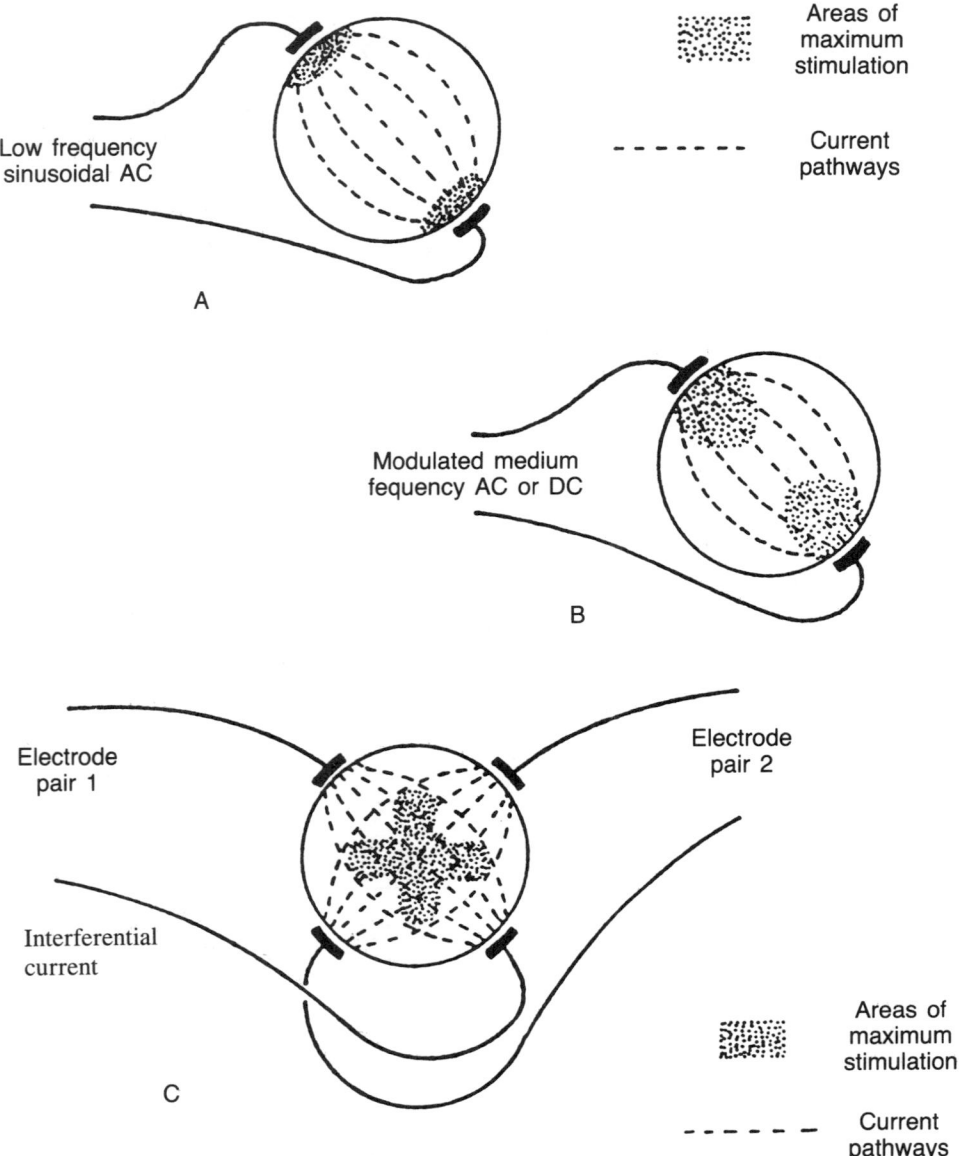

Figure 3 Diagrammatic comparison of the effective penetration of low frequency, medium frequency, and interferential currents. (From Ward A. Electricity, fields and waves in therapy. Marrickville, Australia; Science Press 97, 101.)

5. Stimulation of cellular processes and alteration of cell membrane permeability.

Therapeutic Effects

The therapeutic effects of interferential current are summarized as follows:

1. Decrease in pain
2. Decrease in swelling and inflammation
3. Increase in muscle contraction
4. Increase in local (and remote) circulation

5. Facilitation of healing (bone and soft tissue)
6. Decrease in stress incontinence and urinary frequency.

Suggested Mechanisms for Therapeutic Effects

Decrease in Pain

1. Activation of pain-gating mechanism
2. Stimulation of descending pain suppression system
3. Direct block of nociceptive activity

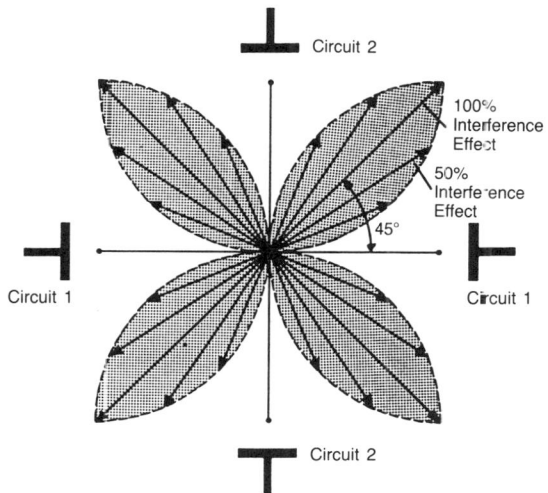

Figure 4 The interferential field. (From De Domenico G. Basic guidelines for interferential therapy, 11.)

4. Removal from damaged area of substances which stimulate nerve endings
5. Placebo effect

Decrease in Swelling and Inflammation

1. Increase in removal of debris and waste products through increased local circulation
2. Increase of cell membrane permeability allowing more extra-cellular fluid to be resorbed
3. Activation of motor nerves will bring about some muscle contraction, enhancing muscle pump effect

Increase in Muscle Contraction

1. Direct stimulation of motor nerves

Increase in Local and Remote Circulation

1. Stimulation of autonomic nervous system (depression of sympathetic activity) leading to vasodilatation in a local area
2. Stimulation of sympathetic ganglia over appropriate area of spine may produce vasodilatation in limbs

Facilitation of Tissue Healing

1. Local increase in circulation, bringing oxygen and foodstuffs, and removing debris and waste products
2. Increase in cell membrane permeability thus decreasing local inflammation, allowing natural healing process to continue
3. Promotes callus formation across fracture site

Decrease in Stress Incontinence and Urinary Frequency

1. Depression of both sympathetic and parasympathetic activity, thus removing "autonomic" bladder emptying reflexes
2. Stimulation of the pelvic floor muscles to assist in control of micturition

Suggested Treatment Parameters

For Pain Relief
Constant Frequencies. At or above 100 Hz (gate control).
Variable Frequencies. 80 to 200 Hz (gate control, but less accommodation); 1 to 200 Hz (increase removal of substances stimulating pain fibers).
Decrease in Swelling and Inflammation
Constant Frequencies. At or above 100 Hz (decreased sympathetic system activity); between 1 and 50 Hz (muscle contraction—muscle pump effect).
Variable Frequencies. 1 to 200 Hz (increased lymphatic and venous blood flow; increased cell permeability); 1 to 10 Hz (increased cell membrane permeability); 1 to 100 Hz (as above, plus increase in vasodilatation).
Increase in Muscle Contraction
Constant Frequencies. Between 20 and 50 Hz (most effective)—stimulates motor nerves at frequency rate within tetany range; between 1 and 10 Hz (fasciculation type contractions).
NB: Even high frequencies (100 Hz) may result in motor contraction if intensity high enough.
Increase in Local Circulation
Variable Frequencies. Between 1 and 200 Hz (vasodilatation); between 20 and 50 Hz (motor nerve stimulation, thus enhancing circulation through muscle pump).
Facilitation of Healing Process
Constant Frequencies. Between 10 and 20 Hz (bone healing).
Variable Frequencies. 1 to 100 Hz (increased blood flow, increased cell membrane permeability, increased foodstuffs, increased waste product and debris removal).
Decrease in Stress Incontinence and Urinary Frequency
Variable Frequencies. 0 to 100 Hz—up to 15 minutes maximum; 10 to 100 Hz—stimulates pelvic floor muscles and autonomic nerves are inhibited; 80 to 100 Hz for 10 minutes—depression of automatic nerve activity.

Dosage

Interferential currents are generally quite comfortable, and the patient should find the sensation to be a pleasant buzzing. The treatment time is arbitrary,

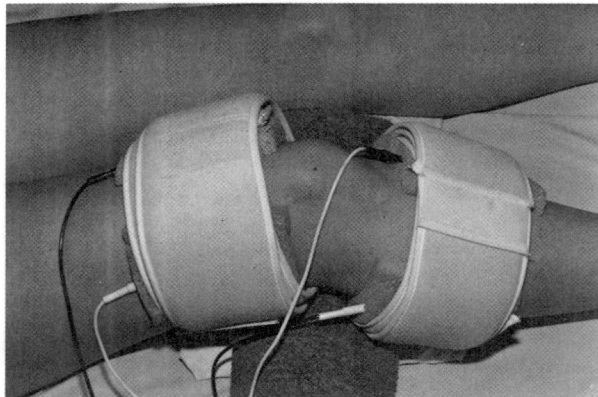

Figure 5   Interferential treatment of the knee region using four plate electrodes.

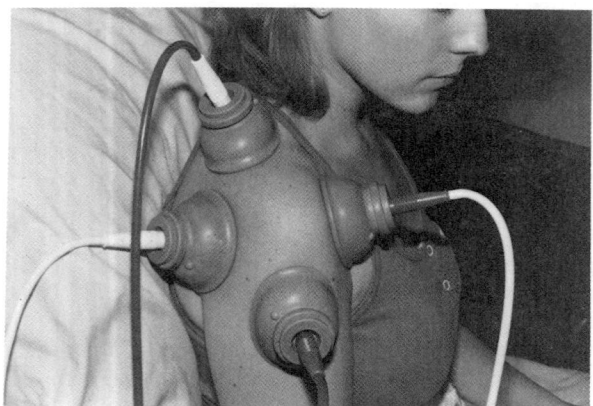

Figure 6   Interferential treatment of the lateral aspect of the shoulder region using four suction electrodes.

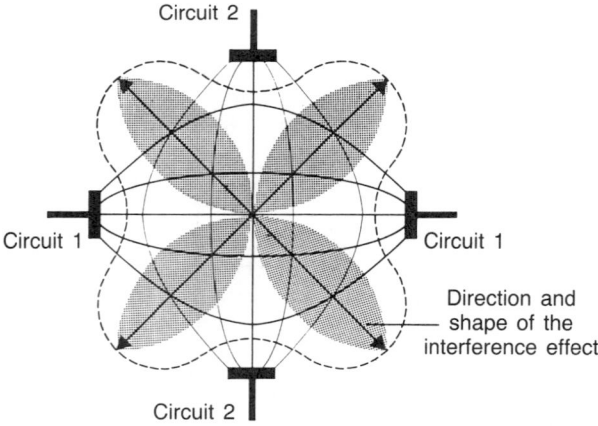

Figure 7   Current pathways and direction and shape of interference effect with interferential therapy. (From De Domenico G. Basic guidelines for interferential therapy, 9.)

and varies from 10 to 30 minutes per treatment session, depending upon the presenting signs and symptoms and desired therapeutic effects.

METHOD OF APPLICATION

Interferential current is normally applied using four metal plate or carbon rubber electrodes. These electrodes are held in position either by bandages or rubber straps (Fig. 5) or by a special suction apparatus (Fig. 6). The two circuits (four electrodes) are arranged in a diagonal manner whenever possible, so that the interferential (interference) effect occurs in the area within the electrode boundaries (Fig. 7). A "tingling" or "buzzing" sensation should be felt predominantly over the area where the major problem is occurring.

The electrodes are covered by a moist pad or sponge before being placed on the skin. It is important that all electrodes and pads be of equal size, otherwise there will be a greater current density under the smaller pad(s), and this may interfere with the required effect.

Many manufacturers have recently developed smaller electrodes for more local applications of interferential therapy. Two of the most common of these are the "single-" and "split-quadripolar" pads. These electrodes are particularly useful in the treatment of

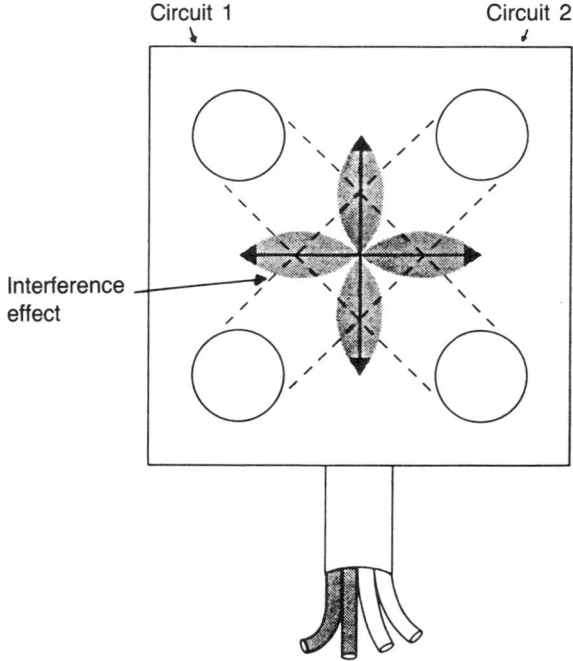

Figure 8   Diagrammatic representation of wiring and interference field of a single quadripolar pad interferential electrode. (From De Domenico G. Basic guidelines for interferential therapy, 31.)

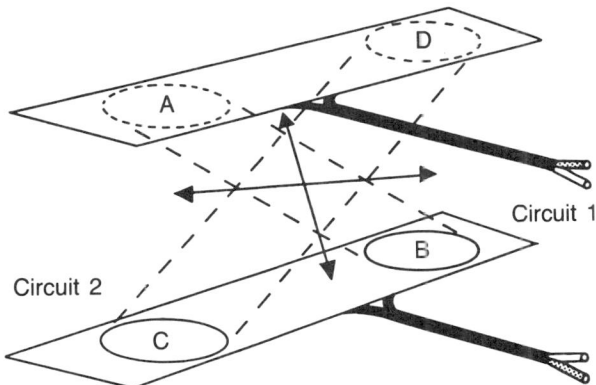

Figure 9 Diagrammatic representation of wiring and interference field of two split quadripolar pad interferential electrodes. Current should only be felt between A and B, and C and D. (From De Domenico G. Basic guidelines for interferential therapy, 36.)

small localized lesions or for the treatment of certain parts of the body that are inaccessible to the use of suction cup or standard sizes of plate electrodes. These electrodes come in various sizes and are wired in such a manner that the interferential effect is felt between the electrodes in the same manner as standard four pole interferential applications (Figs. 8 and 9). These electrodes are usually embedded in a flat rubber plate, which is simply bandaged to the part to be treated, after first moistening the four electrodes (Figs. 10 and 11).

CONTRAINDICATIONS AND PRECAUTIONS

Contraindications

Use of interferential current is not recommended in the following situations or conditions:

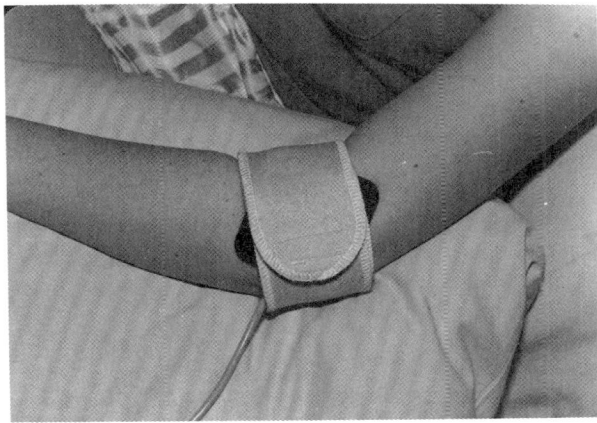

Figure 10 Treatment of "tennis elbow" with a single quadripolar pad.

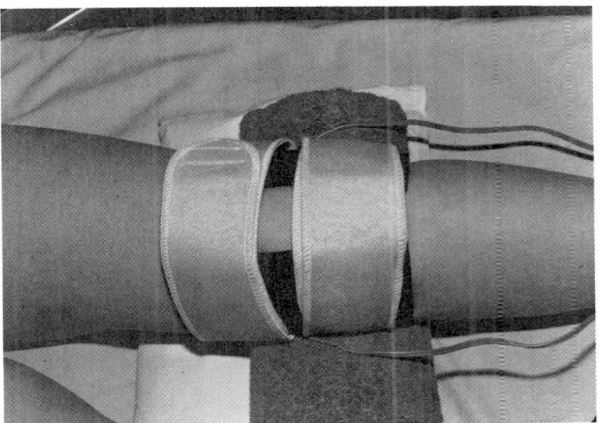

Figure 11 Treatment of knee pain with a pair of split quadripolar pads.

- vascular disease (arterial or venous)
- danger of hemorrhage (in the area being treated)
- malignancy (in the area being treated)
- patients with cardiac pacemakers or cardiac disease
- pregnancy (if treating lower abdomen or pelvis)
- large open wounds
- infective conditions
- unreliable patients (owing to age, language difficulties, mental confusion)
- dermatologic conditions (in the area being treated)
- within 20 to 30 feet of an operating shortwave diathermy machine
- absent cutaneous (light touch) sensation (in the area being treated).

Precautions

Cautionary use of interferential currents is recommended in the following situations or conditions:

- diminished skin (light touch) sensation (in the area being treated)
- over metal implants (in the area being treated)
- when applied to the lumbosacral spine of pregnant women
- over areas with large amounts of swelling
- patients with fragile skin, particularly when using suction cup application.

SUGGESTED READING

De Domenico G. Basic guidelines for interferential therapy. Ryde, Australia: Theramed Books, 1981.
De Domenico G. Interferential "burns." Aust J Physio 1983; 29:vi.
De Domenico G. Pain relief with interferential therapy. Aust J Physio 1982; 28(3):14–18.
De Domenico G, Strauss G. Motor stimulation with interferential currents. Aust J Physio 1985; 31:225–230.

Dougall D. The effect of interferential therapy on incontinence and frequency of micturition. Physiother 1985; 71:135–136.

Ganne JM et al. Interferential therapy to promote union of mandibular fractures. Aust NZ J Surg 1979; 49:81–83.

Mcquire W. Electrotherapy and exercises for stress incontinence and urinary frequency. Physiother 1975; 61:305–307.

Nelson B. Interferential therapy. Aust J Physio 1979; 27:53–56.

Quirk A et al. An evaluation of interferential therapy, shortwave diathermy and exercise in the treatment of osteoarthrosis of the knee. Physiother 1985; 71:55–57.

Savage B. Interferential therapy. Vancouver, BC: Penguin Books, 1984.

Szehi E, David E. The stereodynamic interferential current: a new electrotherapeutic technique. Electromedica 1980; 48:13–17.

Truscott B. Interferential therapy as a treatment for classical migraine: case reports. Aust J Physio 1984; 30:33–35.

Wadsworth H, Chanmugam A. Electrophysical agents in physiotherapy. 2nd ed. Marrickville, Australia: Science Press, 1983.

Ward A. Electricity, fields and waves in therapy. Marrickville, Australia: Science Press, 1980.

INTERFERENTIAL CURRENT STIMULATION IN RECURRENT JAW PAIN

KATHY TAYLOR, M.S., P.T.
ROBERTA A. NEWTON, P.T., Ph.D.

The prevalence of temporomandibular joint dysfunction and myofascial pain dysfunction (TMJ-MPD) syndromes are common. Epidemiologic reports from a number of countries have shown that 50 to 60 percent of people studied demonstrated some type of MPD symptomatology. The typical profile of an individual experiencing TMJ-MPD syndrome is a female within the 20 to 40 year age range. Common patient complaints are pain related to head, ear, neck, TMJ, and tenderness in muscles of the head, neck and jaw. Other signs and symptoms associated with TMJ-MPD syndrome include limited jaw movements, TMJ noises, nonspecific dental pain, pain with mastication, jaw fatigue. Although a multitude of symptoms are associated with this syndrome, pain of a chronic variety is most notable.

Differential diagnosis by a physician, dentist and/or oral surgeon may be necessary to rule out other causes of facial pain. Facial pain may be caused by any number of disorders including, but not limited to, headaches, facial neuralgias, diseases of the salivary glands, ear diseases, brain tumors. Mandibular dysfunction and pain can also result from rheumatic disease, trauma, and congenital abnormalities.

PHYSICAL THERAPY EVALUATION OF TMJ-MPD SYNDROMES

Following appropriate medical and/or dental evaluation, referral to physical therapy for evaluation and treatment can be made. The chief complaint(s) and what influences the chief complaint should be determined. Past history, activities that increase or decrease symptomatology, parafunctional oral habits (clenching, bruxing) and lifestyles are obtained. Measurement of jaw range of motion can be taken with a Boley gauge. Normal vertical jaw opening ranges from 38 to 60 mm, normal lateral jaw deviation ranges from 8 to 10 mm, and normal jaw protrusion ranges from 6 to 8 mm. Vertical mouth opening can also be measured by the patient placing her first two finger widths

of her nondominant hand into her mouth. Less than two finger widths indicates restriction. Active jaw motion should be observed for symmetry of action. Clicking during mandibular function may also be noted. Approximately 80 percent of the TMJ-MPD patients exhibiting symptomatology have clicking and approximately 35 percent of normal individuals and asymptomatic patients exhibit clicking. The Visual Analogue Scale (VAS) for both intensity of pain and affective quality of pain should be given.

Evaluation should then be expanded to include the head and neck region. A postural evaluation of the head and neck can be conducted, as well as examination of cervical range of motion. Postural evaluation should include head and neck alignment and symmetry.

To determine if the chief complaint of pain is of a local and/or referred nature, palpation of the muscles in the region of the TMJ, head, and neck is necessary. The TMJ area should be palpated with the subject in the supine position. Palpation should include the superficial and deep masseter, medial pterygoid, temporalis, TMJ extraorally; and palpation of the temporalis tendon, lateral pterygoid, and intrameatal palpation of the TMJ intraorally. Palpation of the upper trapezius and sternocleidomastoid muscles can be performed with the subject in a seated position. The patient should be asked if the pressure and/or pain is felt where palpation is occurring (local pain) or is felt elsewhere (referred pain).

Results from a comprehensive evaluation of the TMJ region, head and neck assist the clinician in the selection of appropriate physical therapy treatment. Overall goals of treatment are to decrease pain, increase functional mobility, instruct patients in proper body mechanics, and educate and help patients alter parafunctional oral habits, i.e., clenching and bruxing. Physical therapy treatment can consist of a variety of exercises for the jaw and neck, postural correction techniques, relaxation techniques, soft tissue and TMJ mobilization, moist heat, ice, fluoromethane spray, ultrasonography, and electrical stimulation. These treatments are discussed later.

INTERFERENTIAL CURRENT STIMULATION TREATMENT

Interferential current stimulation (ICS), an electrotherapeutic modality was introduced in the United States in the early 1980s. A search of the literature yielded no studies for the use of this modality on patients with chronic jaw pain. Since the modality has been shown clinically to relieve pain, we decided to determine if this form of treatment was effective in our patient population.

We initially evaluate jaw and facial pain patients referred to our clinic. First, the chief complaint and the history of the chief complaint are identified. If pain is the main complaint, the patient is asked to describe the pain as to location, type, what aggravates it, and what makes it better. The patient then marks the intensity of the pain on a visual analogue scale consisting of a 10-cm line labeled at the left end, "no pain," and on the right end, "unbearable pain." Palpation of the TMJs, sternocleidomastoid, upper trapezius, masseter, temporalis, and medial and lateral pterygoids is performed to determine whether the chief complaint can be reproduced and whether the pain is of a local and/or referred nature. Head-neck posture is then observed, primarily examining forward position of the head, slumped shoulders, and rounded back. It is most important to examine head-neck posture in the seated position. We also examine posture with the patient standing. An upper quarter scan is then performed.

With the patient in the seated position, jaw mobility is examined. The patient is then asked to open her mouth. Upon observation, asymmetries, particularly early protraction and lateral deviation upon mouth opening, are noted. Objective measurements of jaw mobility are taken with a Boley gauge. Normal range of jaw opening is 38 to 60 mm, lateral deviation is 8 to 10 mm, and protraction is several millimeters.

If jaw pain is a chief complaint, then ICS may be one treatment choice. The following treatment procedure describes one method of ICS to treat jaw pain.

The subject is placed in the supine position and glasses and bite guards are removed. A Cyborg Quick-Stick Flexible Sensor patch impregnated with aquasonic gel is used as a tetrapolar electrode. The electrode is placed extraorally approximately 1 to 1.5 cm in front of the tragus of the ear covering the approximate region of attachment of the four primary muscles of mastication and a portion of the TMJ.

Waveform parameters for the ICS are set at a sweep frequency of 90 to 100 Hz, with a 6/6 oscillation cycle. Following a 15-minute period, the sweep frequency is reduced to a sweep frequency of 45 to 90 Hz for 5 minutes. The intensity is adjusted to the patient's tolerance so that a minimum of visible facial muscle contraction is produced. We typically use an intensity range from 3 to 7 milliamperes. Following ICS treatment vertical jaw opening is remeasured and the patient completes another VAS. After each treatment we ask the patient to rate present pain to original pain as to better, no change, or worse. Patients are treated for a minimum of three ICS treatments.

The above described technique of ICS to decrease jaw pain and to increase maximum mouth opening was examined in a clinical research study. Forty subjects were randomly assigned to an experimental or a placebo treatment group. The experimental group received three 20-minute treatments of ICS and the other group received three 20-minute treatments of placebo ICS (machine was turned on, but no current was applied).

A one-tailed t-test ($p = 0.05$) was used to analyze the differences between mean jaw pain and mean vertical jaw opening between the ICS and placebo ICS groups. No significant difference was found between ICS and placebo treatment for reduction of jaw pain. Jaw pain for both groups decreased over the three treatment sessions, but there was no significant difference between ICS and ICS placebo. No significant difference was found for vertical jaw opening between ICS and the ICS placebo. Vertical jaw opening for the ICS group improved slightly over the three treatment sessions, but the jaw opening for the placebo group remained unchanged. Each group rated overall level of pain after the final treatment session as to "better, no change, worse" in comparison to their pretreatment pain. Both groups showed a high percentage of improvement and a low percentage of no improvement. Sixteen people (80 percent) in the ICS group, as compared with 13 people in the ICS placebo group (65 percent), perceived they were better following the three treatments. Only one person in each group believed that they were worse, and the remaining individuals did not believe the pain changed.

To summarize, the use of ICS may be an effective, analgesic physical therapy treatment adjunct for patients with chronic jaw pain. The placebo effect of the ICS treatment was shown to have a high degree of therapeutic effectiveness. The effectiveness of the placebo effect should not be underestimated or forgotten. To be able to discern the placebo effect from the effects of electrotherapy, an extended treatment period is needed. When using any treatment modality, the effects of the placebo should be recognized and utilized. Although this clinical study was unable to differentiate the effects of placebo versus actual treatment, the results do warrant the use of ICS as an effective clinical modality for the treatment of patients with recurrent jaw pain.

ALTERNATIVE THERAPEUTIC TREATMENTS

As demonstrated in our clinical study ICS can be used to treat the TMJ-MPD patient population. In our clinical experience, no complications treating TMJ-MPD patients with ICS have been observed, and the current is comfortable and well tolerated. There are several advantages for utilizing ICS: it can be applied easily to a very small region of the jaw with the use of small tetrapolar electrodes; moist heat packs or ice packs can be applied directly over the electrodes; and the electrodes can be placed over metal, e.g., wires for fixation of the jaw, braces, and fillings in the teeth.

There are several disadvantages noted from our clinical experience. Higher intensities of current stimulate the facial nerve, which in turn produces a distracting and sometimes irritating contraction of facial muscles, especially about the eye and lip. The electrodes cannot be applied over much of the belly of the temporalis due to hair overlying the region. When treating men with facial hair, the electrode cannot be effectively applied unless the patient shaves his beard or long sideburns.

Other forms of physical therapy treatment are appropriate for TMJ-MPD patients to interrupt the pain-spasm-pain cycle and to assist with the healing process. When applying any modality remind the patient to relax the jaw so that the teeth are apart.

Moist heat packs can be applied easily to the neck and bilaterally to the jaw. Moist heat can produce an increase in superficial circulation and promote relaxation of tense jaw and neck musculature. Ultrasonography (US) can effectively deliver heat deep into the jaw and neck musculature and over the TMJ region to interrupt the pain-spasm-pain cycle. Medication, such as hydrocortisone, can be effectively transported to the target tissue via phonophoresis. Precaution should be used not to deliver US over the eyes or carotid sinus, thus a smaller head is necessary. US cannot be applied over facial hair, e.g., beards, long sideburns, and hair over the temporalis muscle belly.

Ice packs, ice towels, or ice massage can be easily applied to the jaws and neck to decrease pain. Ice application immediately following heat provides a temperature contrast, which further promotes an increase in circulation. Both moist heat and ice can be incorporated into a home program. Disadvantages of using ice include patient discomfort and initial decrease in relaxation. A possible rebound phenomenon exhibited by an increase in symptomatology may occur at some time following application of this modality.

Fluorimethane spray and stretching of the upper trapezius, sternocleidomastoid muscle, as well as the masseter and temporalis muscles, can be used for both evaluation and treatment. If limited jaw opening is caused by a physiologic holding of jaw musculature, then following application of vapocoolant spray, a major increase in mouth opening occurs immediately. However, if more TMJ and soft tissue stiffness are present, then no significant change in jaw motion will be noted following application of the spray. Fluorimethane can be used effectively to treat trigger points to decrease pain and increase jaw and neck mobility. When using vapocoolant sprays eyes, ears, nose, and mouth need to be properly covered.

Other forms of electrical stimulation such as high voltage pulsed galvanic stimulation (HVPGS) and transcutaneous electrical nerve stimulation (TENS) can be applied to the face and neck. The only electrotherapeutic modality that can be applied inside the mouth is HVPGS using an intraoral probe. If the patient is allowed to hold the probe, control the intensity knob, and assist in finding the correct placement on the temporalis tendon or masseter-pterygoid complex prior to turning on the machine, then a decrease in anxiety (that is naturally experienced by the patient when an electrical current is applied inside the mouth) will occur. A stimulation intensity to patient tolerance and a high frequency are applied for 30 to 60 seconds per stimulation site. Time for stimulation is increased with subsequent treatment sessions. Extraoral electrode placement for both HVPGS and TENS are the same as for ICS. The same stimulation parameters as those for intraoral application with HVPGS are used for extraoral application. TENS may be used as part of a home program. Since most patients choose not to wear facial electrodes in public, an appropriate home treatment schedule should be developed. Electrode placement as described above is appropriate for pain of local origin. If the pain is of a referred nature then the electrodes should bracket the referring trigger point region.

Many exercise regimes can be used to increase range of motion, improve coordination, and promote relaxation of the jaw and neck musculature. Selection of the appropriate program is based upon the goals of the treatment. An overzealous program may be harmful. Clinically, we use general active range-of-motion exercises for the neck and jaw, proprioceptive neuromuscular facilitation techniques, Feldenkrais exercises, tongue exercises, passive and active assistive exercises using tongue blades, and manual mobilization for the TMJ and neck. Relaxation techniques using soft tissue mobilization, biofeedback, patient education on stress management and cassette tapes for relaxation are also used. Postural improvement techniques and exercises for the head and trunk are also emphasized since forward head postures may contribute to increase stress on joints and soft tissue, thereby producing abnormal mechanics and pain about the neck and jaw, as well as possible changes in occlusion of the teeth.

In summary, a comprehensive approach for physical therapy is recommended. Not only are structures associated with the TMJ evaluated and treated, but also head and trunk evaluation and treatment should be included. The physical therapy program should compliment the medical and/or dental programs prescribed for patients with a TMJ-MPD syndrome.

SUGGESTED READING

Bell WE. Clinical management of temporomandibular disorders Chicago: Year Book, 1982.

Ganne JM. Interferential therapy. Austr J Physiotherapy 1976; 22:101–110.

Gelb H. Clinical management of head, neck and TMJ pain and dysfunction. Philadelphia: WB Saunders, 1977.

Greene CS, Laskin DM. Long-term evaluation of treatment for myofascial pain—dysfunction syndrome: a comparative analysis. JADA 1983; 107:235–238.

Hansjurgens A. Fundamental explanation of interferential current. Karlsruhe, W. Germany: Deutsche Nemectron GMBH, 1974.

Lader E. TMJ: clinical and practice management. New York: Vadare, 1981.

DIADYNAMIC CURRENT THERAPY

SANDY RENNIE, M.Sc., B.P.T.

PHYSICS

In 1929, Dr. Pierre Bernard successfully used electrical wave forms knows as diadynamic current to reduce nerve pain. A diadynamic current is a single or double phase rectified pulsed current of sinusoidal wave form.

Current Format

The wave form originates from a sinusoidal current and is rectified to produce two available current formats. Figure 1 demonstrates the original sinusoidal wave form.

MF Current

Through single or half-wave rectification, a monophasic wave pattern is produced. This is termed the mono-phase fixe or MF current, as shown in Figure 2. This 50 Hz half-wave rectified current has a pulse width of 10 milliseconds (ms), has a pulse interval of 10 ms, and delivers 50 pulses per second (pps).

DF Current

Through double or full-wave rectification, a biphasic or diphasic wave pattern is produced. This is termed the di-phase fixe or DF current, as shown in Figure 3. This 50 Hz full-wave rectified current has a pulse width of 10 ms and delivers 100 pps.

From these two basic rectified wave forms, two more currents are available, which are modulations of the MF and DF currents.

CP Current

Module en courtes periodes or CP is a current with abrupt and rhythmic changes between MF and DF currents. Each individual portion of the total current form lasts 1 second before changing to the other current form (Fig. 4).

LP Current

Module en longues periodes or LP is a current with a slow and surged alteration between two MF currents, with one MF current running continuously, and the second MF current surged and shifted through the first MF current, thereby making this phase appear like a DF current. The length of "on" time for each phase depends upon the manufacturer. (e.g., Siemen's Neodynator 725: 5 seconds single MF, 10 seconds double MF [Fig. 5]; Enraf Dynatron 406: 6 seconds single MF, 6 seconds double MF).

The pulse duration of each impulse is generally derived from the mains supply frequency, and is 10 ms for a 50 Hz mains supply, and 8.5 ms for a 60 Hz mains supply. The duration between individual impulses is the same length as the pulse duration, thus the MF current is 10 (8.5) ms on, 10 (8.5) ms off, whereas DF current has no off time (Fig. 6).

PHYSIOLOGIC AND THERAPEUTIC EFFECTS

The physiologic effects of Diadynamic current therapy are not well understood because of the lack of available scientific articles in English journals. The primary therapeutic effect appears to be pain relief, but the exact mechanism is not well understood.

Physiologic Effects

The physiologic effects of diadynamic current are summarized as follows:

1. Stimulation of large diameter (mechano-receptor) nerve fibers
2. Stimulation of A-delta and C-type pain carrying nerve fibers
3. Stimulation of intact motor nerves
4. Increased vasodilatation
5. Stimulation of cellular processes and alteration of cell membrane permeability.

Therapeutic Effects

The therapeutic effects of diadynamic current are summarized as follows:

1. Decrease in pain
2. Decrease in swelling or inflammation
3. Increase in muscle contraction
4. Increase in local circulation
5. Facilitation of healing process

Suggested Mechanisms for Therapeutic Effects
Decrease in Pain

1. Activation of pain-gating mechanism
2. Stimulation of descending pain suppression system

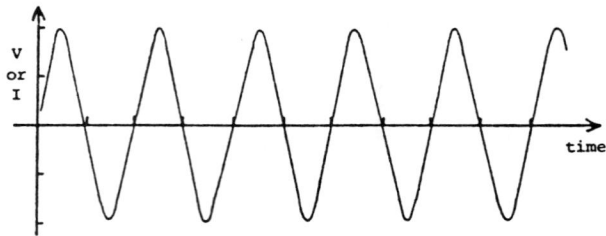

Figure 1 Sinusoidal current. (From Ward A. Electricity, fields and waves in therapy. Marrickville, Australia: Science Press, 1980:37.)

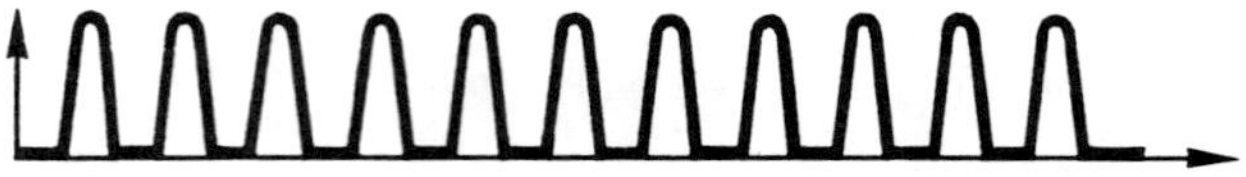

Figure 2 Mono-phase fixe (MF) current. (From Siemens Neodynator 725 Brochure:2.)

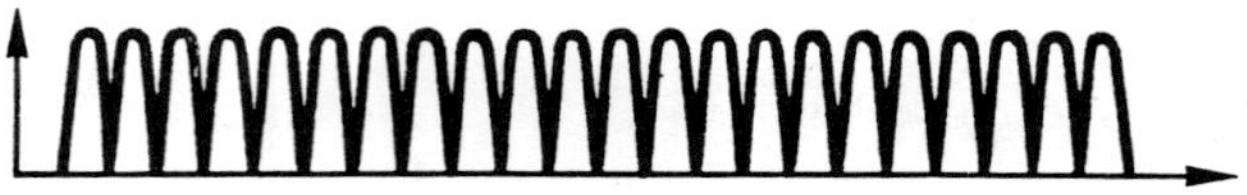

Figure 3 Diphase-fixe (DF) current. (From Siemens Neodynator 725 Brochure:2.)

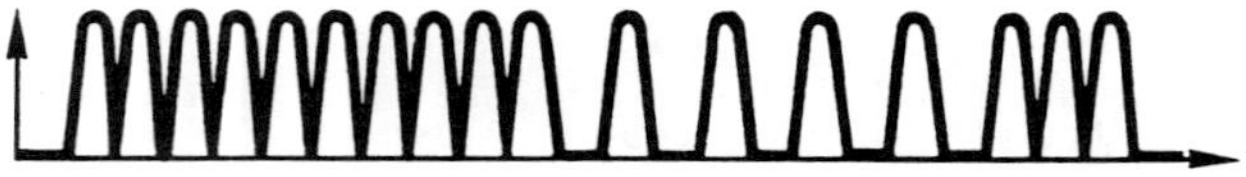

Figure 4 Module en courtes periodes (CP) current. (From Siemens Neodynator 725 Brochure:2.)

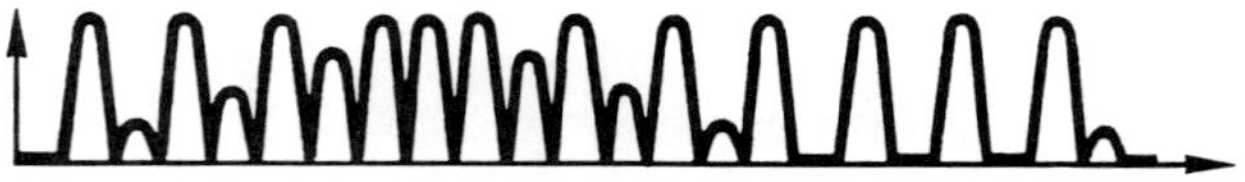

Figure 5 Module en longues periodes (LP) current. (From Siemens Neodynator 725 Brochure:2.)

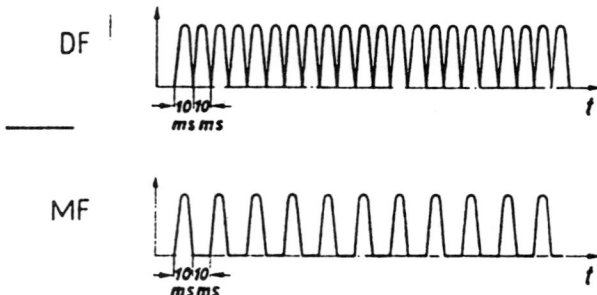

Figure 6 Pulse and interval duration, MF and DF currents. (From Petersmann K. Practical hints for treatment with diadynamic currents, Siemens Electrical Ltd:21.)

3. Stimulation of enkephalinergic pain suppression system
4. Removal from damaged area of substances which stimulate nerve endings (e.g., histamine)
5. Placebo effect.

Decrease in Swelling or Inflammation

1. Increase in removal of debris and waste products through increased local circulation
2. Increase of cell membrane permeability allowing more extra-cellular fluid to be resorbed
3. Activation of motor nerves brings about some muscle contraction, thereby enhancing muscle pump effect.

Increase in Muscle Contraction

1. Direct stimulation of motor nerves

Increase in Local Circulation

1. Stimulation of autonomic nervous system (depression of sympathetic activity) leading to vasodilatation in a local area
2. Release of histamine-like substances in response to monodirectional current flow (electrolytic build-up causes local erythema)

Facilitation of Tissue Healing

1. Local increase in circulation, bringing oxygen and foodstuffs, and removing debris and waste products
2. Increase in cell membrane permeability thus decreasing local inflammation, allowing natural healing process to continue
3. Restoration of natural "polarity" of wound through the passage of interrupted direct (diadynamic) current across or through the wound.

Suggested Treatment Parameters

1. For pain relief
   DF = 30 seconds to 2 minutes
   CP = 2 to 5 minutes, and/or
   LP = 2 to 5 minutes
2. Decrease in swelling and inflammation
   DF = 30 seconds to 2 minutes
   CP = 2 to 5 minutes, and/or
   LP = 2 to 5 minutes
3. Increase in muscle contraction
   MF or DF = as necessary for muscle strengthening
4. Increase in local circulation
   DF = 30 seconds to 2 minutes
   CP = 2 to 5 minutes, and/or
   LP = 2 to 5 minutes

5. Facilitation of healing process
DF = up to 20 minutes, with very low amperage and frequent polarity reversal

Current Description

DF

- used prior to all other diadynamic currents (decrease skin impedance)
- muscles contract at high intensities
- pain is relieved
- patient feels prickling/burning sensation which subsides momentarily

MF

- not used very often
- muscles contract
- some pain relief is experienced
- patient feels strong, penetrating vibration/prickling sensation

CP

- used primarily for pain relief
- muscles contract rhythmically with sufficient intensity
- patient feels buzzing in DF phase, and stronger vibration in MF phase

LP

- pain relief is long lasting
- muscles contract rhythmically with sufficient intensity
- patient feels strong vibration of MF phase which is followed by slowly rising and falling buzzing sensation of DF phase

METHOD OF APPLICATION

Diadynamic current therapy is applied using two pad-type electrodes, one positive and one negative. As with other low frequency currents, the negative electrode gives the most stimulating effect. The positive electrode also has a therapeutic effect, but generally less than the negative electrode. In some conditions, the patient may experience the positive electrode more strongly than the negative electrode.

Choice of Electrodes

Metal plate or carbon rubber electrodes are usually available in three sizes. The choice of which electrodes to use depends upon the *size of area to be treated* and how much one wants to *localize the current*. For example, large electrodes diffuse the current, whereas small electrodes localize current. Small electrodes are also used in the treatment of trigger points. Electrodes

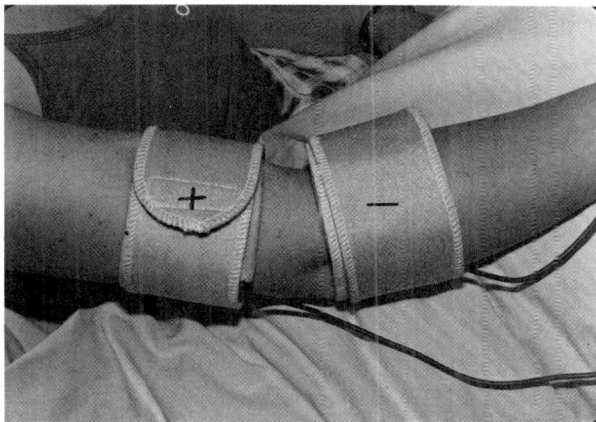

Figure 7 Localized treatment of tennis elbow using two carbon rubber pad electrodes.

should be covered with a moistened sponge about 5 to 10 mm thick.

Placement of Electrodes

For the treatment of a localized pain, electrodes may be placed on either side of the painful area, or one electrode (usually the cathode) may be placed over the painful area and the other electrode placed proximal or distal to the cathode. (Fig. 7, 8)

For joint pain, the electrodes may be placed on either side of the affected joint. (Fig. 9, 10)

For treating trigger points, a small negative (cathode) electrode is placed on the trigger point and the positive (anode) electrode placed two to three cm away in a proximal direction.

Intensity of Current

There are usually two controls for current intensity.

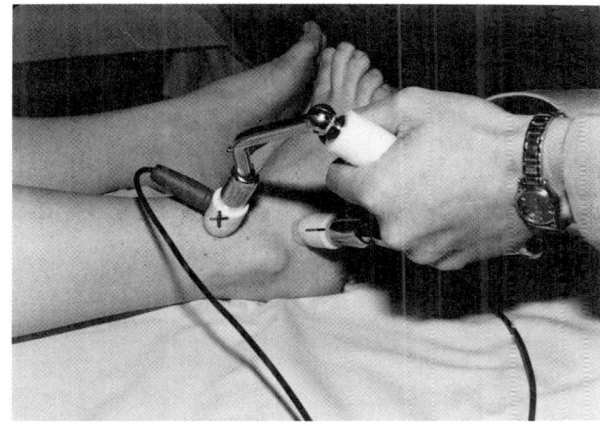

Figure 8 Treatment of lateral ankle pain using a yoke electrode.

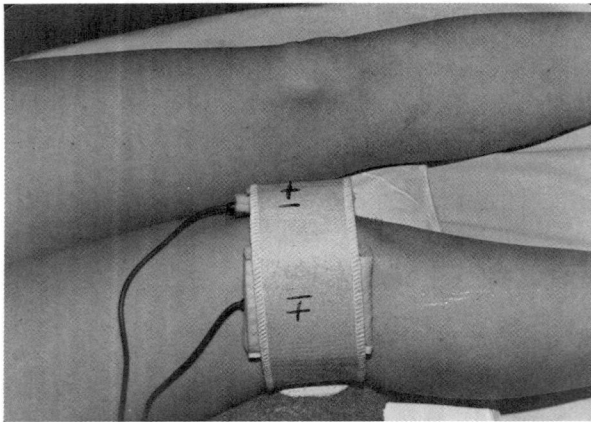

Figure 9 Treatment of patellofemoral joint pain using pad electrodes.

The Basis

The basis represents a direct current of low amperage. Most manufacturers recommend a setting of 2 to 3 mA. This direct current lowers the value of the membrane potential, which results in lower intensities of diadynamic current required during treatment. The intensity of the basis current is set first, followed by the selection of intensity of the diadynamic current. The sensation of the basis current may be felt as a slight itching, prickling, or burning.

Dosis

The dosis represents the intensity control for the four different diadynamic currents. This intensity is adjusted for each patient and should be set *between the threshold of perception and the threshold of pain*. There should be no acute burning or painful sensation. The feeling may be uncomfortable, but should not be painful.

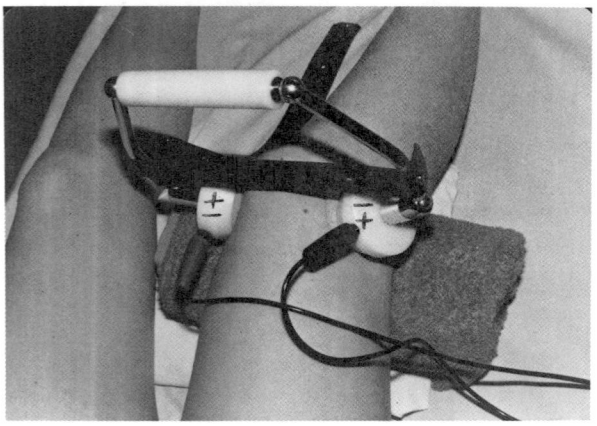

Figure 10 Treatment of knee joint pain using a yoke electrode.

Length of Treatment

The length of treatment is normally not longer than 10 to 12 minutes per area. This is to prevent any skin irritation and to prevent too much accommodation effect. DF is usually applied for 30 seconds to 2 minutes because of its rapid accommodation effect, CP is applied for 2 to 5 minutes, and LP is applied for 2 to 5 minutes.

NOTE: 1. MF current is not often used. The usual treatment format is DF followed by either CP, LP, or both CP and LP currents
2. Polarity should be reversed halfway through treatment to avoid any electrolytic effects under the electrodes. Some diadynamic units have an automatic polarity reversal, others must be done manually.

Number of Treatments

The literature written by Bernard recommends treatment 2 to 3 days in a row, stopping for 1 week, then another 2 to 3 days in a row.

Clinically, it appears to be better to treat 5 days in a row for acute pain, wait 1 week, then another 5 days in a row. For chronic pain, treat for 5 days, wait 2 weeks, then another 5 days. There appears to be no justification for either of these routines in the literature.

CONTRAINDICATIONS AND PRECAUTIONS

Because of the direct current (basis) that may be utilized, and the interrupted direct current (diadynamic dosis) that is used, skin breakdown and burns can occur due to electrolytic build-up under the electrodes. Skin sensitivity should be checked and the patient instructed that no acute burning or pain sensation should be felt.

Contraindications

It is recommended that diadynamic currents not be used in the following situations or conditions:

- not after ice (cryotherapy) in the area being treated
- not after any other pain relieving modality (in the area being treated)
- through the chest wall
- over recent fractures
- over fragile skin
- vascular disease (arterial or venous)
- danger of hemorrhage (in the area being treated)
- malignancy (in the area being treated)

- pregnancy (if treating the lower abdomen or pelvis)
- patients with cardiac pacemakers or cardiac disease
- infective conditions
- unreliable patients (due to age, language difficulties, mental confusion)
- dermatologic conditions (in the area being treated)
- within 20 to 30 feet of an operating shortwave diathermy machine
- diminished to absent cutaneous light touch and hot or cold sensation in the area to be treated

Precautions

It is recommended that diadynamic currents be used with caution in the following situations or conditions:

- over metal implants (in the area being treated)

- when applied to the lumbo-sacral area of pregnant women
- over areas with large amounts of swelling

SUGGESTED READING

Petersmann K. Practical hints for treatment with diadynamic currents according to Bernard. Information brochure. Siemens Electric Limited, Pointe Claire, Quebec, (No date).

Stimulation current analgesia with NEODYNATOR 725. Information brochure. Siemens Aktiergesellschaft, Federal Republic of Germany, (No date).

Ward A. Electricity, fields and waves in therapy. Marrickville, Australia: Science Press, 1980.

Diadynamics. Delft, Holland: BV Enraf-Nonius. Catalogue no. 1424-762.

Practical hints for treatment with diadynamic currents according to Bernard. Pointe Claire, Quebec: Siemens Electric.

Theron E, Vermeulen A. The utilization of transcutaneous electric (diadynamic) nerve stimulation in postoperative ileus SAfr Med J 1983; 63:971–972.

ULTRASONIC THERAPY

CHRISTOPHER J. SNOW, B.P.T., M.Sc.

The therapeutic uses of ultrasound (US) were first developed in Germany in the late 1930s and 40s. Even though unsubstantiated by controlled clinical research, extravagant claims of efficacy helped quickly to popularize the treatment in Germany and many other European countries. While American medical scientists studied the biologic effects of ultrasound in the 1950s and established thresholds for tissue damage, the therapeutic use of ultrasound spread to North America and the empiric reports and claims continued. However, controlled clinical trials to substantiate clinicians claims have been few and far between. There have been less than 30 adequately controlled clinical trials on therapeutic ultrasound in the last 35 years, and over half of those have either reported negative results regarding the benefits of US or were inconclusive. This lack of hard evidence regarding efficacy of US, together with minimal study of the subject by therapists in training (usually less than 10 hours on theory and practice), and poor quality instrumentation (the output of most machines is inaccurate), has produced minimal advancement in the field. In striking contrast, its medical counterpart, diagnostic US, is now an established specialty in its own right, with hundreds of papers published each year. However, this has not stopped therapeutic US from becoming one of the most widely used modalities in physical therapy for the treatment of many varied conditions. What US is, what it is used for, how it is used, and why so little progress is being made in the field are questions briefly discussed in this chapter.

PHYSICS

US is a mechanical wave phenomenon that can only propagate through a medium, such as water. It is usually produced by a piezoelectric transducer that converts a high frequency electrical current to high frequency sound waves. The frequencies of commercial therapy devices range from 0.75 MHz to 3 MHz with 1 MHz being the most common frequency used in North America. One MHz is viewed as a compromise frequency between the need for deep penetration of US into tissue (the lower the frequency the less the attenuation of US and therefore the greater the penetration) and the need to minimize the risk of tissue-damaging transient cavitation (this risk begins to increase significantly in the upper kilohertz range).

When US passes through tissue, it is attenuated. This means that some of the energy of the wave is absorbed by the tissue, whereas the rest is either transmitted deeper into the tissue or is scattered. When US is absorbed in tissue it is converted into heat. The greater the protein (particularly collagen) content of a tissue and the less water content, the greater the US absorption. Relative absorption of 1 MHz US by different tissues can be compared to that of muscle by multiplying by the following factors: bone ($\times 10$); ligament/tendon ($\times 4$); fat ($\times 0.5$), e.g., bone absorbs 10 times more US than muscle.

Propagation of US from one tissue to another can be significantly affected if the acoustic impedances of the tissues are different from one another. The greater the impedance mismatch between adjacent tissues the greater the amount of US reflected and therefore the less US transmitted into the next tissue. The two interfaces where this is most marked is the transducer/skin interface and the soft-tissue/bone interface. The impedance mismatch at the former interface is minimized by the use of a coupling medium. Whereas the latter cannot usually be avoided, it can be used to advantage for certain treatment effects.

US also produces biologic effects by nonthermal mechanisms, such as cavitation and acoustic microstreaming. Cavitation is a complex phenomenon that essentially involves the oscillatory behavior of minute bubbles containing gas or vapor, which can form in insonnated tissue. Transient cavitation is the most destructive form and involves the growth and collapse of these bubbles, thereby producing extremely high temperatures and tissue destruction. However, this form of cavitation is unlikely to occur in tissue at therapeutic intensities (below 4 W per cm^2) and frequencies (above 0.75 MHz) although it can occur in fluid-filled cavities. Stable cavitation involves the formation of bubbles which oscillate in the sound field. This high frequency oscillation can produce microstreaming of fluid with high velocity gradients around the bubbles. Stable cavitation is now thought to occur in mammalian tissue at intensities as low as 80 mW per cm^2. The number of bubbles increases with increasing intensity and treatment time. It is these nonthermal effects of US that are believed to be responsible for observed cell membrane changes and the stimulation of such processes as protein synthesis.

US UNIT PERFORMANCE

Probably the single most important factor limiting real progress in the clinical application of US is the performance of the machine itself. There is no doubt that the majority of US machines in clinical use are out of calibration. In 1981, tests of performance of US units in Manitoba and Northwestern Ontario, found up to 80 percent of units to be inaccurate in one or more of the key parameters of power output, effective radiating area, frequency, and timer accuracy. These results are entirely consistent with every other such study in the world literature dating back to the 1960s.

Although more departments are becoming aware of the need for calibration checks, such checks are usually limited to power output and timer accuracy and are usually only done once a year. Most units need to be checked far more frequently if accurate dosages are to be expected. How often the machines should be checked depends on the machine in question, and can vary from every few months to as often as every day. It does not necessarily depend on the make or model of the unit or even how old it is. It is not unusual to find even brand new units out of calibration.

Since power output is the one parameter most likely to vary, the purchase of an US power meter is essential. A list of companies who sell US power meters can be obtained from the Non-Ionizing Radiation Protection Section of Health and Welfare Canada, Ottawa. Most are easy to use, and a routine calibration check should only take a few minutes. Unfortunately, the way most machines are designed, if the output is found to be inaccurate, the machine has to be opened to recalibrate the unit; this should not be done by untrained personnel. However, if the degree of inaccuracy is known, it can be compensated for by adjusting the power output accordingly. The machine can then be recalibrated at the earliest convenient opportunity.

Because the quality of the machines can be so variable, even within a given make and model, it is strongly recommended that when buying an US machine, you should demand from the manufacturer a calibration report on the unit in question to include the results of tests that measure acoustic power output, effective radiating area, US frequency, and timer accuracy. A manufacturer who has a good quality control program and high performance machines is able to provide this information.

TECHNIQUES OF COUPLING

Therapeutic US cannot propagate in air. Therefore a coupling medium is required between the soundhead and the tissues. There are three common techniques.

Contact Coupling

The most common method of application is to apply the US transducer directly to the skin over the target area. A coupling medium is used to minimize acoustic impedance mismatch between the skin and the sound head, thereby maximizing the transmission of US into the tissues.

Waterbag Coupling

For uneven or irregular treatment surfaces, a waterbag can be used. This requires the filling of a plastic bag with a coupling medium (usually degassed water), and sealing it. The bag is placed over the uneven surface to which it molds. The soundhead is then applied over the bag. For complete coupling, gel is usually applied between the skin-bag and bag-soundhead interfaces. For maximum transmissibility, the plastic should be as thin as possible (e.g., Saran wrap is ideal). Rubber products, even very thin ones, are not recommended because they absorb US resulting in significant US power losses to the tissues

Immersion Coupling

This method is preferred when continuous contact with the skin is not possible (e.g., over uneven surfaces or when the area to be treated is too painful to have the soundhead in direct contact). The part to be treated is submerged in a coupling medium (usually water) and the soundhead is directed at the target area, but need not come in contact with the tissue. Particular attention should be given to aiming the US beam at the target area and keeping a constant distance from the skin surface.

CHOICE OF COUPLING MEDIUM

Commercially available gels have the advantage of having high viscosity and low attenuation coefficients (ideal for contact coupling); and water, which has very low viscosity and, if degassed, a low attenuation coefficient, is ideal for immersion coupling.

Although there have been a few studies that show one coupling medium or another to have a lower attenuation coefficient, there is no clinically important difference in attenuation coefficients of the gels because the thickness of the gel layer during insonation is so small. Therefore, choice of US gel can be based on cost and aesthetic considerations. However, the use of an oil-based coupling medium, such as mineral oil, requires comment because its temperature can affect the temperature distribution produced by US in the tissues. Normally, the highest temperature rise in tissue as a result of US is in the superficial bone and soft-tissue/bone interface. However, it has been shown that mineral oil applied at 24° C causes the highest temperatures in the superficial tissues, whereas if it is applied at or below 21° C, the highest temperature occurs at the soft-tissue/bone interface. This temperature dependance is not seen with water-based coupling media. However, high skin temperatures can still occur, even with water-soluble gels, if the soundhead is allowed to get hot.

Water can be a good coupling medium, but its attenuation coefficient can vary considerably depending on the concentration of dissolved gases in it. In normal tap water significant US energy losses can occur and actual dosage to the tissues can be significantly overestimated. Bubbles seen on the soundhead or the skin during insonation indicates the water needs to be degassed.

This can be done by boiling the water for at least half an hour and keeping it in an air-tight container until cool enough to use. A 2 liter plastic pop bottle is useful for this purpose. They are cheap and keep the water degassed for several days.

A more convenient alternative is available to therapists who work in hospitals that produce their own sterile and distilled water using high temperature and pressure sterilization procedures. This water can contain as little as 1 ppm dissolved oxygen (water can be considered degassed if its dissolved oxygen concentration is less than 4 ppm). To test a hospital's sterile and distilled water for dissolved gas concentration, buy an economical dissolved oxygen testing kit such as that sold by Chemetrics Inc., Calverton, Virginia 22016. It can be purchased for about $30 from any scientific instruments supplier.

APPLICATION TECHNIQUES

The soundhead must be moved continuously over the target area for the duration of the treatment. Movement is required to minimize uneven heating of the tissues due to the uneven intensity distribution in the near field of the US beam. Movement also decreases the risk of the development of standing waves, which have been shown to produce blood flow stasis and platelet coagulation. There are two common moving head techniques.

Moving Head Techniques

Circular motion. This technique involves the soundhead being moved continuously over the treatment area with small overlapping circular motions. It is the preferred technique for treating small areas.

Parallel motion. This technique requires the soundhead be moved continuously over the treatment area in straight, overlapping parallel lines. It is usually used for treating larger areas.

It is unfortunate that in much of the clinical literature, there has been a misplaced emphasis on keeping the soundhead perpendicular to the skin surface and on specific descriptions of how fast the soundhead should be moved. Some still argue that if the soundhead is tilted more than 10 to 15 degrees, the soundwaves are reflected and the treatment is ineffective. If this were so, Doppler US, which uses angles of 45 degrees between the transducer and the skin, would not work. The speed with which the soundhead is moved is not important neither is the angle of the soundhead to the skin. What is important is that the soundhead be directed at the target area, be applied with an even pressure, and in the case of contact coupling, remain in complete contact with the skin at all times.

Stationary Head Technique

This technique involves the soundhead being applied over the treatment area and held stationary for the duration of the treatment. Though there are some who still advocate this technique, most, including myself, do not. Keeping the head stationary significantly increases the risk of tissue damage resulting from hot spots caused by the invariably uneven spatial intensity in the US beam, and also encourages the development of standing waves, which can cause blood flow stasis and platelet damage.

INDICATIONS

Heat and Stretch

US can be transmitted to deep-seated structures without excessive surface heating. US can selectively heat tissue with high collagen content and tissue interfaces, particularly where the acoustic impedance between adjacent tissues is different. Therefore, US is the modality of choice for heating joints, joint structures, ligaments, fibrous scars, myofascial interfaces, nerve trunks, tendons, tendon sheaths, and other soft tissue adjacent to bone.

Since heat increases the extensibility of collagen tissue, US is particularly useful in helping to restore or increase joint mobility in cases such as capsular tightness, irrespective of cause, and in increasing extensibility of tendons. Heating the tissue before or during stretching produces greater residual post-treatment elongation of those tissues than is produced by stretching alone. Elevating the tissue temperature prior to stretch also significantly reduces the amount of tissue damage and minimizes any weakening of the structure that stretching alone could produce.

Care must be taken to apply the US so that a therapeutic temperature is reached and maintained in the target tissues. This is achieved by adjusting the intensity or area of insonnation to maintain sensation just below the pain threshold. If the temperature rise is too rapid, the pain threshold is reached too soon; the heat generated in the superficial bone will not have had enough time to conduct to the adjacent collagenous tissues; and treatment will probably have to be terminated before any therapeutic benefit is realized. If the temperature rise is too slow, the heat is conducted away from the target area faster than it is generated, and the therapeutic temperature range is not reached. For optimal results, a low-load long-duration stretch should be applied to the target tissue while the US maintains the temperature in the therapeutic range for at least 5 minutes. After US is terminated, the stretch should be maintained for up to 10 minutes while the tissues cool.

Other treatments such as mobilizations and active exercises usually follow a heat and stretch treatment to maintain the increased range of motion.

Other Major Uses

US is often used to help decrease joint stiffness, relieve pain and muscle spasms, and assist in the resolution of soft tissue inflammation. To what degree the thermal and nonthermal mechanisms contribute to these effects is still controversial. The scientific evidence suggests that the above conditions can be relieved by other heating modalities and therefore the success of US must be attributable to its thermal mechanisms. However, clinicians claim success in treating these problems with dosages that produce insignificant temperature rises in tissue; thus, the nonthermal mechanisms may in some way be responsible.

Phonophoresis

This is the technique of using US to drive medication through the skin to underlying tissue. The exact mechanism of action is unclear, but could involve permeability changes in the skin, the mechanical effect of the US radiation force and acoustic microstreaming. The most common medications used have been anti-inflammatory drugs such as hydrocortisone and local anesthetics such as lidocaine. The medication is pre-mixed into a coupling cream and is applied using a direct contact technique. In patients for whom injection of the drug is not possible or desirable, phonophoresis is a good alternative.

Wound Healing

There is some evidence to suggest that small doses of US (1 W per cm^2 pulsed 2 milliseconds on 8 milliseconds off for 5 to 10 minutes) can stimulate wound healing in such conditions as varicose ulcers and pressure sores. Whether or not US has similar effects on other tissues remains to be seen. Studies on bone healing have been encouraging, thus suggesting increased rates of healing and fracture strength of up to 50 percent. However, much more animal research needs to be done before human experimentation can be justified. Results on the effects of US on tendongraft healing have shown delayed healing, and so such treatment is not recommended at this time.

DOSAGE STRATEGY

Dosage regimens vary widely even for the same conditions, from 0.1 W per cm^2 Spatial Average Temporal Peak (SATP) for 2 to 3 minutes to US (intensity as high as tolerated) for 10 to 15 minutes. However, this is not surprising because little controlled clinical research has been done on treatment efficacy. Thus in order to justify particular dosages, clinicians rely on clinical experience and, to a lesser extent, on the results from animal and in vitro studies, which has led to two different approaches to dosage determination that depend on whether the therapist believes the desired response to US is attributed to either thermal or nonthermal mechanisms.

Those therapists who believe nonthermal mechanisms are primarily responsible for therapeutic effects, such as relief of pain and decrease in edema, recommend pulsed doses of US in the 0.5–1.0 W per cm^2 SATP range for 2 to 5 minutes. Those who believe the primary mechanism to be thermal use the dosage necessary to produce a mild to vigorous rise in temperature, the level depending on the acuteness of the condition. The only consensus in the literature is (a) the more acute the condition, the lower the intensity and the shorter the treatment duration should be; and (b) the greater the intensity, the greater the temperature rise. Until there are a substantial number of controlled clinical trials involving accurately calibrated equipment and meticulous attention to application techniques, dosimetry of therapeutic US in physical therapy will remain inconsistant.

Therapeutic US has tremendous potential. It has already been established as the modality of choice for heat and stretch procedures. It could be a major treatment modality in some forms of wound healing. However, much more clinical research is needed before we can provide the patient with the most effective treatments possible.

CONTRAINDICATIONS AND PRECAUTIONS

At therapeutic dosages, transient cavitation can more readily occur in fluid-filled cavities; therefore, US should not be applied to areas such as the eye, the dural sac surrounding the spinal cord, or the pregnant uterus. At therapeutic intensities, the insonnation of the pregnant uterus could also be detrimental to the fetus. US should not be applied to the reproductive organs because they are particularly sensitive to heat. Therapeutic doses have produced sterility in animals and man. Consequently, although US to the testes is currently contraindicated in physical therapy, its effects on spermatogenesis are presently being studied as a possible form of male contraception. Another interesting area of current research is the use of US and other forms of heat in the treatment of malignant tumors. However, until more is known about the benefits and risks, US should not be applied to malignant tissue.

US should be applied with extreme caution, if at all, over areas of impaired pain or temperature sensation, because of the risk of severe burns. High doses should also be avoided over areas of poor circulation because of the decreased cooling ability of the tissues, and in conditions such as thrombophlebitis because of an increased risk of thrombus formation. Although some have cautioned against applying US over growing bone because of the possibility of inhibiting growth and bone damage, there is no evidence to indicate that therapeutic doses applied with a moving head technique have any effect on bone growth.

CONCLUSION

In conclusion, there is no question that US has significant biologic effects and, therefore, has great therapeutic potential. US is an established heating modality with advantages such as superior depth of penetration, selective heating ability, and excellent beaming properties. However, poor machine performance, little academic study of the subject, and a marked lack of controlled clinical trials to establish effective treatment protocols has prevented significant advancement in the field. Until these problems are acknowledged by physical therapists and corrected, US will continue to be widely used, but not necessarily in the most efficacious way.

SUGGESTED READING

Hashish I, Harvey W, Harris M. Anti-inflammatory effects of ultrasound therapy: evidence for a major placebo effect. Br J Rheumatol 1986; 25:77–81.

Lehmann JF, De Lateur BJ. Therapeutic heat. In: Lehmann JF, ed. Therapeutic heat and cold. 3rd ed. Baltimore: Williams & Wilkins, 1982:486.

Rivest M, Giraldi CQ, Seaborne D, Lambert J. Evaluation of therapeutic ultrasound devices: performance stability over 44 weeks of clinical use. Physiotherapy Can 1987; 39(2):77–86.

Williams AR. Ultrasound: biological effects and potential hazards. Toronto: Academic Press, 1983.

Ziskin MC, Michlovitz SL. Therapeutic ultrasound. In: Michlovitz SL, ed. Thermal agents in rehabilitation. Philadelphia: FA Davis, 1986:141.

Therapeutic ultrasound. 1. Physiotherapy 1987; 73(3):100–115.

Therapeutic ultrasound. 2. Physiotherapy 1987; 73(4):154–168.

HEAT AND ICE IN MUSCULOSKELETAL DISORDERS

JACQUELINE HARVEY, M.C.S.P.
DALE STASZEWSKI, B.Sc.(PT)

The aims of physical therapy in the management of disorders of the musculoskeletal system are to relieve pain and muscle spasm, to improve joint mobility and muscle power, and to maximize the patient's functional level. The application of heat or cold, together with a therapeutic exercise program, will help achieve these goals. This chapter discusses the use of superficial heat and cold in the management of inflammatory and degenerative arthritis and in some orthopaedic conditions.

Clinicians and researchers have found that the application of superficial heating agents relieves pain, muscle spasm, and joint stiffness, and increases blood flow. The application of cold also decreases pain and muscle spasm, and decreases inflammation and bleeding following trauma.

A detailed description of the mechanisms by which these effects are achieved is beyond the scope of this chapter. The following two paragraphs summarize briefly the findings described in Lehmann's *Therapeutic Heat and Cold*.

The application of heat is thought to relieve pain by reducing secondary muscle spasm, by acting as a counter-irritant or by increasing blood flow in tension syndromes. Superficial heat stimulates the exteroceptors in the skin, which may result in decreased muscle spindle excitability, allowing muscle relaxation. The application of either heat or ice may interrupt the pain/spasm cycle. Some researchers have also demonstrated that heating increases the speed and decreases the resistance of joint movement.

The application of cold can relieve pain by acting as a counter-irritant, by relieving protective muscle spasm, and by depressing the excitability of nerve endings. The application of ice packs lowers the intramuscular temperature, which is thought to lessen muscle spindle sensitivity and thus reduce muscle spasm. The application of cold also reduces inflammation and post-traumatic bleeding by vasoconstric-

tion, either by reflex action or by direct cooling of the blood vessels.*

While the application of either superficial heat or cold is effective in relieving pain and muscle spasm, cold penetrates to deeper tissues and has a longer lasting effect than that of superficial heat.

Although superficial heat may be provided in several forms, including chemical packs and fluidotherapy, this chapter deals with the application of heat in the form of hydrotherapy, wax baths, and moist hot packs. The cooling agents to be discussed include ice packs, ice massage, and contrast baths.

THERAPEUTIC APPLICATION OF HEAT

Whirlpool

Deep whirlpools permit submersion of feet and ankles, whereas shallow ones are best suited for hands, wrists and elbows. The Hubbard tank is large enough to allow total body immersion and is contoured to permit movement of all four extremities. It is equipped with an overhead hoist to transport the patient by stretcher into and out of the tank.

Heat from a whirlpool is transferred by convection, with the degree of heating controlled by the temperature of the water. Most of the heating occurs in the skin and most superficial tissues. The water temperature of the Hubbard tank is kept at 100° F (37.7° C) and that of the standard whirlpool at 110° F (43.3° C). Treatment time is usually 20 minutes.

The advantage of the use of a whirlpool is that it simultaneously allows heating of the parts being treated with range of movement exercises, which are further facilitated by the buoyancy of the water. Most patients claim a degree of pain relief and demonstrate a greater ease of movement while in a whirlpool. However, observation by the therapist of the movement being obtained is sometimes difficult when the limb is immersed in bubbling water.

Unless the whirlpool and agitators are sterilized prior to each patient's use, those parts of the skin that have open areas should not be submerged because of the risk of infection. With total body immersion, as in the Hubbard tank, heat loss occurs via the head only. This can result in a rise in body temperature with water temperature above 100° F (37.7° C). Total immersion should therefore be used with caution for cardi-

---

* Lehman JF. Therapeutic heat and cold. Baltimore: Williams & Wilkins, 1982.

ac, diabetic and pregnant patients, and those who suffer from multiple sclerosis and adrenal suppression.

Wax Baths

A mixture of paraffin wax and mineral oil is kept in a thermostatically controlled bath with the temperature at 126° F. (52° C). The mixture is used as a method of heating wrists and hands, and in some departments, ankles and feet.

The heat from paraffin wax is transferred by conduction and, in the most commonly used dip method, is thought to heat skin and superficial structures. It is thought that this must include some periarticular structures of the joints of the digits that have little overlying tissue. The patient is instructed to dip the hand and wrist into the wax seven to ten times. The part is wrapped in paper then Turkish towelling for a period of 20 to 30 minutes.

Wax baths should be used with caution in elderly patients, whose skin has become thin, and in those who have a loss of fatty and muscle tissues, as some are unable to tolerate the temperature of the wax.

Due to the risk of infection, parts of skin that have open areas should not be submerged in wax. Patients with advanced scleroderma, where there is fixed narrowing and obliteration of digital arteries, should not use the wax bath.

Hot Packs

Hot packs are silica-gel filled canvas packs, which are kept in the hydrocollator tank with the water temperature not exceeding 170° F (77.6° C). They are used to heat areas of the spine and large peripheral joints.

The heat from a hot pack is transferred by conduction with most of the heating occurring in the skin. The degree of heating depends on the thickness of towelling between the pack and the part being treated. Any water from the pack, which makes contact with the patient's skin, will rapidly transfer the heat by conduction to the skin, thereby increasing the risk of burns.

The advantage of the use of hot packs is that a number of joints can be treated simultaneously, the pack can easily be removed for observation of skin reaction, and the areas being treated are accessible for exercise following removal of the packs.

Special care should be taken when treating elderly patients and those with a reduction in fatty and muscle tissues. Extra towelling and checks on skin reaction are indicated for these patients.

THERAPEUTIC APPLICATION OF COLD

Ice Packs

Ice packs are made by wrapping ice shavings in moistened towels, the size and shape appropriate to the area being treated.

The pack is then wrapped around or placed on the affected structure. The duration of the treatment depends on the patient's reaction to cold, the effect being sought, and the thickness of subcutaneous fat of the part being treated—thickly covered areas require longer treatment time. In practice, the desired effects are usually obtained within about 10 minutes.

Some advantages of using ice are that it is usually readily available, inexpensive, and easily applied in the clinic or at home.

If compression is being used with ice, care should be taken to avoid pressure over superficial nerves. Skin sensation must be intact and hypersensitivity to cold noted.

Ice Massage

Water can be frozen in a small paper cup or on a popsicle stick for ice massage. This method of cooling is effective in the treatment of pain and inflammation in soft-tissue injuries, particularly when symptoms are localized to a small area. A subjective reduction in pain is the reaction sought. Analgesia can usually be achieved within a few minutes, particularly for superficial structures. The patient's skin reaction is easily observed with this method.

CONTRAST BATHS

Two tanks are required, one containing water at 108° F. (42° C), the other with water at 64.4° F (18° C). The part being treated is alternately immersed in the hot then the cold, beginning and ending with the hot. Total treatment time is 20 to 30 minutes, with 3 to 4 minutes in the hot and 1 minute in the cold. This can be preceded with a few minutes in the hot tank.

This treatment method is indicated for reducing pain, stiffness, and swelling in the wrist, hand, ankle, and foot in inflammatory joint disease or following removal of a cast.

The disadvantage of using contrast baths is the inconvenience involved in using two tanks and the difficulty the patient may have in lifting the lower extremity, in particular, from one tank to the other.

Contraindications

The use of these forms of heat is contraindicated where there is impaired sensation, impaired circulation, post trauma—where hemorrhage is apparent or suspected—in comatose patients, or over malignancies. These cooling agents should not be used where circulation or skin sensation is impaired or for patients who are hypersensitive to cold.

Practical Uses of the Modalities

Disorders of the musculoskeletal system that are frequently referred to physical therapy are (1) mechanical and degenerative disorders of the lumbar spine, (2) postural and degenerative cervical syndromes, (3) postoperative knee procedures, (4) soft tissue injuries, (5) inflammatory joint disease (polyarthritis, spondylitis), and (6) osteoarthritis of peripheral joints.

Low Back Pain

Acute strains and acute exacerbations of degenerative disease of the lumbar spine are often initially treated with a short period of bed rest, medication, and advice on correct positioning. When physical therapy is instituted, but where there is still pain, marked muscle spasm and loss of mobility, the application of an ice pack to the lumbar region with the patient in the supported prone position often provides relief of symptoms.

For less acute episodes, for the elderly patient or for those with a poor tolerance to cold, the application of a hot pack also reduces pain and muscle spasm. However, the effects, are not as long-lasting as those of cold. The patient is positioned in side-lying, hips and knees flexed, with a pillow between the knees. The hot pack can be held in place with a pillow or sheet. Lying directly on a hot pack increases the risk of burns.

Complaints of "stiffness" often persist long after muscle spasm has been eliminated. Although this form of heating is superficial, the comfort provided by hot packs often facilitates stretching exercises. Once a modified long-sitting position can be tolerated, an adequately covered hot pack can be placed in the lumbar region and controlled stretching exercises started with the hot pack in place after a few minutes of heating.

Cervical Syndromes

Acute episodes are often treated with a collar and medication only, as at this stage any form of physical therapy can aggravate symptoms.

If marked muscle spasm is still apparent when physical therapy is initiated, the application of an ice pack, when tolerated, may afford dramatic relief.

The patient should be seated in a comfortable, supported position. The ice pack is then applied to the paraspinal and upper trapezius muscles. Ice should not be applied over the carotid vessels.

For subacute conditions, for those patients who cannot tolerate ice, or for those with tension syndromes, the application of a hot pack will relieve pain and muscle spasm. The patient may be positioned in supine with a pillow beneath the knees. The cervical spine is kept in a neutral position with a small pillow or folded sheets under the occiput.

Very gentle heating may be provided in the form of a "warm collar." This is made by folding two dry towels in half lengthwise, thus creating a four-ply thickness. The middle 6 to 8 inches of a third towel is immersed in the hydrocollator and wrung out. This towel is then wrapped in the four-ply dry towelling and applied like a soft collar so that the warmth is delivered to the posterior aspect of the neck.

This method of applying superficial heat is always well tolerated, can be applied in any position and is easily used by the patient at home. It retains its heating effect for about 15 minutes. Even this mild form of heating should not be applied over the anterior aspect of the neck if any pathology involving the carotid vessels is suspected (e.g., carotid stenosis).

Postoperative Knees

Depending on the extent of the surgery, the approach, and the duration and position of immobilization postoperatively, the therapist will be dealing with various degrees of pain, joint effusion, stiffness, muscle inhibition, and weakness of the lower extremity.

An ice pack applied to the knee in a supported position would be the first choice to reduce these symptoms. It can be placed on the anterior surface or wrapped loosely around the joint. The skin should be examined after a few minutes if there is a loss of sensation around the scars. The temporarily reduced effusion and analgesia provided may allow the patient to begin range-of-motion and strengthening exercises. At the same time, the lessened inhibition permits the patient to begin activities involving the whole lower extremity.

Throughout the course of treatment of most postoperative conditions of the knee, ice is the modality of choice even for a small degree of swelling or pain, and is generally well tolerated.

In later stages of rehabilitation, if a small flexion contracture persists, 20 minutes in the whirlpool may be a beneficial prelude to stretching and mobilizing. The patient, who is permitted full weight bearing can stand with his back to the jets, supporting himself with a hand on either side of the tank. With some weight bearing through the affected leg, shortened hamstrings can be stretched by active contraction of the quadriceps.

Soft Tissue Injuries

Pain, edema, and inflammation, which occur with ligament sprains, muscle strains, bursitis, and tendinitis may be alleviated with the use of ice. Cooling also reduces the tendency to bleeding in acute injuries. To reduce edema, ice may be applied with compression and elevation of the affected limb.

Ice can be very effective in the treatment of tendinitis. For example, a painful medial arch, caused by tibialis posterior tendinitis, can be relieved by stroking with ice. The patient can sit with the affected ankle resting on the opposite knee for the treatment. For Achilles tendinitis, ice massage or the application of an ice pack to the tendon, with the patient prone and a pillow under the shin, may be used.

Most patients with tennis elbow experience a degree of pain relief following the application of ice, especially in the acute phase. When an uncomplicated elbow fracture has been immobilized in a back slab or sling, the patient may benefit from the application of an ice pack prior to range-of-motion exercises.

After the arm or leg has been immobilized in a cast following a fracture or severe ligament sprain, there may be shortening of the tendons, tightening of muscles and capsules, and some edema. If these symptoms are localized, ice packs serve to reduce the pain and swelling and may, in turn, allow freer movement prior to exercise and mobilizations.

For example, after the removal of a Colles fracture cast, patients who have only localized pain and stiffness in the wrist may benefit from the application of an ice pack prior to exercising. Many patients, however, complain of painful, stiff elbow, wrist, thumb, and finger joints. This may be the effect of protective positioning as well as the result of other minor soft tissue injuries sustained at the time of the fracture. When many joints are involved, the counterirritant effect and the buoyancy of the whirlpool may allow the patient to begin exercising in the water. If there is significant edema, contrast baths may be preferred.

The same principles apply to casting of the lower extremity. Muscle atrophy and proprioceptive deprivation, possibly as a result of reduced weight bearing through the limb, present a greater need for early reeducation. Elevation and the application of ice packs to the ankle or knee help to reduce the swelling and permit the patient to begin exercises and gait training.

Many athletes suffer from various degrees of overuse syndromes. For example, runners may develop recurrent inflammation of the distal iliotibial band. Ice can be effective in reducing pain and swelling here and is also used to minimize muscle pain after exercising.

Inflammatory Joint Disease

In inflammatory joint disease there is an increase in intra-articular temperature, which is thought to promote the activity of destructive enzymes. The appli-

cation of deep heating modalities, which may further increase the joint temperature is, therefore, thought to be contraindicated.

The application of ice packs and superficial heating agents, which decrease pain and muscle spasm, are the modalities chosen to facilitate therapeutic exercise programs.

During acute stages of inflammatory joint disease, involved joints demonstrate increased temperature to touch, marked effusions, and decreased mobility. In many cases, the use of superficial heating agents on such joints results in increased pain and decreased ability to move.

In these instances, an ice pack manufactured from crushed ice wrapped in a damp towel and applied to the affected joint decreases pain, protective muscle spasm, and swelling, thus permitting greater ease of movement.

Acute flexor and extensor tenosynovitis of hands (which is common in rheumatoid arthritis) and acute Achilles tendinitis (a manifestation of ankylosing spondylitis) both show a favorable response from the application of an ice pack.

Elderly patients, even during acute stages of inflammatory joint disease activity, have a poor tolerance to the application of ice. The use of ice is contraindicated in those patients with Raynaud's phenomenon.

Where there is pain and limitation of movement of many joints of all extremities, treatment in the Hubbard tank permits simultaneous heating and mobilization of all affected parts. This method of treatment requires less energy on the part of the patient and is less time consuming for the therapist than applying other modalities to numerous joints.

In subacute or more chronic stages of inflammatory joint disease, affected joints have normal temperature to touch and small or no effusions. Where there is still limitation of movement, a superficial heating agent will aid in facilitating exercise programs.

With the patient in lying position, a hot pack applied to involved large joints prior to exercises decreases pain, spasm, and stiffness. Flexion contractures are common in inflammatory disease of elbows and knees. Provided the inability to gain full extension is not caused by a marked effusion, a hot pack applied to the flexor aspect of these joints together with extension exercises will demonstrate a reduction in the contracture. The same affect can be achieved by submerging the elbow in a whirlpool.

As there is meant to be little significant heating of muscle or soft tissue articular structures from either modality, one must assume that extension is facilitated by relaxation of the flexor group of muscles.

Either wax baths or whirlpools are used to heat affected wrists and hands. The advantage of the former is that once the wax is applied, the patient can be lying down for the application of suitable modalities to other involved joints. The advantage of the latter is that exercises are performed while the heating is taking place.

Tightening of intrinsic muscles and ligaments and capsules of proximal interphalangeal joints is thought to contribute to the development of some rheumatoid hand deformities. Following the application of wax or whirlpool there appears to be increased extensibility of these structures, which facilitates the exercise program aimed at minimizing these deformities.

Subacute or chronically inflamed joints of feet and ankles can be heated and mobilized in a whirlpool. While this method of treatment offers pain relief and increased ease of movement, the observation of the degree of movement being obtained is difficult. Patients with severe disease have difficulty climbing on and off the high stool required to submerge feet and ankles in deep whirlpool.

For patients with spondylitis, the application of a hot pack to the affected cervical spine in conjunction with range-of-motion exercises can result in decreased pain and stiffness. Its application seems less effective when applied to dorsal and lumbar spines. Most patients claim greater relief from a warm shower in the early morning when stiffness is most pronounced, and where some mobilizing exercises can be performed, than from being in one position for 20 minutes for the application of a hot pack.

Patients with severe disease, which may also affect hip and shoulder joints, benefit from a therapeutic exercise program in a heated pool.

Osteoarthritis of Peripheral Joints

In degenerative joint disease, though recent evidence has shown enzyme activity in joint cartilage, many of the pathologic changes that occur are mechanical. Elevations in temperature discernable by touch, and effusions, when present, are usually small. Joints affected by this disease process show few adverse effects and gain a favorable response from the application of heat.

While deep heating modalities are frequently chosen in the management of this disease process, the application of superficial heating agents is useful in reducing muscle spasm in degenerative disease of the spine, and pain and stiffness in osteoarthritis of peripheral joints.

The most common sites of osteoarthritis of peripheral joints are hips, knees, proximal and distal interphalangeal joints and first carpometacarpal joints of the hands and first tarsometatarsal, talonavicular and midtarsal joints of the feet.

The deep seated hip joint, which is covered by large muscle and often fatty masses, gains little relief of pain and stiffness from the application of a hot pack. When practical, mobilization in the Hubbard tank is of greater benefit.

A hot pack applied to an affected knee joint with the patient supine offers some short-term pain relief and in many cases facilitates mobilizing and strengthening exercise programs.

The use of wax baths to treat degenerative joint disease of the hand and the use of whirlpools to treat the feet offer relief of pain and, in the early stages, decreased stiffness.

There appear to be few indications for the use of ice in the management of osteoarthritis. However, the application of an ice pack is appropriate when there is exacerbation of degenerative disease of the knee joint, which demonstrates increased temperature and an effusion.

There is no evidence to suggest that the application of heat or cold alters the pathologic changes that occur in disorders of the musculoskeletal system. They do, however, appear to give relief of symptoms and aid in rehabilitation.

Generally, for acute conditions the application of ice in the management of osteoarthritis. However, the application of an ice pack is appropriate when there is exacerbation of degenerative disease of the knee joint, which demonstrates increased temperature and effusion.

SUGGESTED READING

Kottke FJ, Stillwell GK, Lehman JF. Krusen's handbook of physical medicine and rehabilitation. 3rd ed. Philadelphia: WB Saunders, 1982.

Lehmann JF. Therapeutic heat and cold. 3rd ed. Baltimore: Williams & Wilkins, 1982.

Riggs GK, Gall EP. Rheumatic diseases: rehabilitation and management. Stoneham, MA: Butterworth, 1984.

Scott WN, Nisonson B, Nicholas JA. Principles of sports medicine. Baltimore: Williams & Wilkins, 1984.

PAIN MANAGEMENT

ROLE OF THE PHYSICAL THERAPIST IN PAIN TREATMENT CENTERS

CLARICE M. DOLIBER, M.S., R.P.T.

Pain is the chief concern that brings the majority of patients to seek medical care. Chronic pain, defined as a problem of several months duration that has not been responsive to conventional medical therapies, is a complex malady that can affect every aspect of life. Physical therapists and other health professionals have used many approaches to chronic pain treatment. These approaches include nerve blocks, cordotomies, dorsal column stimulators, exercise, massage, mobilization, myofascial release, cold, heat, relaxation, transcutaneous electrical nerve stimulation (TENS), biofeedback, pharmacology, psychotherapy, and operant and behavioral conditioning. Though these treatments have been successful with some chronic pain sufferers, many continue to suffer unrelenting pain. For more information about some of the aforementioned approaches, the reader can refer to several other chapters in this book. This chapter focuses on the role of the physical therapist in treating chronic pain in pain treatment centers and the elements of this treatment that can be used for chronic pain treatment in other milieus.

The concept of a multidisciplinary team approach to the treatment of pain was first implemented after World War II. Since that time, hundreds of pain treatment centers have been developed in the United States. Recent publications have professed the success, measured by patient surveys, of these patient treatment centers in chronic pain treatment. Most pain treatment centers are located in hospitals or medical centers and can provide care on an inpatient or an outpatient basis. The most common types of pain treated at these centers are cervical pain, low-back pain, headache, nerve root injury, and myofascial syndromes. Selection criteria for patients varies widely among pain treatment centers, though most select patients who have experienced pain for a minimum of 6 months.

The physical therapist is a key member of the multidisciplinary treatment team. Other team members usually include physicians (frequently psychiatrists), psychologists, nurses, social workers, occupational therapists, and biofeedback specialists. Recreational, movement, and art therapists are often members of the multidisciplinary team.

Because chronic pain affects every aspect of life, the multidisciplinary team approach used by pain treatment centers is of primary importance in the treatment of chronic pain. Since most patients do not seek this type of treatment setting until they have tried numerous conventional therapies, most have been experiencing pain for much longer than 6 months (usually 2 to 3 years).

The multidisciplinary team has several goals in treating patients with chronic pain. The major goals are to increase activity level, to decrease pain behavior, and to decrease drug intake. Other goals include improving the self-concept, and increasing the range of motion or strength. Since pain is a subjective phenomenon that is difficult to quantify, the goal of pain reduction is only valid in terms of reducing the effect of pain on the patient's life. Hence, treatment needs to be directed towards both the physical and psychological aspects of chronic pain. Since it would be impossible to separate one aspect from the other, both need to be addressed by the multidisciplinary team in a well coordinated manner. Team members need to meet weekly to ensure continuous collaboration of their specialized approaches. These team meetings help to avoid the unnecessary overlap and limited treatment scope that can occur when patients seek isolated clinical specialties.

The most common physical therapy treatments used at pain treatment centers are group and individualized exercise programs, relaxation training, TENS, instruction in body mechanics, and biofeedback. Patient and family education are a large part of the physical therapist's role at these centers. Education in proper body mechanics and pain reducing techniques (such as ice, heat, TENS, stretching, relaxation, or exercise) to be done independently or by family members, and reviewing guidelines for activity levels are important aspects of treatment. Family education is also an important component of treatment as any change in behavior influences and is influenced by the family.

Behavior modification is used as an adjunct to the treatment of the patient with chronic pain by all members of the multidisciplinary team. Changing the patient's attitude towards pain is important and leads to the eventual reduction of the pain experience. For some pain sufferers, pain may be used in place of needed social skills and may remove many burdensome responsibilities. Therefore, reinforcement of healthy, socially-appropriate behavior is a significant part of treatment.

Physical therapists treating chronic pain patients in settings other than pain treatment centers utilize many of the same treatment techniques as previously listed; however, the goals of treatment differ greatly. When a physical therapist is the only health professional treating a patient with chronic pain, the goals of treatment are generally to decrease or eliminate pain, and to identify and reduce (or eliminate) the physical dysfunction causing the pain. Physical therapists treating patients who have had pain for longer than 6 months need to be sensitive to the effects of this long-term pain. Some form of stress management or relaxation training should be incorporated into the traditional treatment program. If the physical therapist does not have the skills to do this, a health professional, who who is skilled in this area should be consulted. The physical therapist also needs to recognize when there is a great disparity between the objective measure of physical dysfunction and the subjective report of pain. This finding may indicate the presence of chronic pain syndrome, which would warrant further evaluation by a multidisciplinary team.

Many health and non-health professionals differentiate between "real" pain and "imagined" pain. However, physical therapists should not use this type of terminology when referring to pain. Pain is a subjective phenomenon elusive to our objective measures. It is important to treat it as such, addressing physical dysfunction, pain control, and referring to or consulting with other appropriate professionals as indicated. Regardless of cause, be it physiological, psychogenic or a combination of the two, the pain is real to the patient. The multidisciplinary team approach used at pain treatment centers is indicated for some of our patients and may be their only hope of relief.

SUGGESTED READING

Aronoff GM, Wilson RR. How to teach your patients to control chronic pain. Behav Med 1978; 21(7):29–35.

Berns J. Team approach to chronic pain. Health Soc Work 1978; 3(2):182–192.

Cairns D, Thomas L, Mooney V, et al. A comprehensive treatment approach to chronic low back pain. Pain 1976; 2:301–308.

Chapman CR. Psychological aspects of pain patient treatment. Arch Surg 1977; 112:767–772.

Gorsky BH. Chronic pain: a management plan based on experiences in a pain clinic. Postgrad Med 1979; 66:147–154.

Seres JL, Newman RI. Results of treatment of chronic low back pain at the Portland Pain Center. J Neurosurg 1976; 45:32–36.

ACUSTIMULATION IN MUSCULOSKELETAL DISORDERS

ROY P. WALMSLEY, M.Sc.

Acustimulation can be defined as a method of applying a small electrical stimulus to the skin, preferably through the acupuncture points although this is not mandatory. The first technique for applying acustimulation in treatment of pain from a musculoskeletal origin is the method for which the neurometer was originally designed and intended; a method called Ryodo-raku. The second method is the method developed basically through trial and error for use in the clinic.

RYODO-RAKU

The neurometer is a device capable of measuring electrical conductivity as well as applying an electrical stimulus (Fig. 1). When the electrical conductivity of the skin is measured over the body surface against an indifferent electrode placed in the hand, certain spots show better conductivity than others. These spots are referred to as Ryodo-ten points, which simply means better electroconductive points.

Several factors that can affect the electrical conductivity of the skin need to be considered when taking measurements. Factors such as the existence of skin lesions, edema, perspiration, and skin temperature. The influence of perspiration and uneven contact of the active electrode to the skin can be overcome by using a saline-soaked cotton electrode. As skin resistance is so unstable, measurements should be taken within a few seconds of the electrode application on unprepared skin, i.e., untreated and uncleaned.

Most Ryodo-points are seen at or close to the traditional acupuncture points. Lines linking these points called Ryodo-raku, correspond reasonably well to the traditional meridians. Thus twenty-six Ryodo-raku meridians are found over the entire body. Two are located on the midline of the body, one in front and one on the back; while each extremity has six meridians. The meridians in the upper extremities are labelled H1 to H6, whereas the lower extremity meridians are called F1 through F6.

Technique

From the numerous points on each meridian the therapist selects one specific point to represent that meridian. Thus six representative spots are chosen for each extremity to measure the electrical conductivity through the electrode applied to that point. The voltage employed is 12 v and the amperage set to give a full scale deflection on the meter at 200 microamps (μamp) when the active and indifferent electrodes are placed in direct contact. The different spots located around the wrist and ankle are depicted in Figures 2A, B, C, and D.

When dealing with a cervical dysfunction the therapist would take the six "H" measurements; with a lumbar dysfunction the "F" values would be recorded. Comparing these measurements can provide valuable information. If dysfunction is present, it is common to find that one measurement is grossly higher than the other five. Nakatani, the originator of this method of assessment and treatment, attributes this to an autonomic system imbalance. From a clinical viewpoint, the abnormally high measurement usually is found over the dermatome associated with the spinal dysfunction, e.g., H1 is found over the lateral side of the anterior aspect of the wrist and is associated with the C6 dermatome. Consequently, the C6 and 7 spinal segmental area for dysfunction would be looked at more closely if the H1 point was high. Prior to a subsequent treatment session, measurements can be taken through the Ryodo points and any abnormally high value reverting to a reading more closely resembling the other values for that extremity—which signify alleviation of the dysfunction at the spinal level—could be noted.

Nakatani stipulates that the therapist should take values over all twenty-four points, calculate their mean and standard deviation, and then pay particular attention to only those points outside of one standard deviation from the mean. Because this method is somewhat inconvenient in the clinical setting, not to mention time consuming, a more convenient method is employed. On a graph measuring 11 cm high on the Y axis representing the amperage in microamps and the X axis representing the different points, points greater than 1.4 cm from the mean are the relevant points. (Such graph paper is available to go with the neurometer). Thus the therapist simply draws a horizontal line through the mean and parallel to the X axis and then another one 1.4 cm above this line. Those points outside this range (usually only one point) are the ones with abnormally high values.

Treatment consists of stimulation through the

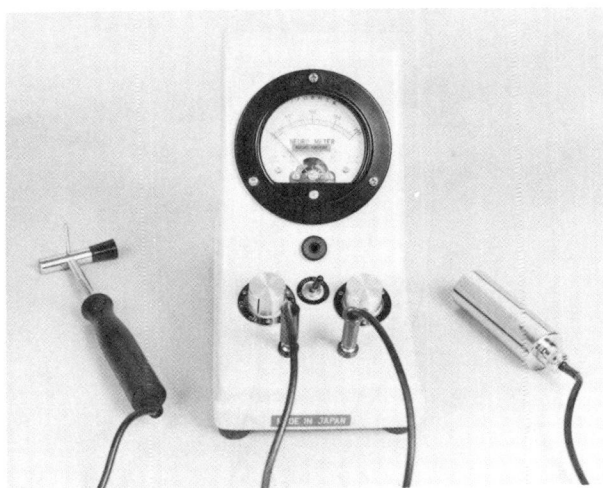

Figure 1 The neurometer plus the indifferent and stimulating electrodes. (Institute of Ryodoraku, Osaka, Japan.)

meridian with a high representative point in comparison to the other points.

Treatment can be administered through a needle electrode supplied with the machine, or through the small electrode mounted at right angles to the measuring electrode (Fig. 3). Treatment consists of inserting the needle through the skin and passing a 200 μamp current for a few seconds to points along the particular meridian. Five or six points are chosen per meridian. If the other electrode is employed, stimulation is simply given to the skin.

Stimulation is given in conjunction with other forms of physical therapy, usually manual therapy, for example the mobilization techniques as advocated by Maitland.

DIRECT STIMULATION

The neurometer, or another such device, is used in a manner entirely different from that which it was first intended. Skin resistance measurements are taken only if there is a need for further information than that gleaned from the selective tension examination. We use the device purely as a treatment device rather than a diagnostic tool.

Using the point stimulator, an electrical stimulus is applied in one of several ways.

Muscle Spasm

For a patient with protective muscle spasm, a stimulus for 5 to 7 seconds is administered directly to the muscles in spasm; this is repeated four or five times. The effect can be assessed by the patient's perfor-

mance of some task, which can be evaluated in comparison to a previous performance.

Since a single muscle in a state of spasm is seldom, if ever, seen, and usually a collection of related muscles is in spasm, one would stimulate throughout the series of muscles. For example if spasm were throughout the cervical musculature, stimuli would be applied over the side of the neck through four or five spots bilaterally. By treating in this manner, the amount of muscle spasm can be reduced in a matter of a few minutes, i.e., however long it takes to simulate four or five spots and to reassess. This not only allows for an increase in active movement, but has the added beneficial effect of making the area more amenable to manual therapy techniques. The affected spinal segment can then be more readily mobilized or manipulated. It could be argued that cryotherapy has a similar effect, but the difference is the time factor.

Treatment Soreness

Immediately following manual therapy the patient may experience a certain amount of treatment soreness. If this be so stimulation is simply given directly to the painful area again for a few seconds at a time to four or five spots, depending upon the extent of the soreness. For example, following a manipulation the patient may experience a residual soreness, this can be easily alleviated by giving localized stimulation for a few seconds over the particular spinal segment.

Radiating Pain

When treating a patient with radiating pain the stimulus can be applied throughout the course of the pain. Five or six spots are picked, depending upon the extent of the pain, and are stimulated for a few seconds each. The patient is reassessed immediately and treatment is repeated.

Localized Pain

Pain over an extensive area not associated with nerve root irritation, for example, localized pain from direct trauma, pain from a localized inflammatory reaction (e.g., supraspinatus tendinitis, joint pain, or a painful amputation stump), can all be treated by acustimulation. In each instance, stimulus is applied directly to the painful area as described for the treatment of radiating pain.

When treating such patients a word of caution is advised. Appreciate that treatment is simply directed towards alleviating the symptom of pain, not altering the pathologic state that caused the pain. In instances of acute inflammatory reaction—for example, in patients suffering from rheumatoid arthritis or immedi-

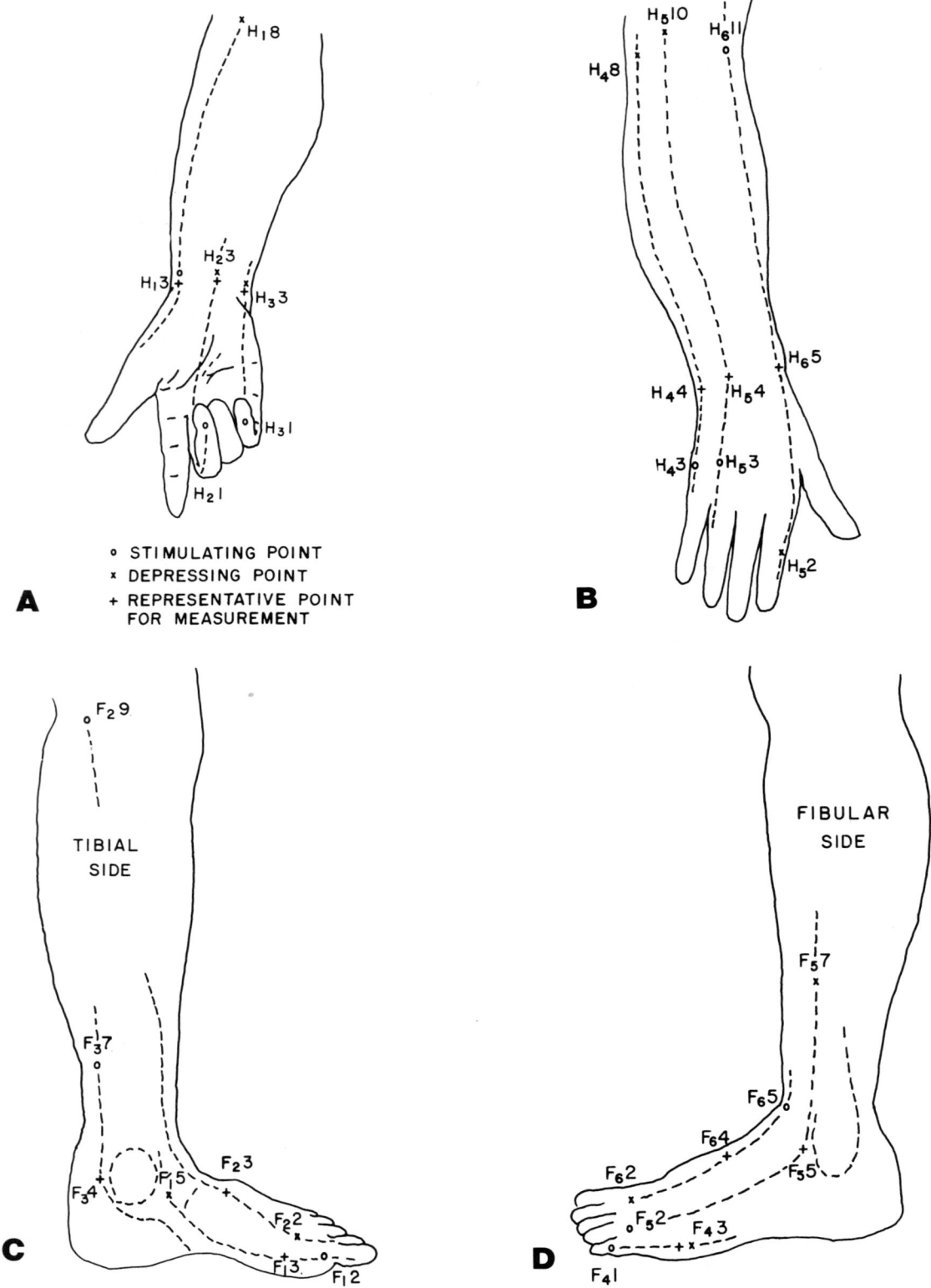

- o STIMULATING POINT
- x DEPRESSING POINT
- + REPRESENTATIVE POINT FOR MEASUREMENT

Figure 2 Representative Ryodo points on the limbs: *A*, anterior wrist; *B*, posterior wrist; *C*, medial aspect of lower leg; *D*, lateral aspect of lower leg.

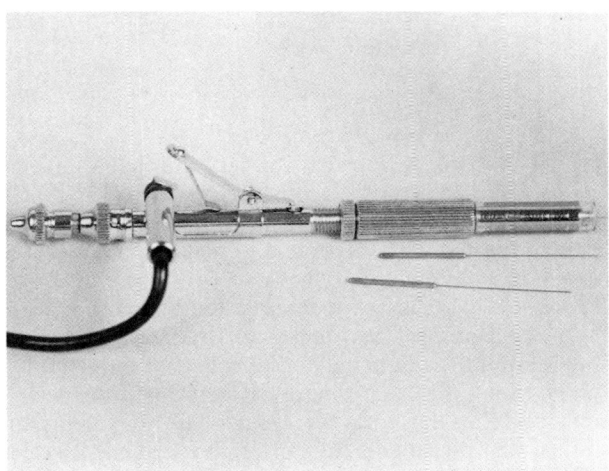

Figure 3 Needle electrodes.

ately following an athletic injury—the pain could be masked by applying this form of therapy yet the pathologic state would remain. Without pain the patient is liable to cause further damage to already traumatized tissues, thereby aggravating the condition. Therefore, this form of therapy is not advocated in circumstances where joint or tissue damage could ensue if pain were alleviated. A typical example of this is the use of acustimulation as a first-aid measure on the athletic field or in the gymnasium. Another ex-

ample is for the treatment of pain associated with chondromalacia patella. Pain can readily be reduced or even alleviated altogether in patients who have this condition. However, if strenuous activity is allowed too soon the symptoms will not only return, but can be more severe than previously.

Acustimulation is an effective and quick form of therapy for alleviating pain and localized muscle spasm found in patients with musculoskeletal problems. The time factor is an important one when working in a busy outpatient clinic. Time may not be available to select and apply electrodes, such as is needed for transcutaneous electrical nerve stimulation (TENS), yet the results with acustimulation are apparent immediately. The indications for this form of therapy, though similar to TENS, are not the same. Experience has taught us to use TENS for patients with a long-standing chronic type of pain and acustimulation for the acute type of pain found in patients with more recent traumatic or pathologic conditions.

SUGGESTED READING

Gunn CC. Motor points and motor lines. Am J Acupunct 1973; 6(1):55–58.

Gunn CC, Milbrandt WE. Tenderness at motor points. A diagnostic and prognostic aid for low-back injury. J Bone Joint Surg 1976; 58A(6):815–825.

Masayoshi H. Ryodoraku treatment. An objective approach to acupuncture. Osaka, Japan: Japan Ryodoraku Autonomic Nerve Society, 1975:1–4.

ACUPUNCTURE, ACUPRESSURE, AND TRIGGER POINT THERAPY

JUDITH A. BRADLEY, B.Sc., P.T., M.C.S.P.

Acupuncture is becoming increasingly popular in the world of physical therapy as a treatment modality for pain and inflammatory conditions. Training varies from self study and short continuing education courses to study of several years duration in Chinese traditional acupuncture. As a treatment modality it has great appeal as even with short training the results can be dramatic and the risks minimal.

CHINESE TRADITIONAL ACUPUNCTURE

Chinese traditional acupuncture has a history of over two millenia and was founded upon astute observation and clinical experience. It differs markedly from western allopathic medicine in that it is based upon a philosophy of life energy or vital force. The basic tenet is that all human beings are energized by a vital force known as Chi or Qi. This force flows through the body in meridians or channels in a predictable and rhythmic fashion while the person is in good health. External forces such as cold, damp or heat, or internal forces, such as emotions or food, may cause excess or deficiency of energy in a particular channel. This causes disease or dysfunction in the organ or body part connected with that channel. To normalize the circulation of Chi, a needle is inserted into a specific point or points.

Such a surprisingly simple concept is supported by an extremely complex system of diagnosis and treatment requiring detailed understanding of the inter-relationship of body functions and knowledge of the laws of acupuncture. These laws are applied to restore energy balance and thus physical, mental, and spiritual wellbeing to the individual.

WESTERN ANATOMIC ACUPUNCTURE

Anatomic acupuncture, such as is taught in short courses, is usually based upon western allopathic diagnosis and the choice of points is made, by the selection of the anatomic structure to be stimulated or by a cookbook recipe, i.e., points that have an empirical value in certain diagnostic categories. The point, selected for its anatomic value, may be within a particular dermatome, myotome, or scleratome or located on a particular nerve or nerve root, motor point, blood vessel, tendon, or musculotendinous junction.

For example, the point Gall Bladder 34 distal to the head of the fibula may be selected for the stimulus effect along the lateral peroneal nerve and the recurrent nerve to the knee for relief of hip or knee pain rather than for an energetic effect on the Gall Bladder (GB) meridian.

Most of the research of acupuncture in the western world has been in the field of pain relief and anesthesia based upon allopathic diagnosis. There have been very few studies of treatment of medical conditions by traditional acupuncture methods.

Comparison of Chinese and Western Acupuncture

The philosophical basis of the two methods varies markedly in that the traditional acupuncturist views the individual as an integrated whole, whereas the allopath separates the individual's symptoms into categories and treats them separately.

In acute conditions of traumatic origin, there is very little difference in the techniques and point selection of the two methods although the Chinese traditional acupuncturist would also treat any underlying energetic disturbance caused by the injury. Both methods also stimulate local spontaneously tender points, which the Chinese call "Ah Shi" points.

It is at the interface of superficial, acute conditions and chronic systemic conditions that the different levels of training and philosophy are significant.

In traditional terms, when a condition becomes chronic it implies a disruption of energy flow and disturbed function of the organ involved. This results in other changes in the body, such as elimination, respiration or circulation, that the allopath does not connect with the presenting chronic problem. Because of the traditional acupuncturist's comprehensive view of the body he or she will not attempt to treat chronic conditions by individual symptoms, treating some (for which the patient is referred) and ignoring others, such as is the tradition in physical therapy.

In order to understand the connection between supposedly unconnected symptoms the therapist must be willing to make a paradigm shift that allows for the possibility of a system of circulating energy. This is not necessarily an easy task as current scientific study has so far been unable to measure it consistently. It is also not helped by the seemingly unscientific and poetic language used by the Chinese to describe the concept. However, with a willingness to receive information in an unfamiliar mode and with personal experience one may find the energy concept tenable. To treat all symptoms in an individual by conventional physical therapy means or even by anatomic or "cookbook recipe" acupuncture is a lengthy process and often goes beyond the scope of physical therapy practice.

As can be seen by the clinical examples given in Table 1, treatment of complex conditions can become much more effective and efficient by more specific and appropriate selection of acupuncture points based on an understanding of traditional acupuncture.

TREATMENT SELECTION

My clinical practice is primarily comprised of patients with musculoskeletal disorders that have been resistant to other forms of therapy.

Treatment sessions are 1 hour long and my approach is essentially "hands-on," drawing on experience in acupuncture and craniosacral therapy. My training in traditional Chinese acupuncture was 6 to 8 hours per week for 1 year with a Chinese acupuncturist. This introduced me to concepts and theories, without having to make the claim of being an accomplished traditional acupuncturist.

When it is indicated, I refer patients to a skilled acupuncturist concurrently with my treatment program.

It should be noted that the system of treatment selection described represents my approach and not neccessarily that of all acupuncture practitioners.

See Table 1 for a comparison of point selection.

Acute Conditions

Anatomic acupuncture is my treatment of choice for acute inflammatory conditions. The more specific one can be about the diagnosis, and thus selection of points, the more effective the treatment. For example, the points chosen for supraspinatus tendinitis where stimulation of the suprascapular nerve is required (S1 12 or L1 16) are not the same as for subdeltoid bursitis where stimulation of the axillary nerve is required (TW 14). (Points are named by abbreviation of the organ name to which the channel belongs. Please refer to an acupuncture text if you are not familiar with the channels). Daily treatment is ideal in acute conditions.

Simple Chronic Conditions

In simple chronic conditions, such as sciatica or osteoarthritis of the knee, in a person who is otherwise symptom free, good results can be achieved by

including commonly used acupuncture points, which the Chinese have shown to have a systemic effect (Table 2).

The effectiveness of some of these points can be explained anatomically, but for the most part their effect has been proven by experience. The parasympathetic and sympathetic switches are western anatomic terms used to describe points which appear to have an effect on the autonomic nervous system. The sympathetic switches are particularly useful in sympathetic dystrophy or chronic pain states where ischemic changes are present. Treatment response, which compares favorably to other physical therapy methods, can be achieved by this method. The question of whether this method restores balance to the energetic system remains unanswered. Treatment is once or twice a week.

Complex Chronic Conditions

In cases such as (1) the chronic complex example in Table 1, and (2) the following case, the individual symptoms are viewed as part of a total pattern, which is significant in Chinese Traditional Diagnosis.

This case would most probably involve the liver meridian system and would be confirmed by pulse and other observation diagnostic methods. Anger or frustration causes blockage of energy flow along the Liver and Gall Bladder meridians and their deep pathways. These encompass the head, low back, and abdominal regions and so include the physical symptoms as well as the emotional dynamics. Chronic disturbance in the Liver system would also cause secondary problems in Stomach and Spleen meridians but these will often be corrected by treating the underlying imbalance in the Liver and Gall Bladder meridians (see Table 1).

Other Conditions

Acupuncture is effective in conditions such as duodenal ulcers, stress and anxiety, asthma, hypertension, and smoking cessation. These conditions may be treated after consultation and specific referral from the physician who then monitors and alters dosage of medication according to response. Treatment for smoking cessation can be effective in reduction of withdrawal signs if the patient has made a definite commitment to stop smoking.

Acupuncture has also been used to induce labor and to control labor pain. Research on the use of acupuncture in cardiopulmonary and neurologic conditions is limited, but there are indications of its efficacy.

STIMULATION

Needles may be stimulated manually, by heat such as moxa, or by an electrical stimulator such as a TNS

TABLE 1 Comparison of Point Selection According to Treatment Approach

Condition	Anatomic	Cookbook
Acute Supraspinatus tendinitis	LI 16—Suprascapular nerve (between Acromium & Spine of Scapula SI 12—Suprascapular Nerve (Supraspinous Fossa) Paraspinal at C5 level	LI 16 (Between Acromium and Spine of Scapula) LI 11 Distal Pt for shoulder (Lateral Side of Flexed Elbow) ST 38 (Between Tibia and Fibula at approx. mid point of Lower Leg) GB 34 (Ant. and Inf. to Head of Fibula
Lumbar sprain	UB 25—Paraspinal L 4/5 GV 3—Interspinal L 4/5 GB 30—Sciatic Nerve (between Sacrum and Grt Trochanter) UB 40—Sciatic Nerve (Popliteal Fossa)	UB 23 (Paraspinal L 2/3) UB 40 (Popliteal Fossa) SI 6 (Styloid Process of Ulnar) SI 3 (MCP 5th) DU 26 (Junction 2/3 rd of Upper Lip) EX 21 (Adjacent to Vertebral Spine) ints
Simple chronic Osteoarthritis of Shoulder	LI 15—Rotator Cuff Tendon (Ant. and Inf. to AC Jt) TW 14—Axillary and Circumflex Nerve (Posterior to Acromium Process) LI 11—"Sympathetic Switch" (Lateral Side of Flexed Elbow) Paraspinal at C5 Level	LI 15 LI 11 TW 5 Distal Point (Dorsal Aspect of Forearm) LI 4 (Between Thumb and First Finger) Extra 28 (Dorsum of Hand in Web Between Fingers
Complex chronic 60-year-old female presenting with: Common migraine—bi-monthly. Rt frontoparietal and retro orbital pain Occipito frontal headache—constant Nonspecific aching—right side of neck and right arm Laminectomy L 4/5 15 years ago Occasional sciatica left leg radiating to the calf Cold feet left and right Nonspecific low back ache Constipation and abdominal distension most of adult life Depression and repressed anger in marital situation Duodenal ulcer	GB 20 UB 10 Liver 3 ST 36 LI 4 DU 15 UB 25 GB 30 LI 11 H 7	GB 20 TW 5 LIV 3 LI 4 DU 15 GB 14 Extra I UB 60 UB 10 Extra 21 UB 23 UB 40 UB 54 UB 25 GB 30 GB 34 UB 57 P 5 ST 36 UB 21 P 6 SP 4 SHU (points)

TABLE 1

Traditional Acupuncture	Acupressure	Trigger Points	
As per cookbook plus Ah Shi points	Along the course of the large intestine (LI) meridian LI 4 LI 11 LI 16	Infraspinatus (SI 11) Supraspinatus (SI 12 LI 16) Scaleni (ST 12) (Plus nonacupuncture points)	
As per cookbook plus Ah Shi points	Along the course of urinary bladder meridian	Quadratus Lumborum (UB Pts. GB 26 Liv 13) (Plus nonacupuncture points) Iliopsoas (SP 12 Extra 15) Gluteus medius (Sacral UB points)	
Disease of Wind Cold and Damp Middle stage Common Ah Shi points— LI 15 LI 14 SI 11 SI 13 (Supra Scapular Fossa) SI 10 (Lateral Scapula) LI 14 (Deltoid Insertion) Late stage—Restricted Movement LI 15 1 DU 14 (between C7 and T1) GB 21 (middle fibers trapezius) LI 3—Difficulty Raising the Arm TW 3—Restricted ADD. SI 3—Restricted ABD. LU 9—Restricted INT. ROT. Local points Extra 2 GB 8 UB 2 GB 20 GB 14 Distal points Liv 3 GB 41 34 37 30	Ah Shi points of neck and shoulder girdle LI 4 TW 5 LI 11 GB 21 LI 16 SI 9	Biceps (Nonacupuncture points) Infraspinatus (SI 11)	
	Along the course of the GB and liver meridian Liver Alarm Point—UB 18 GB Alarm Point—UB 19 UB points along vertebral column	Sterncleido mastoid Temporalis	Migraine
		Frontalis Occipitalis Postcervical muscles Suboccipital muscles	Occipitofrontal headache
		Gluteus medius Psoas Quadratus Lumborum	Lower back pain
		Gluteus Minimus Piriformis Trapezius	Sciatica
		Scaleni Biceps Laser or needling to laminectomy scar	Neck and arm pain

stimulator with needle attachments. Frequencies of below 4 Hz are reported to produce beta endorphin, and frequencies above 4 Hz presumed to work by the gate control theory—although neurotransmitters such as serotonin may be implicated.

In traditional acupuncture, strong stimulation is recommended in acute conditions and minimal stimulus in chronic conditions. Low intensity-infra red laser is effective for stimulation of acupuncture points.

STERILIZATION

In order to insert needles, it is essential to be competent in the technique and fully informed on aseptic precautions and possible complications. Needles must be sterilized by an approved method because of the increasing occurrence and public concern about AIDS. Patient's needles may be stored and used separately, or disposable needles may be applied. The Public Health Department can be requested to perform random swabs of needles to ensure maximal protection.

SELF-TREATMENT

All patients are asked to contribute to the healing process by following a program of exercise, relaxation, imagery, and/or stimulation of acupuncture points by pressure, vibrator, TNS, or heat. Local heating can be effectively applied by dipping a metal rod, such as the handle of a gum massager, into a cup of hot water and repeatedly applying it to the point.

ACUPRESSURE

Acupressure, as the name implies is simply pressure upon acupuncture points or along meridians. The points selected are either acupuncture points chosen according to anatomy or traditional acupuncture, trigger points, or spontaneously tender points (Ah Shi points).

There are also various forms of acupressure known as Shiatsu, Do-in, or Tui Na in which the whole meridian system is stimulated in a systematic way. The advantages include (1) acceptance to the patient as many are needle phobic; (2) the reassurance of physical touch; (3) the immediate feedback to the therapist about the state of the tissues; and (4) self or family treatment potential.

The stimulus applied may either be deep pressure on trigger points or Ah Shi points, which are in muscle, circular massage over acupuncture points, or kneading along the course of the meridian. When performing acupressure, it is important to be sensitive to the changes in the tissues. Too strong a pressure causes the patient to resist, thereby causing unpleasantness for both people and slowing results.

A cooperative agreement is the best arrangement; the patient can help by deep breathing and "relaxing into" the pain rather than by "pulling away" from it. A large part of the disagreeable sensation of pain is that the sufferer feels like a victim and does not know when it will stop. If the patient feels an element of control, the sensation is less disagreeable.

The therapist may also ask the patient to hold an image in mind, such as a ball of wax melting, or sinking into a bed of feathers, or any other image that assists in completely relaxing into the sensation.

Different systems suggest sustaining pressure from 3 to 10 seconds. It has been found most effective to sustain pressure for as long as it takes to feel a softening of the tissues. Pressure can be applied by the thumbs, keeping the arms straight and using body weight to apply the pressure—although where possible using a flexed elbow to avoid strain on the hands. Softening a muscle trigger point can also be hastened by shortening the involved muscle until it is completely slack and by maintaining pressure for 5 to 10 seconds or until a release is felt.

For stimulation of acupuncture points that are not muscle trigger points, a small circular massage can be applied over the point 8 to 10 times. For example, in a home treatment program, such as for chronic rhinitis or sinusitis, the patient can apply the treatment at each point GV 24.5, St 0.2, UB2, and L1 20 twice each. To encourage regular compliance, the treatment can be linked to a daily routine, such as cleaning the teeth, or after meals.

Acupressure as a home treatment program is beneficial as it encourages patients to take care of themselves and can also involve a family member in a helpful manner.

TRIGGER POINT THERAPY

Trigger points have been described as palpable bands or small circumscribed hypersensitive regions in muscle and connective tissue from which impulses arise and by an as yet undetermined mechanism produce referred pain.

The more commonly known labels that have been used to describe the points are fibrositis, fibromyositis, muscular rheumatism, and myalgic spots.

Dr. Janet Travell has recorded the consistent nonsegmental pattern of referred pain produced by pressure on myalgic spots; she also developed the term Trigger Point. This indicates that myalgic spots act like the trigger of a gun to produce an effect at a distant target, known as the reference zone.

Myofascial pain describes pain arising from muscles and their fascial coverings and attachments. It may occur independently or as a component of the following accompanying signs:

1. Presence of trigger points
2. Disturbed sleep pattern and/or fatigue

TABLE 2   Commonly Used Acupuncture Points

Ll 4	For headaches and facial pain—"sympathetic switch" upper limb
Ll 11	For elbow and shoulder pain—"sympathetic switch" upper limb
TW 5	For neck and arm pain
Sl 3	For pain in neck and scapula region
H 7	For anxiety—"Parasympathetic switch" upper limb
Liv 3	For migraine headaches—"sympathetic switch" lower limb
St 36	For general tonic purposes—"sympathetic switch" lower limb
GB 34	For pain along the gall bladder meridian and knee
St 44	For toothache and facial pain along the stomach meridian
Sp 6	For all gynecologic problems—"parasympathetic switch" lower limb
GV 14	For neck and shoulder problems and balance of Yang meridians
Ren 4	For gynecologic problems and balance of Yin meridians

3. Autonomic disturbance such as cold, perspiring skin
4. Sensitivity to changes in barometric pressure.

Normal stresses and strains produce slight tissue damage that usually heals; however, if healing does not occur, areas of hyperexcitability or structural change in muscle may form.

These are called latent trigger points, and the individual may be unaware of their existence for many years as their afferent discharge is subthreshold. Factors that predispose an individual to the formation of latent trigger points are alcohol ingestion, fatigue, and chilling.

Precipitating factors, such as additional abnormal strain, circulatory disturbance, infection, or chronically poor posture, may be sufficient to activate latent trigger points, thus producing an active trigger point.

Active trigger points may be perpetuated by factors including emotional states such as psychogenic tension, conversion hysteria and anxiety, and abnormal endocrine function, chronic focus of infection, and dietary deficiencies. Failure to resolve these factors results in perpetuation of the trigger point mechanism.

Concurrent pathology, such as nerve root compression, and visceral and joint disease, may also cause activation or perpetuation of trigger points. Afferent discharge from a compressed nerve root or diseased joint may cause facilitation of a spinal segment, thus activating a latent trigger point within the same segmental distribution. Conversely, pathologic changes in joints and viscera may actually be caused by effects such as hypoxia, ischemia, and immobility.

Trigger points are a common source of pain following decompression surgery. Many clinicians have felt the frustration of a patient who still complains of pain even months after supposedly successful decompression surgery. In these cases, trigger points that had been activated by the trauma of a disc lesion may be the source of pain and mimic sciatica.

Trigger points may be differentiated from other local tender points in muscle by easily tested characteristics. These include palpable tight band in muscle; tender spot within palpable band; reduced range of stretch of involved muscle; mild weakness of involved muscle; and referred pain produced by pressure, stretch, or strong contraction

An intriguing aspect of trigger points is that their associated pain pattern does not adhere to any known anatomic pathway, but is reproducible in different individuals with remarkable conformity. For example a trigger point in infraspinatus has a pain reference area over the anterior aspect of the shoulder, and a trigger in gluteus minimus refers pain to the calf.

Treatment of myofascial pain by the use of trigger points is extremely simple and effective, once the correct trigger point has been isolated. Travell has produced charts and an excellent book, which clearly shows each trigger point and its referred pain zone.

It is possible to stimulate the trigger point in a number of ways. These include deep pressure; ultrasonography; massage with an ice cube; dry needling with a hypodermic or acupuncture needle; and laser therapy.

These techniques should be followed by completely stretching the muscle. Reciprocal inhibition technique can be used to increase the stretch. The patient is positioned to isolate the muscle accurately and minimal manual resistance is given to isometric contraction followed by relaxation and slow stretch.

Another method developed by Travell is to spray the area from trigger point to reference zone with fluorimethane spray while at the same time stretching the muscle to its fullest length. The spray causes a transient cutaneous stimulus and cooling, which overcomes the muscle's resistance to stretch, and is best followed by moist heat and a home stretching exercise program. Injection of procaine into the trigger point is also commonly used with effect. An effective combination involves fluorimethane spray, pressure, and acupuncture needling.

In chronic pain states where primary and secondary pain are difficult to distinguish, the use of fluorimethane spray is helpful. This can be applied for relief of trigger points in multiple muscle groups, such as in the neck and shoulder region. After inactivation of trigger points the original cause of pain and dysfunction is more readily discovered.

Needling is performed by inserting the needle into the trigger point until the patient feels a deep sensation, which may be painful. At this point the needle is tapped and the therapist then waits until the patient no longer feels the deep ache, and the therapist feels a release of the "grabbing" feeling around the needle. The needle is then removed and the muscle stretched.

The patient is treated two or three times a week and a home program of exercise, stretches and moist heat is included. Heat can be applied by a plastic-covered heating pad with a damp cloth against the skin. The therapist may also teach relaxation and breathing exercises. In subsequent treatments, the therapist reevaluates the patient's report of pain and tenderness of trigger points. It may be necessary to repeat the treatment for a particular trigger point several times or secondary trigger points, which also require treatment, may be revealed. Therapists are familiar with trigger points in the trapezii, rhomboids, and quadratus lumborum; however, the trigger points in sternocleido mastoid, scaleni, and iliotibial tract are equally common. Treatment of trigger points often gives relief in cases that have been resistant to other forms of therapy. It is appropriate to discuss the treatment of scars even though they are not strictly trigger points. Scar tissue is a common and frequently ignored source of myofascial pain either locally or at a distance. The exact mechanism is not known, but it is possible that it may be due to neuroma formation, which causes an aberrant input into the central nervous system or due to a restriction of glide of layers of fascia. Scar tissue can be stimulated by either therapeutic laser or by "peppering" the scar with an acupuncture needle (i.e., brief insertion along the length of the scar) and mobilized by deep massage. The patient can be taught to continue mobilization at home.

SUGGESTED READING

Cerney JV. Acupressure—acupuncture without needles. New York: Simon & Schuster, 1974.

Lewith GT, Lewith NR. Modern Chinese acupuncture. Wellingborough, UK: Thorsons, 1980.

O'Connor J, Bensky D, transl. Acupuncture—a comprehensive text. Shanghai College of Traditional Chinese Medicine. Seattle, WA: Eastland Press, 1981.

Travell JG, Simons D. Myofascial pain and dysfunction—the trigger point manual. Baltimore: Williams & Wilkins, 1983.

CRANIAL OSTEOPATHY AND CRANIOSACRAL THERAPY

JUDITH A. BRADLEY, B.Sc., P.T., M.C.S.P.

Cranial bone movement was first recognized as an important physiologic phenomenon by Dr. William Sutherland in the early 1900s. Dr. Sutherland was an American osteopath who believed that function could be determined by observation of anatomic design and biomechanics. This led him to view the cranium in a new light as the anatomic structure of the sutures seemed to be designed for movement (which was contrary to current anatomy teaching). By self-experimentation using a helmet and clamps he claimed that he was able to produce and relieve nausea, dizziness, personality changes and pain by alteration of pressure on different regions of the head.

Sutherland suggested that the cranial bones and sacrum, and the dural membrane system that connects them formed an entire system. By manipulation of this system he suggested it was possible to directly influence central and autonomic nervous system function and to indirectly influence the endocrine system via the pituitary gland.

The therapeutic value of this work was accepted by only a small group of osteopaths who continued research on these theories both clinically and in the laboratory.

Several therapeutic methods have developed from this original concept and are being taught widely to health professionals in North America and Europe.

Craniosacral therapy is a system of cranial osteopathy which was developed by John Upledger. As this is the field in which I received most of my training, the emphasis of this chapter is on this method.

CRANIOSACRAL RHYTHM

Research by Upledger and Karni, Michigan State University, has shown that there is indeed a rhythmic movement in the range of 6 to 12 cycles per minute, in the living cranium. The movement of each suture is only about 10 to 25 microns, but the summation of these movements is in the region of 1 to $1^1/_2$ mm. This subtle movement can be felt by the hands of a trained practitioner. This is supported by evidence of collagen fibers, nerves, and blood vessels within the sutures which imply a mobile structure.

There are several theories about the origin of this movement; the production and resorption of cerebrospinal fluid (CSF) being the most commonly accepted, but as yet this remains to be proved.

THE CRANIOSACRAL SYSTEM

Components of the system are as follows:

1. Meningeal membranes;
2. Bones to which they attach; cranium, cervical vertebrae 2/3, sacrum, and coccyx;
3. CSF and all structures related to production and resorption of CSF.

The dura forms the periosteum of the floor and vault of the cranium and, as it descends through the spinal canal, is attached only at the foramen magnum, C2/3 and S2 before blending with the periosteum of the coccyx. The intracranial dura forms a horizontal membrane (tentorium cerebelli) and a vertical membrane (falx cerebri and cerebelli). This membrane system affords passage of cranial nerves and blood vessels.

The hypophyseal infundibulum, which suspends the pituitary gland from the hypothalamus, is surrounded by the diaphragma sellae, which blends with the attachments of the tentorium cerebelli and is therefore influenced by any abnormal tension transmitted through it. Disruption of the integrity of the horizontal membrane system may therefore affect pituitary function.

In health there are no impediments to the mobility of the bones and dural membrane system. As the head widens and narrows so the sacrum flexes and extends. The rhythm is of strong amplitude, normal rate and is reasonably symmetrical throughout the head and body. There is relatively unimpeded venous and lymphatic drainage and cranial circulation, normal pituitary function and undisturbed passage of the cranial nerves.

However, there are many opportunities for restriction of this system. A restriction in osteopathic terminology is called a "lesion."

Restrictions

Osseous restrictions. Bones of the head and face, vertebral spine and sacrum and coccyx.

Membrane restrictions. Dural membrane system and entire myofascial system of the body.

These restrictions are most commonly caused by the following:

1. Trauma
   • Birth trauma—particularly long or difficult labor and the use of forceps
   • Direct trauma—blows to the head, whiplash, heavy falls on feet or buttocks
   • Dental trauma—mechanical forces of extractions and fillings, inappropriate or ill-fitting orthodontic appliances, e.g., braces, bridges, false teeth
2. Habitual postural strain, trauma and disease of the myofascial system
3. Viral infections and/or high fever
4. Psychological stress, debilitating illness, nutritional deficiency

Restrictions can cause pain and dysfunction in the body or head as a result of impaired circulation, autonomic dysfunction, and cranial nerve entrapment.

For example, rotation of the temporal bones may be caused by injuries such as whiplash or dental trauma. In whiplash the mandible is also subject to sudden contraction of the sternocleidomastoid which can exert a force on the mastoid process of the temporal bone causing it to rotate. Temporal bone rotation caused by dental trauma may also occur from forced extraction of a lower tooth. The major nerves which pass through or near the temporal bone are acoustic, facial and greater petrosal nerves and the semilunar ganglia of the trigeminal nerve. The internal carotid artery, internal jugular vein, and occipital artery are also influenced by temporal bone rotation. Tinnitus, vertigo, Bell's palsy, memory and "slow-thinking" problems, as well as headaches, migraine, or facial neuralgia, can be expected as a result of this lesion.

A "restriction" of the coccyx or sacrum may cause head pain by exerting an abnormal pull on the dura. A heavy fall on the buttocks can be the cause of a headache of unknown etiology. "Release" of the sacrum and coccyx can relieve the headache.

Restrictions in the myofascial system influence the mobility of the craniosacral system. Many times the restriction is at a distance from the site of the pain or dysfunction in much the same way that a tight guy rope of a tent is responsible for stress on the material around the pole. The aim of treatment is to locate the restriction (tight guy rope) and release it, thus restoring balance to the myofascial tissues (tent). The fascia system of the body is in effect a continuous sheet extending from head to toe containing pockets and tubes to allow for the presence of viscera, muscle and bone.

Evaluation

Restrictions are identified by evaluation of disturbance in the body's subtle movements felt by the therapist. While at first it is hard to believe that one can feel what is happening at the sacroiliac joint by lightly assessing a rhythm at the feet, it is surprising how quickly this skill can be learned and relied upon.

With no prior knowledge of symptomatology I have frequently assessed patients and had my findings confirmed by previous musculoskeletal assessments by other therapists. In addition, I have been able to determine which restriction is having the largest effect on the body and locate other influences that have not been noted by more conventional assessment.

Each of the bones of the head has a normal physiologic motion. For example, internal and external rotation of the temporal bones and side bending and rotation of the sphenoid. The bones are tested for motion restriction and restrictions of membrane mobility are noted.

Treatment

Although techniques vary according to the method of cranial osteopathy, the aim of all treatments is to restore movement to the craniosacral system.

In craniosacral therapy the therapist uses perception of the response of body tissues as a guide and releases the restricted tissues using a force below that which initiates a "defensive" response of the body. For example, the sacrum is decompressed from the fifth lumbar vertebra by a force of about 25 mg (i.e., about the weight of a 25¢-coin) keeping below the level at which muscles contract to prevent the motion.

The first stage of treatment of the head and sacrum is to free all osseous restrictions. The bones can then be used as handles to directly influence the dural membrane system to which they adhere. Free mobility is normally attained by moving the bone into its restricted pattern and waiting for it to release rather than by moving it directly into the corrected position.

The effect of such gentle, almost imperceptible movement is extremely powerful.

Indications for Treatment

Conditions which may be expected to respond to craniosacral therapy are as follows:

1. Headaches and migraine
2. Temporomandibular joint (TMJ) dysfunction
3. Musculoskeletal pain
4. Tinnitus
5. Memory problems
6. Facial neuralgia and tic doloreux

Babies and Children
1. Autism (including a variety of neurologic disturbances)
2. Cerebral palsy
3. Strabismus
4. Learning and behavior problems
5. Scoliosis

6. Colic, respiratory difficulties, and suckling dysfunction

Craniosacral therapy is only indicated in these conditions when there are positive findings in the craniosacral system. The therapist treats the positive findings in each individual rather than following a protocol for a specific condition.

Treatment frequency varies according to specific needs, but I generally treat for 1 hour twice a week until I have made major changes and then reduce to once a week. After the sytem appears to be stable I cease treatment for 1 month and then reevaluate and continue treatment if indicated.

Patient acceptance of this therapy is very high. Side effects can be sleepiness or a recurrence of an old pain pattern. The latter is usually a positive therapeutic sign and is only transitory while the patient's body is adapting to a less restricted pattern.

Some explanation is perhaps required in the case of brain dysfunction, cerebral palsy, scoliosis, and behavior and learning problems.

Brain Dysfunction

In a double-blind study craniosacral evaluation of 63 children with the diagnosis of autism, all exhibited a restriction of the dura in a horizontal plane. Results of treatment of autistic children are variable but are always indicated as even small improvements can make a big difference in the life of the child, parents, or institution workers. Self-abusive behavior is abated or greatly reduced, thumb sucking ceases, and the child becomes more sociable and displays spontaneous emotion. Thumb sucking may actually be an attempt on the child's part to mobilize the cranial base by exerting hard pressure through the roof of the mouth. If one considers the anatomy of the maxilla, vomer, and sphenoid, it is reasonable to assume that this may offer the child some relief for the tight feeling in the head.

In post mortem studies of children with cerebral palsy a fibrotic ring underlying the coronal suture was found. When this restriction is present the results of mobilization can be very dramatic leading to return to normal function in some cases.

Idiopathic Scoliosis

A cranial lesion may be the originator of idiopathic scoliosis. In physical therapy we are familiar with the concept of adaptational curves but have assumed that they stop at the craniocervical junction. In the light of the craniosacral concept it is reasonable to expect that there is yet another curve at the sphenobasilar junction (the junction of the sphenoid and occiput) to which the rest of the spine is adapting. (Dental maxillary bracing, which crosses the midline, may create a lesion or exacerbate an existing lesion.) If this is corrected early enough some alleviation or prevention of further deformity is achieved.

Learning and Behavior Disorders

Learning and behavior problems can be helped quite significantly or even resolved in cases where a cranial lesion is present. The most common lesions in children with reading difficulties are occipitomastoid compression and internal rotation of temporal bone, most commonly the right. Hyperkinesis can be caused by chemical and food intolerances or psychosocial influences, but there is also a group with compression of the occipital condyles which, (if they will lie still long enough to be corrected) respond completely to release of the restriction.

Birth injury is extremely common. The cranium (mostly cartilage) undergoes severe stress during the passage through the birth canal as it moulds to accommodate the shape of the pelvis and the forces exerted upon it. Normally the action of crying and sucking is sufficient to correct any minor lesions, but sometimes this correction does not occur and the child goes into adulthood with a compromised craniosacral system and the symptomatology which this implies. Infants who have difficulty suckling or swallowing, have repeated colic, respiratory difficulties, or repeated vomiting, often have cranial lesions that can be corrected in approximately one to five sessions.

Treating infants and children requires very subtle palpation and should only be practiced by those with considerable experience in treating adults.

Whenever possible I treat the child, while asleep, in his or her own home. I am able to follow this unorthodox practice as I live in a small community where professional boundaries are less restrictive and where personal safety is not a consideration. I find this to be the most effective as, although it is possible to work on a wriggling child, it is much easier if he or she lies still. Frequently the child with a lesion is restless and will wriggle and grind his or her teeth during sleep but as treatments progress they sleep deeply and teeth grinding ceases.

Case Study 1

A four year old girl who was first born of twins. She was an "unhappy" baby, unable to sleep or make eye contact at the normal age. As she grew she became allergic to several foods, was withdrawn and shy, cried with frustration four or five times a day, had poor motor coordination and always felt tired. Her twin by comparison was normal in all respects.

I examined this child while she was asleep and found marked restriction of cranial rhythm in contrast to her twin sister lying next to her who had full range and amplitude.

The left occipital condyle was markedly compressed, the left temporal bone was internally rotated and the sphenoid was side bent with the right wing high. I spent approximately $1^1/_2$ hours treating her and achieved approximately 60 percent correction. Treatment was directed at releasing the sacrum and the cranial lesions. The next day her parents noticed a dramatic improvement. She ran to the door to meet visitors, played with the other children in the bathtub, jumped in and out of a cardboard box with both feet, and ate pizza without getting a skin reaction, all of which she had never been able to do before. I treated her twice more achieving minor releases. She remained at this markedly improved plateau for 4 months until I was able to return to her community to treat her again.

I treated her four more times for approximately 45 minutes each time and gained 95 percent improvement of her craniosacral mobility. She was then able to play normally with the other children, tumbling in the snow from the toboggan and the cries of "Wait for me" have become a memory. I conjecture that her injury was caused in utero as there was some difficulty with her head position during late pregnancy and labor.

Case Study 2

Thirty-five year old woman complaining of left low back pain of an aching character with pain upon flexion and occasional pain upon coughing or sneezing, radiating pain to left groin region, and pain in left side of neck radiating to shoulder. She has pain and watering of left eye with ptosis, increasing in occurrence and severity over the last 5 years. Onset of opthalmic pain was sudden 15 years ago, and all neurologic tests proved negative. She also complained of a weak and recurrently sprained left ankle following a sprain 20 years ago and had major dental work 6 years ago.

In the first session, I decompressed her lumbosacral junction and released fascial restriction in the left lower quadrant of the pelvis. I obtained fascial release of her thoracic diaphragm and thoracic inlet and mobilized C7/T1 C 2/3 and occipital condyles. The left condyle did not release.

This gave her several hours of relief only. Two days later I corrected her left sacral rotation and continued to gain mobility in the upper lumbar and thoracic fascia.

She then went on a hiking trip for 1 week and has since had no back pain although her face and eye were more painful.

In the next session I "unwound" her left talus and leg and inserted acupuncture needles into local ankle points. "Unwinding" is a method of releasing myofascial restrictions by moving a body part in the direction indicated by the pull of the tissues. The body leads the movement to a position where the restriction will release. I adjusted her left first rib, which was subluxed and mobilized the following cranial restrictions:

1. Left occipital compression.
2. Internal rotation left temporal bone.
3. Left fronto sphenoidal restriction.
4. Sphenoid rotation with high wing on right, and
5. Left TMJ compression.

She received two more treatments directed primarily at the cranial lesions with 80 percent symptom relief. However, cranial mobility is still restricted and so treatment should continue until full mobility is restored.

My impression is that the origin of her problems was at the time of spraining her left ankle, the force of which was transmitted through the body causing sacral and vertebral displacement and myofascial imbalance. This probably added further stress to an already present cranial lesion, perhaps from birth or earlier trauma or it may have caused the original cranial injury. Pain occurred 5 years later when the body was no longer able to adapt to the restricted pattern. The dental trauma added further assault to an already impaired cranial mechanism and made the opportunity for self correction very remote.

Craniosacral therapy offers an alternate and comprehensive approach to patient care.

If one can accept that there are subtle movements in the body and head and that changes can be made by equally subtle means the therapeutic significance becomes obvious. It is not so strange, albeit unfamiliar, to think that the body knows best how to heal itself. Craniosacral therapy offers a medium by which we can learn the language of the body by listening with our hands and encourage its inherent self-healing tendencies by subtle and appropriate intervention.

SUGGESTED READING

Magoun H. Osteopathy in the cranial field. Meridian, 1 Southerland Cranial Teaching Foundation.

Magoun H. Entrapment neuropathy of the central nervous system. J Am Osteopath Assoc 1968; 67(1):643–652, (2)779–787, (3)889–898.

Upledger JE. Craniosacral therapy. Vol. I & II. Seattle. WA: Eastland Press, 1983 and 1987.

DEVELOPING PRACTICE

MOTIVATING OLDER PERSONS

OSA LITTRUP JACKSON, Ph.D., P.T.

- Have you noticed how your own motivation to participate in an activity can vary depending on the people and circumstances that are involved?
- Would you agree that you can impact the motivation of a person with whom you are working?
- Is it important for the patient to be motivated to participate in his or her own care and self growth?

If you answered yes to these three questions, it is likely that the motivation of you and your patients are key considerations in every clinical activity that you initiate. Motivation is defined as "the act or process of motivating," and motive is defined as "something (as a need or desire) that causes a person to act." Synonyms for motivation are incentive or drive.

The key clinical questions are as follows:

1. How does a person's motivation get destroyed and/or distorted
2. What are the differences between internal and external motivation
3. What is the checklist used by the clinician to initiate their own motivation to work
4. What is the clinical approach to the patient who chooses resistance or remains unmotivated
5. How does the clinician facilitate the client to create internal motivation—precise self talk
6. What is the timing involved in working with the resistant patient, and
7. How can the clinician assess the therapeutic effectiveness of an intervention designed to support self directed behavior in the patient?

The ultimate goal is patient motivation that leads to action and participation in activities that will enhance an individual's quality of life. The clinical intention is to cause the patient to choose to work on his or her own behalf. However, the clarity of the therapeutic intention can be distorted by the following: patient, family, significant others, payment policies, and institutional policies.

One could swim straight away if one could eliminate all the parasitic acts and perform only those movements that propel one in the direction wished. The expert swimmer produces only those movements that are wanted, and herein lies his skill. His action corresponds to the clear motivation and to that only.—Feldenkrais.

This chapter is meant to create an initial checklist for the clinician to examine if the therapeutic interactions have been focused in such a way that all activity supports and enhances the potential for patient motivation. The discussion about motivation applies to all patients, but it is especially significant for the elderly. From the age of 60 to 80+, there are enormous changes in a person's life. The majority of changes are a natural part of growing older, such as retirement from full time employment, loss of occupationally-related roles (as provider, leader, decision maker for self and/or others, and so forth), death of peers, friends, and often a spouse, brothers and sisters, as well as parents and changes in finances. If the body is to perform as desired when a person ages, the human body calls for more regular and precise maintenance due to normal age-related changes. The age-related bodily changes create a demand for regular maintenance activities (from dental flossing to conscious choice of amount and type of food and exercise). The interrelated factors of normal aging call for the older individual to adapt to many changes. The goal of adaptation is for each individual to develop a meaningful and uniquely satisfying life.

Regardless of age, for every human being there is a limit to the number of changes a person can adapt to over a specific period of time. The elderly who come for rehabilitation commonly have experienced a large number of major changes in the past few months, and they often show warning signs of low adaptive ability (i.e., problems falling asleep or staying asleep, preference for predictable schedules, irritability, nervousness, anxiety). As a part of the initial evaluation, patients who seek rehabilitation need to examine their level of motivation and their inherent drive to do for themselves. Because the elderly as a group are more likely to enter the rehabilitation process under considerable stress, they need precise therapist-patient interaction to support and enhance the individual patient's urge to do for himself or herself.

How does Motivation get Destroyed or Distorted?

Motivation to act and to achieve is molded and shaped from birth. If one happens to live in a family that is able to see "the possibilities" and to visualize "positive outcomes," then an individual learns one way of looking at the events that occur in everyday living. This kind of approach utilizes doubt as a stimulus for purposeful action, thereby presenting the classic case of seeing the glass half full and not half empty. Some people grow up in a family that literally scripts individuals to believe that they are victims of circumstance and consequently have no control over their lives. This kind of family tends to place value judgments on each other with statements like "you should have," "you must," which indicates a negative value judgment of the self. The individual coming out of that kind of home approaches life events with no clear sense of control. The self talk of a patient or client—the private internal dialogue that is carried on all the time—is the first clue to the basic motivational scripts that are currently cuing the actions of an individual patient. It is therefore possible for a patient to experience a severe illness (i.e., a major stroke) and, because he has an internal script that says he has no control and a nagging sense of inadequacy, the patient arrives at rehabilitation with his sense of internal motivation already distorted and/or destroyed.

Another contributing factor to the destruction or distortion of a patient's motivation is the family member or clinician who is in a hurry. Such contacts often presume that the patient's sense of reality and values are the same as theirs. In addition, they may inadvertently judge themselves as best able to decide what is best for the patient, neglecting to ask what are the key things on the patient's mind at that moment. The result can be that the patient in the wheelchair refuses to try to feed himself. The patient at that moment chooses the route of resistance, thereby openly expressing that there is no motivation to participate in the activity, at least under the conditions of that interpersonal interaction. As a clinician if I then say, "this patient is not motivated," I make a value judgment that can be interpreted to mean the following:

1. I, the clinician, know what is best for you
2. I, the clinician, do not care about your sense of reality since I did not take the time to inform, educate, or build a conceptual bridge between your sense of reality and mine
3. I, the clinician, am the locus of control, and you the patient need to do as I tell you, and
4. I have overlooked what you are motivated to do

for some reason (sense of needing to hurry, personal bias, etc.).

The third major contributor to the destruction or the distortion of motivation is simply cross motivation as applied to the design of the health care delivery system. One example of cross motivation is that what is best for the institution financially is not always best for the individual patient. If possible, the majority of elderly patients prefer to undergo rehabilitation while living in their own home, yet there continues to be a heavy national investment in institutional care instead of in-home care.

A patient who is not motivated is a person who is dealing with cross motivation. For motivation to lead to action, the individual patient needs to be self determined, and in nearly every situation, it is possible to nurture the innate human quality described as motivation. The art of human interaction lies in the recognition of the momentary failure in the interaction between clinician and patient. The patient may react to this failure by refusing to cooperate and acting withdrawn. The ability of the clinician to adapt to the individual needs of the patient at each moment is the key to the clinical outcomes. As the patient changes moment to moment, the clinician needs to keep the clinical focus on the desired outcome (mutually agreed upon by clinician and patient). Therapeutic interaction needs to be fluid and to accommodate the need for increased control by the patient as he or she outgrows the role of "patient or client" and returns to self-determination. The clinical problem of motivation occurs in part because clinicians may cling to their own conceptualization of what is best for the patient and demand that the patient accommodate their view of the world. The entire goal of rehabilitation is to prepare the patient for independence and self-determination and then for the clinician to consciously step out of their way and encourage the patient to make his or her own decisions.

What are the Differences Between Internal and External Motivation

The rehabilitation professional (physician, nurse, physical or occupational therapist, or social worker) can provide input to the patient that either affects their motivation over a short period of time (hours, days, weeks) or over an entire lifetime. Short-term motivation is labeled external and temporary. The example to consider is the cheerful professional who leads the patient by encouraging, praising, and cheering the patient toward success. The external temporary motivation provided by the high energy clinician can influence the patient to make a change; however, it cannot (a) make the change for the patient, or (b) keep the patient from drifting off course when the motivator is out of the room. The external motivator (i.e., the high energy clinician), has good intentions, inspiring words, and credible ideas. The problem is that when the clinician goes home, so does the patient's motivation. The patient may progress or achieve certain functional goals, but it is being done with someone else's energy—it is not that of the patient.

Shad Helmstetter states that "since the real meaning of the word motivation is 'to put into motion,' it seems to me that most of us would rather decide for ourselves what should put us 'into motion' than have someone else decide for us." Internal motivation is the only kind of motivation that lasts. It is the internal coach (internal dialogue) that is able to charge up the individual and to keep him or her going. Patients would never need someone to prod or push them since the script is written in. Internal motivation is the process that clears out negative and destructive self talk and replaces them with positive and inspiring ideas. The key factors in an environment that fosters the growth of self-motivation or internal motivation are as follows:

1. a sense of self esteem (feeling positive about oneself and a sense of personal adequacy
2. a personal sense of purpose, and
3. a sense of self-determination (a perception of control over one's life).

The goal of each member of the rehabilitation team needs to be to encourage the patient by our every action to become a self starter and a doer.

Checklist to Initiate a Motivation to Work

As any member of the rehabilitation team chooses to work, there is an initiation of specific self talk. The basic concept acknowledged at some level is the belief that there is the self-determination to make changes (positive modifications) within their actual work setting.

The therapeutic interaction is viewed as an ongoing experiment. The patient presents with a set of needs and problems. The clinician works actively to provide input and to modify therapeutic intervention so that it is maximally suited to each patient. If the clinician is going to guarantee the ability to support the individual patient's motivation, the therapeutic intervention is not mechanical repetition of fixed tasks, but rather the use of all patient feedback (kinesthetic and emotional) to adapt and to refine the therapeutic intervention to be ideally suited to the patient (as is possible).

Approach to the Unmotivated Patient

The overall goal of clinical intervention is to enhance as much as is possible the potential for patient motivation. As conceptualized in Figure 1, this in-

volves a process of building a "bridge of trust" between the patient and the clinician. The desired outcome of the interaction between the patient and the therapist is that patients begin to act, to take action, to participate in any and all activities of daily living, and to choose to work on their own behalf. Each action initiated by the clinician assures the patient that the bridge of trust is safe and predictable and that the clinician's intent is ongoing and consistent. The clinician needs to take predictable actions to develop a climate of acceptance and understanding as follows:

Step 1

As a part of the initial evaluation, time is taken to encourage the patient to share his or her concerns. The rationale is that if the individual patient is upset, worried, anxious, or angry, the limbic system prevents easy retrieval of our abilities for use as they are needed. It is a normal result of limbic system activity to distort the ease of retrieval of basic concepts and abilities when a person is emotionally upset, and it results in patients appearing less capable than they truly are.

Step 2

As a patient begins to feel at ease with the clinician and the therapeutic environment, the limbic system supports a natural access to an individual's potential. It has been stated that a genius is a person who uses less than 6 to 10 percent of his or her brain power. The clinical implication is that nearly every patient has some hidden potential or some underdeveloped or latent abilities. The early part of the therapeutic process involves helping the patient to sense and begin to believe as well as to feel that there is within them untapped potential. One clinical example that consistently works well is how we, as human beings, move. Why do I habitually fold my hands with the left (or right) thumb on top? What if I begin to change even small things like how I sit? It is usually easy to acquaint an individual patient with his or her habits of movement and open up the sense that each of us can *choose* new options. The habits of how we rest, sit, or fold our hands are choices that have become automatic over time. The important concept that this brings up is that the individual patient can choose new options and can start with small and manageable steps on the road to independence.

Step 3

As a clinician, my foremost intention during every moment of interaction with the patient is to encourage the patient to choose to work on his or her own behalf. The psycholinguistics (awareness of the interaction between emotional response, attitudes, and

Motivation – Action – Participation – Patient chooses to work in own behalf

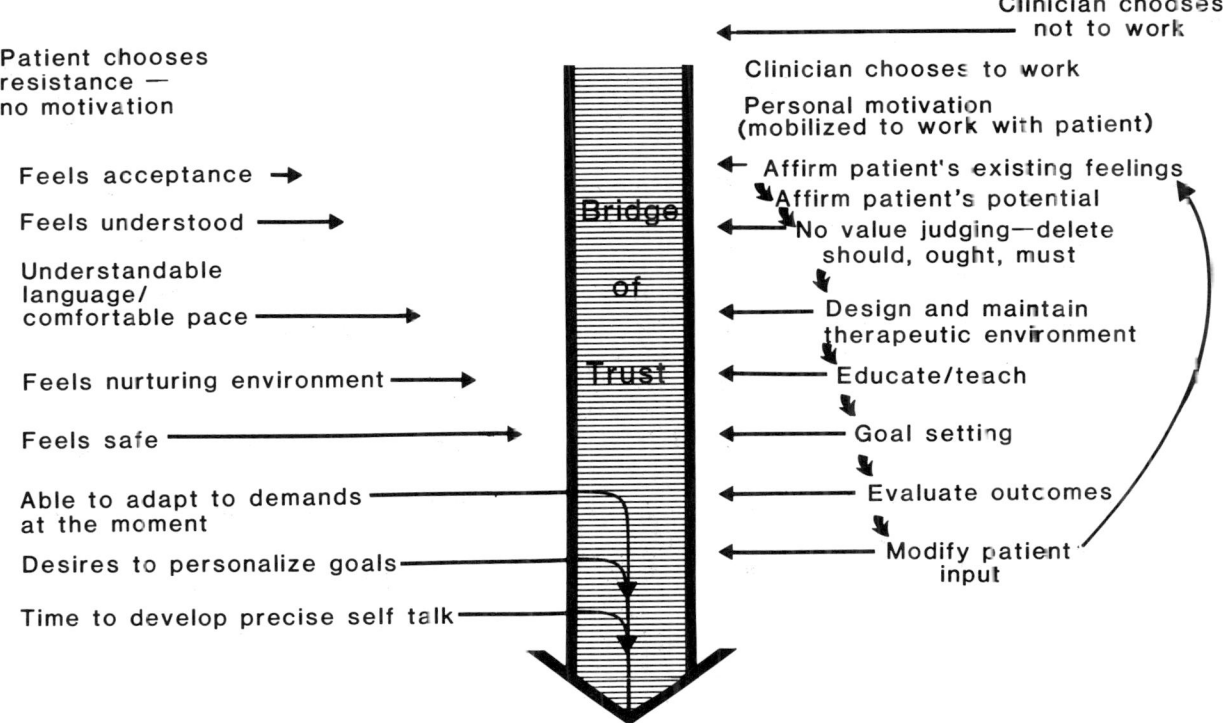

Figure 1   Enhancing the potential for patient motivation.

choice of words) of patient interaction calls for a conscious choice of words that avoids behavior that is value judging. A person who is value judging tends to make use of words like *should, ought,* and *must* while communicating with another person. Therapeutic interaction calls for verbal dialogue and self talk to build upon concepts of self directed behavior and choice; therefore, a substitution of the words should, ought, and must with *need, want,* and *consider* is called for. The choice of words is a conscious way to place the motivator internally in the patient.

The patient asks "what should I be doing"? The clinician helps the client to redirect and develop an internal motivator by asking and by helping the client to learn how to feel—"What feels best for you"? "Which motion feels easiest"? "How far can you move without pain"? The outcome for the patient is to develop an internal sense of "what I need to consider . . . in safely managing myself." The unspoken message to the patient by the clinician is as follows: 'I believe in your ability to develop control over your body." Psycholinguistics are of course used within the realms of safety, that is, in emergencies the words should, ought, and must may be temporarily appropriate and intended to get the patient safely to begin to work toward knowing his body.

Step 4

The clinician consciously creates a therapeutic environment for the patient. Modifications of environment that put the patient at ease may include such things as choice of words, construction of language, pace of interaction, as well as the more traditional professional adaptations.

The goal is to create in the patient a sense of being safe and a feeling that interaction with the clinician is a nurturing experience (i.e., it promotes a sense of self worth and acceptance).

The by-product of creating a therapeutic environment is that the patient is constantly invited to use the skills that are now being developed. The therapeutic environment presumes a daily interaction between team members, which facilitates carry over between professionals, (that is to say, PTs and OTs, orienting nursing staff, family, or meaningful others. These team members can provide safe follow-up that ensures new skills are used either on the nursing unit or in the home setting).

Step 5

The natural step, which can create carry over from the professional environment to the patient's real life setting, is patient education of the family, and the staff. A major part of this process is to teach the significant persons in the patient's world (family, friends, and nurses aides) the goals set for patients and how they as individuals can help the patient to achieve them. The process at this stage is to assist patients to develop a trust in their own ability in order that they might adapt to unforeseen demands. (An example being that of the patient who has practiced a transfer presuming that the person guarding him or her feels confident. Suddenly, one particular evening there is a new nurse's aide who says she is not comfortable doing this. In this situation, how can the patient get to bed safely with both motivation and sense of self intact?)

Step 6

As a patient begins to adapt in situations that by design are less and less ideal (more like real life) outcomes made are evaluated and modifications made to improve the overall experience. At this time, the patient is encouraged to personalize life goals and to broaden the focus beyond the pure medical or rehabilitative setting. To assist the patient, the entire cycle from Step 1 to 6 is continued on an ongoing basis to assure that patients feel at ease and can work in their own way (within reason) to develop latent abilities.

Precise Self Talk

As a major part of the ongoing process of discharge planning, ideally there is time set aside to develop precise self talk. This work can be done in many ways—on an individual basis or in small groups, using journal writing or verbal exchange. The patient is asked to examine the following issues on an ongoing basis: (1) Do you see yourself as half empty or half full? (2) Do you focus on what you can't do or do you celebrate and enjoy what you can? The goal is not to deny any losses, but rather to place emotional energy on a positive, self-supporting activity that can lead to fulfilling outcomes. This part of motivation building is likely handled differently in each clinical setting and can be the responsibility of one team member or a key component that is reinforced by all professionals, patients, families, and friends. The key to a long-term positive outcome is ongoing repetition of constructive self talk. Support groups led by other patients or nonprofessionals are used in some areas with great success.

Timing of Intervention

Timing of intervention demands answers to the following questions: Do you like being rushed? Did you overlook an important detail?

In our real life, timing is the key to effective in-terpersonal interaction. Two factors are critical if the urge to do for oneself is to be encouraged. First, each individual, especially the elderly, need to feel there is adequate time to try. As a group, the elderly commonly would rather not try, if it is not perceived that there is time enough to be successful. The gift of having enough time to feel at ease with the environment, the people, the activity around you, at ease with yourself, is a key component of the therapeutic process. Clinical specialists in geriatrics are the group of professionals who, in time, will mold clinical practice in hospitals and in other parts of the rehabilitation system to meet the unique needs of the elderly. The elderly can make enormous gains in rehabilitation when therapeutic intervention is individualized and takes place at a pleasant pace for each patient.

The second aspect of timing involves the time to note the details, the kinesthetic experience, and the emotional sense of the experience. The goal is to use every available channel to create long-term retention of new concepts and abilities. Each individual has one primary learning style (either kinesthetic, auditory, or visual). Taking the time to reinforce new concepts through other neurologic pathways tends to anchor the experience and to improve retention. Taking the time to process is something that we must do in many real life situations just as a computer must.

The human brain, like a computer, has a limit and can experience moments of overwhelming input. The ability of the rehabilitation community to accept modifications in pace by the elderly to work at an individually comfortable pace allows personalization of rehabilitation.

Signs of Therapeutic Effectiveness

- It is a patient who breathes a sigh of relief or joy, relaxes in the moment, and then begins to participate.
- It is a patient who can adapt and has the strength to define their own pace based on what they feel is best for them.
- It is a patient who can relate to the limitations of the health care delivery system with a sense of self-determination and an urge to work on their own behalf and with a sense of purpose—to make the system work even better in the future.
- It is a patient who talks about today and enjoys this—the only moment of life that any individual can really feel.

In summary, the clinician works to help the individual patient find the *urge* to do for themselves. The patient needs to believe at some level that improvement is a possibility. As the clinician meets each individual patient, it is a unique interaction molded by the patient's perception of reality. Motivation to do for ourselves develops under very specific conditions and at a pace that feels right to each patient. The clinical ability to facilitate motivation is an art that is a key in geriatric rehabilitation.

SUGGESTED READING

Bandler R, Grinder J. Reframing. Utah: Real People Press, 1982.

Cameron-Bandler L, Gordon D, Lebeau M. Know how—guided programs for inventing your own best future. San Rafael, CA: Future Pace, 1985.

Feldenkrais M. Elusive obrious. Cupertino, CA: Meta Publications, 1983.

Helmstetter S. What to say when you talk to yourself. Scottsdale, AZ: Grinale Press, 1986.

Jackson O. Physical therapy of the geriatric patient. New York: Churchill Livingstone, 1983.

Murray RB, Huelskotter MMW. Psychiatric/mental health nursing: giving emotional care, 2nd ed. Norwalk: Appleton & Lange, 1987.

Speads C. Ways to better breathing. Great Neck, NY: Felix Morrow Publisher, 1986.

MAINTENANCE OF MOBILITY IN THE ELDERLY

ANTHONY A. VANDERVOORT, Ph.D.

Safe, confident mobility is a precious aspect of health for the elderly individual who strives to remain active and independent.

A highly-motivated 70-year-old lady has been receiving physical therapy following fracture of the right femur, caused by a bicycling accident. Healing is normal, and the lady shows excellent compliance with therapy to the point where the injured leg is now comparable to the other side. The patient describes a very active lifestyle, which she and her husband pursue together, and asks the therapist to outline an exercise program to maintain her mobility at a high level.

The therapist may be approached by such people or their advocates to implement a program of exercises for maintenance of mobility. In such cases, emphasis is on prevention of loss of function, rather than on treatment of a specific condition. Prevention or delay of dependence in an elderly person living in the community is being vigorously promoted as a key component of the health care system today, and the physical therapy professional can take a leading role in this promotion. A particularly important target group for such initiatives is senior citizens in their sixth and seventh decades, or the "young elderly." An approach to the assessment and management of the geriatric patient referred for physical therapy is provided in the next chapter. In this chapter, factors which influence mobility of the elderly are reviewed with attention to issues regarding physical training programs.

FACTORS INFLUENCING MOBILITY OF THE ELDERLY

Normal upright ambulation, which young adults take for granted, is in fact a very complex function involving many body systems working in unison. An organizational chart for discussion of the many requirements for safe confident mobility is presented in Table 1.

Musculoskeletal Support System

Beginning with the body's framework, a proper gait clearly depends on an axial skeleton and a symmetrical limb structure that have the strength to support muscular action. However, the aging process weakens bone through the processes of osteoporosis and osteomalacia. This problem is particularly prominent for postmenopausal women. Prevention, or at least slowing of the rate of bone loss through weight-bearing activity, appears to be an important intervention, which is dealt with in detail in a separate section of this book.

Joint flexibility is a second prerequisite for mobility. The awkward lopsided walking pattern of an elderly person who is protecting an osteoarthritic hip serves to illustrate the necessity for smooth and painless articulation. It has been reported that healthy elderly people show considerable range of movement in the leg joints; therefore, pronounced stiffness and inflexibility can be considered as a disease-based ailment. Can it be prevented? This is a difficult question to answer unequivocally, given the complex etiology of joint dysfunction. However, one may speculate that moderate activity tends to sustain the maintenance of articular surfaces, ligaments, and the joint capsule. On the other hand, hard stress on these structures from excessive exercise patterns may precipitate joint deterioration. Given this fact, walking is much preferred over jogging for most senior citizens, particularly when an individual has been inactive, has some arthritic symptoms already, or is obese. Elderly people may need to be taught the value of stretching routines and the proper way to do them. For some, such instruction may be the first they have heard in several decades! There is good evidence that a program of calisthenics can significantly improve the flexibility of seniors.

A firm base of support must be present for secure mobility, but footcare is sometimes overlooked in a health regimen. It is encouraging to see the increase in numbers of older men and women wearing proper footwear for exercising and this must be stressed to all age groups. Boots and shoes with a poor fit or slippery sole may not only be uncomfortable to walk in, but also dangerous, and fashion should always give way to function. Blisters, bunions, ingrown toenails, and sore arches can also cause a tentative footfall pattern and such problems must be cleared up before a mobility maintenance program can be effective.

Muscular contraction provides the torque to control joint rotation precisely in smooth movement patterns. The normal aging process causes a progressive decrease of strength in old age as a result of a loss of nerve and muscle cells from the motor system. Yet this aging effect can be amplified by inactivity, and a program of resistance training may be utilized to

TABLE 1 Requirements for Safe, Confident Mobility

Musculoskeletal support system
    Symmetrical, solid limb structure
    Flexible, pain-free joints
    Adequate foot support
    Symmetrical, effective muscle strength
Sensory input regarding posture and gait
    Visual acuity to assess relation of body to environment (including obstacles)
    Vestibular monitoring of body orientation
    Proprioception from muscles, joints, and skin
Central neurological coordination
    Awareness of environment and impending hazards
    Competent motor planning consistent with capability
    Coordination of agonist-antagonist muscle actions
    Reciprocal interaction of limbs
Cardiorespiratory function
    Efficient response to metabolic needs of exercising muscle
    Autonomic control of blood pressure during postural changes
Environmental characteristics
    Adequate time to reach destination
    Absence of obstacles and sudden changes in surfaces or slopes

maximize the potential of aged muscle. Should strengthening exercises be isometric, concentric, or eccentric? Although isometric muscle contraction has the advantage of simplicity, caution is advised when prescribing such exercise for the elderly, because of its potent stimulus to increase blood pressure and, hence, to put stress on the cardiovascular system. If isometrics must be used, the muscle contraction should be limited to a few seconds at a time. In our experience eccentric exercise against a machine is difficult for nonathletes to learn and should be supervised closely; otherwise, there is some possibility of muscle and joint soreness, which quickly leads to a loss of motivation. Eccentric muscle contraction does have the advantages of simulating some of the natural lengthening maneuvers, which muscles make in normal locomotion, and of producing high tension.

For home or group exercise routines concentric muscle work is often the best choice for preventive programs. Simple exercises can be prescribed involving convenient items such as sandbags, spring devices, or dumbbells. Individuals can keep track of their progress by noting the amount of weight lifted, resistance overcome or the number of repetitions possible at a given intensity. Some exercises can be done in a sitting or recumbent position so that there is no danger of losing balance.

Sensory Input Regarding Posture and Gait

The upright stance of humans is precarious because of the high ratio of the height of our center of gravity to the area of our base of support. We rely heavily on three main sources of sensory input—vision, vestibular information and proprioception—to assess our balance constantly during standing and ambulation. Since postural control and instability are dis-

cussed in detail in another section of this book, some highlights of the topic relative to the elderly and prevention are provided here.

Vision has a powerful stabilizing influence on posture; this can be demonstrated when attempting to stand on one leg with eyes closed. Visual input also plays a major role in detecting progress during ambulation and when perceiving obstacles. It is thus important to have the maximum acuity possible by using proper corrective lenses, having adequate lighting and utilizing any environmental cues available. Any mobility maintenance program must emphasize the need for the elderly to use caution in or to avoid any situation where vision is limited, e.g., getting up in the night without putting a light on. Vestibular input is also utilized to maintain balance by providing information about body orientation and by acting as part of the vestibular-ocular reflex in maintaining visual fixation. Rapid or extensive turning movements leading to dizziness should be avoided in activity programs and it should be remembered that people with ear infections or sinus congestion may be very susceptible to falls.

Proprioception also forms an integral part of our postural control system. Although there is evidence that some loss of proprioceptive input occurs in the very old, as demonstrated by reduced ability to detect joint position and by slowed, muted tendon reflexes, there are also reports that "young elderly" groups who maintain vigorous activity patterns show little age-related differences from young adults In a manner similar to muscle strength ability, proprioceptive ability also appears to be regulated by the motto "use it or lose it." The elderly should be encouraged to include safe balancing exercises in their activity program. Those with postural instability may need specific exercises in a physical therapy clinic to regain a sense of equilibrium and confidence before attempting unsupervised exercise.

Central Neurologic Coordination

Common to many falls is the factor that, before the accident, a person was hurrying or was distracted and unaware of an impending hazard. Clearly the more active people are, the more susceptible they become to this type of event; epidemiologic surveys have noted that the young elderly are at considerable risk of falling. Hopefully, if such an event is experienced it does not cause any trauma, but rather serves to remind the senior citizen that footing and balance should be continually monitored. Alzheimer's disease is an example of a disease condition that creates a tendency to fall—because of inattentiveness and loss of short term memory, which may cause people to forget about obstacles in their path.

Maintenance of mobility in older people may also require some acceptance (on their part) of age-related decreases in motor capacity. Because of weakening muscles, sluggish reflexes, or stiff joints, they may no longer be able to carry a large load safely up and down steps. In this case, prevention involves assessing functional limits and helping the elderly individual set realistic activity goals. Although this may seem like common sense, it should be remembered that old habits die hard and that we tend to ignore or minimize such physical disabilities; for example some seniors are reluctant to use a cane instead of limping in an unstable manner. The therapist may thus be challenged to keep an older patient active, but exercising within safe limits, especially when prescribing unsupervised home programs.

Motor programming involves regulation of muscle stiffness on both sides of the joint, as typified by the three burst pattern of agonist-antagonist-agonist firing observed when a limb is moved to a target. It is important to maintain muscle balance across elderly leg joints with exercises to promote coordinated use of both antigravity and more phasic muscles. This is particularly true for the ankle dorsiflexors, which must get the foot turned up briskly at the right time in the gait cycle to avoid stubbing the toes. It is noteworthy that, whereas the resistance that this muscle group must overcome (as a result of foot weight plus passive stiffness of the antagonist) does not decrease with aging, the strength and contractile speed of the dorsiflexors is reduced significantly in the average elderly person. A final point regarding CNS coordination of mobility is that exercises should include reciprocal limb actions that simulate the alternate contraction pattern of gait, e.g., bicycling and "scissors" type calisthenics.

Cardiorespiratory Function

The profound increases in blood flow to vigorously contracting skeletal muscle serve to maintain its ability to generate tension for extended periods. However, the capacity for oxygenating and delivering blood to the tissues is diminished in the average elderly person and fatigue may lead to incoordination of movement. Many studies have now shown that this capacity can be dramatically improved in the elderly by endurance training programs. There are many options available to the therapist when prescribing aerobic activities. The aim is to get a large part of the body's muscle mass contracting rhythmically in low intensity efforts maintained for 15 minutes or more. Bicycling, walking, jogging, skipping, rowing, and swimming are examples of activities that can be easily quantified and applied where there is space and equipment. It is important to include a warmup and cooldown period in any aerobic exercise period, regardless of time limitations. These principles of exercise programming are outlined in Table 2 under the headings of Design, Mechanics, and Safety.

TABLE 2   Principles of Preventive Exercise Programs for Mobility Maintenance

Program design based on T.A.P.E. principle
  T.—*Test* individual thoroughly for current functional level
  A.—*Assess* for areas of decreased competence
  P.—*Program* to enhance mobility
  E.—*Evaluate* at a regular intervals to provide feedback
Program mechanics based on F.I.T.T. principle
  F.—*Frequency* of program should be three or more times per week
  I.—*Intensity*—warmup, sustained training period, cooldown
  T.—*Time* of each session is about 20 to 40 minutes
  T.—*Types* of exercise should be varied and appropriate to needs
Program safety based on S.A.F.E. principle
  S.—*Supervise* during learning period
  A.—*Allow* adequate time for task completion and rest periods
  F.—*Forgetfulness* causes accidents—avoid distractions and know medication side-effects
  E.—*Environment* should be as hazard-free as possible

Autonomic nervous control of cardiorespiratory function serves to maintain the blood supply to the brain during changes in posture. For example, when we stand up from a sitting or lying position, blood pressure temporarily falls due to the effects of gravity on circulation, and healthy baroreceptors quickly respond with a signal to increase cardiac output. However, this postural hypotension effect can cause fainting if the autonomic response is muted by prolonged bed rest or medication and it is necessary to check this function before implementing an exercise program for the elderly. A drop in systolic blood pressure of greater than 20 mm Hg upon standing is one rule of thumb used to identify people at risk of syncope.

Environmental Characteristics

A final consideration in the maintenance of mobility is to try and make locomotion as safe as possible (see Table 2). Examples of such a strategy are as follows: allowing extra time for the older individual to cross a street rather than rushing at an unsafe speed; installing firm handrails at the proper height along steps; eliminating obstacles, such as unsecured rugs, in the home; and encouraging elderly people to walk indoors at malls in winter when sidewalks are slippery. Another preventive approach involves using signs and color cues to denote changes in slope or surface of a pathway. Half of the falls that elderly people suffer are attributed to "accidents,"—the slips and trips that are usually avoidable.

Medication may also create a tendency toward unsafe mobility in the elderly. Commonly used drugs, such as alcohol, antihypertensives, antidepressants and sedatives, can affect blood pressure and state of consciousness. The therapist needs to know what an individual is taking and to offer counseling on what sort of precautions are required to avoid falling during activity. It should be remembered that old people may undergo frequent changes in medications and that they do not usually metabolize drugs at the same rate as young adults.

SUGGESTED READING

Burdman GM. Healthful aging. Englewood Cliffs, NJ: Prentice-Hall, 1986.

Jackson O, ed. Physical therapy of the geriatric patient. New York: Churchill Livingstone, 1983.

Vandervoort AA, Hayes KC, Belanger AY. Strength and endurance of skeletal muscle in the elderly. Physiother Can 1986; 38:167–173.

Walker J. Exercise and aging. NZ J Physiother 1986; 14:8–12.

Whipple RH, Wolfson LI, Amerman F. The relationship of knee and ankle weakness to falls in nursing home residents: an isokinetic study. J Am Geriatr Soc 1987; 35:13–20.

MANAGEMENT OF THE GERIATRIC PATIENT

ANTHONY A. VANDERVOORT, Ph.D.
NANCY S. MICK JONES, B.Sc.(PT), M.Sc.

Geriatric patients are becoming more numerous in physical therapy settings.

Following her children's concern that she is no longer coping independently in her own apartment, a frail, 85-year-old woman has been admitted to hospital for geriatric assessment. Previous history includes a right CVA 5 years ago, which resulted in mild symptoms of left hemiplegia; hypertension now controlled by medication; osteoarthritic deterioration of the right hip joint, and cataract surgery. Referral is made to the physical therapy department regarding the patient's poor balance and fear of falling.

The number of people in our population over the age of 80 years is rapidly increasing and will continue to do so as the "baby boom" generation moves into the twenty-first century. This group will expect a high level of health care that includes physical rehabilitation that maximizes function and independence regardless of age. Contrary to the vigorous, active "young elderly" population (aged 65 to about 75), the very old suffer from advanced chronic diseases, which create complex physical problems for therapists to deal with. Issues in the management of this latter age group are the focus of the following chapter. The common characteristic of geriatric patients is multiple dysfunction in several body systems caused by the combination of an age-related decline in function and increasing incidence of such diseases as osteoarthritis, arteriosclerosis, and dementia. Therapists dealing with this type of case are challenged to make comprehensive assessments and then appropriate treatment plans based on performance objectives that stress independence in activities of daily living.

EFFECTS OF AGING ON FUNCTION

Aging is an inevitable process that leads to a progressive decline in many body functions. Although scientific debate has gone on for many years over the mechanisms of aging, there now appears to be some consensus that humans are programmed genetically to age, and eventually to die, within a fixed lifespan of approximately ten decades. Thus, the ideal life is one of vigor from birth until very old age, and in fact, the majority of old people do remain relatively healthy and independent. The inevitable loss of function varies considerably among individuals, but some trends based on average levels of performance at different ages can be discussed. The functions presented are just those most likely to be assessed by therapists and a more comprehensive list can be obtained from textbooks on geriatric care.

Musculoskeletal System

Muscle mass, and hence strength, appears to be well maintained throughout middle age, and it is not until after the age of about 60 years that men and women experience significant declines in performance. A healthy, well-motivated 85-year-old lady would be expected to have only about half the strength of a young woman. When assessing and when setting treatment goals for geriatric patients, it should always be remembered that *standard reference values must be age-matched*.

Similar observations have been made on bone composition and joint flexibility that aging causes alterations in the levels to be expected when assessing old people. Loss of bone tissue is particularly important in females, thus leading to a high rate of osteoporosis and a tendency to fracture bones during falls. Joint range of motion (ROM) is reduced in the elderly because of increased stiffness of elastic tissue and loss of voluntary strength for overcoming this passive resistance to joint movement. However, extreme limitation of ROM should not be expected at any age, and such a finding indicates an abnormality.

Neurologic System

Age-related decreases to be aware of in peripheral neurologic function include a slowing of nerve conduction in both sensory and motor nerves; a loss of acuity in the senses, e.g., vision, hearing, and proprioception; absent or sluggish tendon reflexes. In the central nervous system, aging causes a loss of cells from many regions of the brain and the spinal cord. The redundancy of the nervous system prevents this loss from creating significant deficits of cognitive functioning in most elderly people, but subtle changes do exist. For example, speed of information processing in a choice reaction time test is slowed.

Disease of the nervous system causes much disability in the elderly, particularly that stemming from cerebrovascular, Alzheimer's, and Parkinson's disease. Associated with the motor and cognitive deficits of these disorders may be bladder and bowel incontinence, a problem which may resolve as the patient becomes more oriented to the environment and as mobility is increased with physical therapy. A final point about the nervous system is that depression is a common psychological reaction to personal aging (and disease) that may interfere with a patient's motivation to comply with prescribed therapy.

Cardiorespiratory System

Aging causes a marked reduction in circulatory and pulmonary function. Such changes as decreased maximal heart rate, reduced ability to vasodilate arteriosclerotic blood vessels, and declining maximal breathing capacity limit exercise tolerance in the elderly patient. An additional important consideration is the increased incidence of hypertension in the elderly; hence, isometric type exercise, which is a potent stimulus for raising blood pressure, must be used cautiously with geriatric cases. The profound effect of bed rest on the cardiorespiratory system may cause severe fatigue when exercise is taken after a long period of immobilization. Resumption of activity as soon as possible following illness or operation is thus advocated, but even then progress may be slow in reaching therapeutic goals.

ASSESSMENT

Due to the fact that aging affects all body systems, geriatric assessment needs to be broad in scope. General information is needed on lifestyle prior to hospital admission and his or her level of function in various daily activities. Any aids required for these activities should be known. Previous medical history and medication record should be checked. If possible the physical assessment should be carried out with the occupational therapist present to obtain a more complete picture. The assessment should include information on the following systems:

Musculoskeletal

Remembering that for the geriatric patient functional capabilities are of utmost importance, ROM of all upper and lower extremity joints should be examined. Any asymmetry or gross restriction should be noted. A slight overall decrease in range tends to be the normative finding. Neck and trunk movement should also be checked. Stiffness in these areas may affect ability to attain a sitting position from recumbency independently and vice versa. As mentioned, muscle strength decreases in the elderly patient. Again this should be assessed not strictly as a quantitative value, but rather as an indicator of functional ability,

e.g., it is more important to note whether the patient can stand up from a sitting position than whether the quadriceps are a grade 3^+ or 4^-. Very often a patient may appear to have sufficient strength to complete a task, but (due to any number of other factors) cannot. For this reason, when assessing function, the musculoskeletal and neurologic systems must be viewed as interdependent.

Neurological

Specific areas to check in the geriatric patient are (1) sensory—including touch, temperature discrimination, and proprioception, (2) motor—including coordination, muscle tone, and balance, (3) and cognitive. The status of the sensory system indicates the amount of afferent information the CNS is receiving and how this may be affecting ability to carry out specific tasks. It also highlights any potential problem areas and situations that need to be handled with caution; for example, any areas of decreased sensation should be watched for potential breakdown caused by pressure and/or irritation. All functional mobility activities should be examined with regard to motor sequencing, balance, and safety. Posture should be noted in various positions, in addition to the effect it has on ability to complete a task or maintain a position. Abnormalities in posture may be musculoskeletal or neurologic in nature. It is important to ascertain level of awareness, ability to comprehend verbal commands, memory, motivation, and reliability. These all have a significant bearing on the overall function level and the capacity to undertake therapy.

Cardiovascular

In general, the overall capacity for activity should be assessed. Cardiac status and any fluctuations in blood pressure in relation to changes in body position should also be noted. Besides supplying a baseline, this information is necessary for planning an effective, safe treatment regime within realistic limits for each individual.

TREATMENT

The treatment plan is based on the specific findings of the assessment and the objectives for the patient and, therefore, varies with the individual. In contrast to younger adults, the geriatric patient also has some limitations, as a result of aging effects, for which allowances must be made. The most obvious limitation is that of endurance. There may also be multiple problems requiring treatment. When this is the case, the treatment regime should be designed to maximize the number of problems treated with the

TABLE 1 Levels of Independence

Level*	Indications
Independent	No verbal or physical assistance to complete a task is required
Standby assistance	As above, but someone should be present during task (i.e., not completely safe)
Verbal cues	A verbal reminder is required at some point during task
Minimal assistance	Hands on assistance is required at some point during task
Moderate assistance	Hands on assistance is required for 50% or more of task
Maximum assistance	Patient is totally dependent on assistant(s) to complete task

* These may be colour-coded or numbered and placed beside a particular task to indicate level of assistance needed for a number of tasks. This key should also be readily available for Nursing to consult. (Note that this code does not indicate at what point or how assistance is required.)

minimum of exercises, i.e., choose exercises that combine aspects of strength, range, coordination, and balance. Have the treatment take place in the most convenient location—which may not necessarily be the physical therapy department since travel time to and from may be tiring. There are several other general points that should be kept in mind when planning a treatment program. These include the following:

1. A daily routine—a program structured so that patients may orient themselves is both beneficial and functional. Morning is more often the appropriate time of day for this.
2. Stress independence—have patients do whatever they can for themselves. Every functional activity performed is treatment. Have a chart posted by the bed to indicate the amount of assistance required for various activities (Table 1).
3. Choose appropriate aids—safe and functional mobility is a priority objective. Choose aids that best accomplish this objective and stress that only a properly fitted aid should be used (Table 2). Remember proper footwear is very important for the ambulatory patient.
4. Modalities for pain relief—often the geriatric patient benefits from some form of heat applied to a stiff or painful area. Pool therapy is also useful as it provides a warm, buoyant medium for exercise. Sensory and circulatory status should be considered prior to application of any modality. In addition, certain medications may alter the effect of the modality.

TABLE 2 Mobility Aids

Type	Indication	Advantages	Limitations
Cane single	Minimal assistance required mainly for gait correction	Light, easy to take along up and down stairs	Not much support if patient tires, or terrain becomes slippery
Cane quad	More support than single cane; only one upper extremity can be used	As above—slightly heavier and more cumbersome	Needs to be placed properly on ground otherwise easy to tip
Walker wheels	More assistance required than with cane alone; patient tires easily with cane	Good support on most flat terrains; collapsible so easy to transport; easy to teach use; easy to attach bags, etc.	Patient must have use of both upper extremities; not good on carpet, not good for stairs, etc.
Walker no wheels	As above	As above; good on most flat terrains including carpets	As above; not as easy to teach use
Crutches axilla forearm elbow	Forearm crutches are useful with limited hand use	Forearm supports can be adapted to a walker—adequate support without using the hand	All require good upper limb and trunk strength and good balance—generally recommended in the geriatric patient
Wheelchair	For the patient who wishes to be very mobile (i.e., shopping, sightseeing) yet cannot walk long distances	Comfortable, safe, convenient for longer travel; more independence	Expensive, more difficult to transport, requires assistance from another person unless able to push on own or chair is electric

5. Team approach—be aware of the assessment findings and treatment regimes provided by other health professionals. The team approach ensures that all problem areas are identified and that the most appropriate treatment is selected.
6. Maintenance of joint range of motion and muscle strength—this is particularly important for the nonambulatory patient to facilitate maximum functional ability, nursing care, and patient well-being.

Discharge Planning

There are many factors to consider when a patient is preparing to leave the hospital setting. The physical therapist's role is important in these preparations in supplying information regarding functional abilities and tolerance. Home care physical therapy should be involved if there is any question regarding the living situation and the need for adaptations to the home. There are many community services that can be called upon to assist in enabling the patient to function at home.

Contraindications

The main precautions to be aware of in the geriatric patient relate to individual physical conditions that may require exercise modification. The major areas to be aware of are cardiac, alterations in blood pressure, sensory deprivation (including proprioception), strength decrease, and reaction time delays. Medications can also have an effect on the outcome of treatment and specific drugs should be checked out in regard to this, particularly if medication list and schedule are undergoing continuous changes and assessment during the hospitalization.

SUGGESTED READING

Brocklehurst JC, ed. Textbook of geriatric medicine and gerontology. 3rd ed. Edinburgh: Churchill Livingstone, 1985.

Coren A, Andreassi M, Blood H, Kent B. Factors related to physical therapy students' decisions to work with elderly patients. Phys Ther 1987; 67:60–65.

Jackson O, ed. Physical therapy of the geriatric patient. New York: Churchill Livingstone, 1983.

Lewis CB. Aging: the health care challenge. New York: FA Davis, 1985.

Tinetti ME. Performance-oriented assessment of mobility problems in elderly patients. J Am Geriatr Soc 1986; 34:119–125.

OSTEOPOROSIS AND EXERCISE

BARRIE PICKLES, B.P.T., M.S.

PATTERNS OF BONE LOSS WITH AGE IN MEN AND WOMEN

The bones of normal older persons are less dense than those of younger individuals. Both the organic and the inorganic components of bone are progressively reduced with age. When this age-related bone loss is excessive, the situation is termed involutional osteoporosis. This term is more appropriate than either "senile" or "postmenopausal" osteoporosis. Although the majority of sufferers are elderly women, the problem is not restricted to either older people or to females.

In males, from the age of 35, there is a regular loss of bone at an average rate of approximately 0.5 percent per year. In females, loss of bone also occurs at this rate between the ages of 25 and 50, increases to between 2.5 and 3.0 percent per year, between the ages of 50 and 65, and reverts to the slower 0.5 percent per year rate of loss after the age of 65. At all ages, the bones of females are less dense than those of males of similar age, with the difference in bone density between the sexes widening with increasing age.

In males of all ages, and in females over the age of 65, similar reductions occur in the density of both cortical and trabecular bone. In contrast, postmenopausal loss of bone in women appears to affect the trabecular bone selectively, with the horizontal trabeculae showing the greatest reduction in both thickness and number.

Any reduction in bone density weakens the bone. Where loss of horizontal trabeculae has occurred, considerable loss in bone strength is evident, resulting from the loss of the cross-bracing support normally provided by these structures. Osteoporosis achieves clinical importance when the density and mechanical strength of the bones has been reduced to such an extent that the weakened bones may fracture when minimal trauma is applied. The existence of osteoporosis is related frequently to fractures at the lower end of the radius (Colles' fracture), the upper end of the femur, and in the vertebral bodies. Until or unless such fractures occur, the condition is usually symptomless.

Often an unsuspected reduction in bone density is revealed as the result of radiographic screening during routine medical examinations.

The typical patient who suffers from, or is predisposed to, involutional osteoporosis is an older Caucasian woman, of slight build, with sedentary occupation and interests, whose diet includes a high proportion of protein, and who has smoked moderately to heavily over a long period of her life.

BONE DENSITY AND PHYSICAL ACTIVITY

A general relationship between the bone mineral content (BMC) in the axial skeleton and the general physical performance capacity of older men and women has been clearly established. It has also been shown that the BMC of the lumbar vertebrae correlates closely with both the force of maximum voluntary contraction (MVC) of the back extensor muscles and the cross-sectional area of the muscle belly of the psoas major. A similar strong correlation also exists between physical work capacity and BMC of bones in the lower limb and trunk. These findings serve to emphasize the importance of general physical activity in the maintenance of bone density.

In the bones of the upper limb, this relationship is less clear. Although a weaker relationship between these factors exists in the dominant upper limb, no consistent findings have been reported for the nondominant side. The lack of consistent correlation between forearm BMC and working capacity suggests that BMC in the upper limb bones may be more dependent on the local demands of physical activity, rather than on general physical work capacity.

Two separate mechanisms—muscle activity and weight bearing—have been identified as being important in the maintenance of normal BMC.

In normal subjects who are confined to bed, the performance of exercises, from a supine position on a bicycle ergometer for up to 4 hours per day, has no effect on the rate of calcium loss. Rapid decalcification has also been reported in the bones of astronauts during weightless space flights—even though a stringent program of exercises was performed during these flights.

Weight bearing alone, although helpful, is not necessarily adequate either. Patients with poliomyelitis affecting muscles of the calf, who were involved in a program of standing on the affected limbs for up to 3 hours per day failed to demonstrate any increased density of the bones in the affected calf and foot, although an increase in BMC was shown on the unaffected side. In another study, a program of 3 hours per day of quiet standing proved to be sufficient to induce a slow decline of an elevated calcium excretion rate in normal subjects who were otherwise confined to bed.

From these findings, it appears that adequate amounts of both compression of bone and simultaneous activity of the overlying muscles are necessary to prevent loss of BMC and to stimulate bone growth. Involutional osteoporosis develops when this combination of factors is lacking over a prolonged period. In other words, the maintenance of weight-bearing activities throughout life would appear to be a vital factor in reducing age-related bone loss to a minimum in normal adults.

The performance of weight-bearing activities and resisted exercises places a variety of stresses and strains on the bones. These forces—compression, strain, torsion—create small micropotentials in the connective tissue within the bone, through the operation of a piezoelectric effect. Other micropotentials (flow potentials) are created in the bone tissue as the result of an increased rate of flow of blood through the vessels in the bone, which is caused by intermittent contraction of the overlying muscles.

The micropotentials resulting from the piezoelectric and flow effects each appear to be inadequate to produce any significant effect on the bone when applied separately. However, when the micropotentials from these two sources are combined, both the secretion of procollagen by the osteoblasts and the deposition of bone crystals and calcium salts in the bone matrix are stimulated.

BONE DENSITY AND FRACTURES

If a comparison is made between radial bone density and the rate of forearm bone fractures at different ages, different patterns emerge for men and women. In males, no significant increase in the fracture rate occurs during life, even after the age of 65 when the density of the bone is significantly reduced. In females, on the other hand, a significant increase in the forearm bone fracture rate begins at the age of 45 and continues thereafter.

A closer inspection of these data reveals two points of particular interest. First, the appearance of a significant increase in the fracture rate of the forearm bones in women precedes the appearance of a significant decrease in bone density by a 5- to 10-year period. Second, the appearance of a significant increase in the fracture rate of forearm bones occurs in women at a time when the hydroxyapatite density in the radial cortex averaged 680 mg per milliliter; however, in males over the age of 65, whose average hydroxyapatite density varies between 620 and 650 mg per milliliter, no increase in fracture rate is found.

An examination of density of the vertebral spongiosa during aging in women with and without vertebral compression fracture shows that those who sustain such a fracture have, on average, a considerably lower spongiosa density than those who do not suffer fracture. However, the spongiosa density of some women without vertebral fracture is well below that of a substantial proportion of the women who have suffered fracture.

It would appear reasonable to infer from these data that (a) no simple relationship exists between bone density and fracture rate in either the axial or appendicular skeletons; (b) it is not possible to designate any particular bone density as a threshold level for fracture; and (c) factors other than bone density are important determinants of whether a fracture will result from the application of a given force.

PRODUCTION OF EFFECTIVE HYDRAULIC SUPPORT BY MUSCLE CONTRACTION

In a number of in vitro laboratory experiments it has been shown that bone tissue may fail when compression forces lower than those developed during normal activities are applied. It has been claimed that during normal activities bones are protected from damage and are strengthened hydraulically by the pressure exerted by the intramedullary fluids contained within them. Evidence has also been presented to demonstrate that bone marrow pressure is closely related to the force of contraction of the overlying muscles.

When bones are compressed, some of the blood contained in the cancellous endosteal bone and some of the other fluids from the marrow cavity are forced out of the bone through small foramina in the bone surface. If the surrounding muscles are relaxed or paralyzed there is little or no impedance to this outflow; consequently, the bone marrow pressure remains unaltered.

On the other hand, if the surrounding muscles are in a state of contraction at the moment the compression forces are being applied to the bone, the outflow of fluid through the foramina is reduced or stopped completely, depending upon the degree of contraction of the overlying muscles. If escape of fluid from the medullary cavity is reduced or prevented, bone marrow pressure is increased.

Any increase in bone marrow pressure changes the mechanical properties of bone The presence of fluid at an increased pressure in the marrow cavity absorbs some of the potentially damaging and destructive forces that would otherwise fall on the bone tissue when compression is applied. Indeed, compression forces, which might otherwise result in fracture, may be dissipated and resisted by the increased hydraulic support created by strong and timely contraction of the surrounding muscles.

It follows, then, that the risk of fracture from the application of a given force depends upon an interaction between bone density and the ability of the surrounding muscles to develop an effective degree of hydraulic support.

ABILITY TO GENERATE EFFECTIVE HYDRAULIC SUPPORT IN MALES AND FEMALES

Four generalizations are often drawn from an examination of studies on the strength of skeletal muscle in the elderly. First, there is a progressive loss in strength with age. Second, the pattern of strength loss is similar for all muscle groups, whether they be proximal or distal, or located in the upper or lower limbs. Third, by the seventh decade, the average maximum voluntary contraction is at least 20 percent lower than in young adults, and fourth, males and females appear to experience similar aging changes in their muscles.

Whereas the muscles of males and females appear to experience similar aging changes insofar as the progressive reduction in maximum voluntary contraction over time is concerned, the effect of this reduction on the ability to develop effective hydraulic support and, consequently, on fracture rates, is more pronounced in women whose bone density and muscle strength (at all ages) is lower than that of men of similar age.

In the biceps brachii, for example, the average force of the reported maximum voluntary contraction in females is 288 N, compared with 573 N for a matched group of male subjects. When body weight is taken into account, the maximum voluntary contraction per kilogram of body weight in females is 4.71 N, as compared with 7.27 N for males. These data clearly show that the potential for development of effective hydraulic support to bones in females is considerably less than in males.

The rate of force development during a muscle contraction in males is 1.5 to 2.0 times faster than in females; the reasons underlying this difference are not clear at this time. However, it does appear reasonable to infer that, since the time taken to generate a maximum voluntary contraction of muscles (and, consequently, to develop an effective level of hydraulic support to the bone) is greater in females than in males the risk of fracture is higher in females.

Differences between males and females in both the strength and speed of muscle contraction may explain, at least in part, why the fracture rate for a given bone is invariably higher in women than in men in situations where the bone density in the two groups is the same.

SUGGESTED READING

Alffram P, Bauer G. Epidemiology of fractures of the forearm. J Bone Joint Surg 1962; 44A:105–114.

Bell DG, Jacobs I. Electro-mechanical response times and rate of force development in males and females. Med Sci Sports Ex 1986; 18:31–36.

Brewer V, Meyer BM, Keele MS, Upton J, Hagan RD. Role of exercise in prevention of bone loss. Med Sci Sports Ex 1983; 15:445–449.

Kumar S, Davis PR, Pickles B. Bone marrow pressure and bone strength. Acta Orthop Scand 1979; 50:507–512.

Meema S, Meema HE. Involutional (physiologic) bone loss in women and the feasibility of preventing structural failure. J Amer Geriatr Soc 1974; 22:443–452.

PREVENTIVE ROLE OF THE PHYSICAL THERAPIST IN THE MANAGEMENT OF OSTEOPOROSIS

BARRIE PICKLES, B.P.T., M.S.

The physical therapist may be involved in the management of osteoporosis in two basic types of situations—the preventive role and the therapeutic role. This chapter considers the preventive role.

POPULATIONS AT RISK OF OSTEOPOROTIC FRACTURE

Three groups of women have been shown to be at particular risk and are as follows:

1. Women who seek medical care for problems associated with menopause and who are found to be losing bone at an excessive rate at that time. Considerable variation is found in the rate at which postmenopausal women lose bone. Whereas the average rate of bone loss in this group has been reported to be 1.0 to 1.5 percent per year, some women show losses of 3.0 percent per year or more. Moreover, those whose bone loss is excessive in the immediate postmenopausal period are likely to continue to lose bone at a faster-than-average rate thereafter. Obviously, if the faster rate of bone loss is not halted, the weight-bearing bones will be weakened to a critical degree within a few years.

2. Middle-aged women who sustain a Colles' fracture. It has been clearly established that the bone mineral content (BMC) in both the axial and appendicular skeletons is lower, on average, in women who have sustained a Colles' fracture than in age-matched normal females. This difference is particularly apparent in those women who sustain this fracture on their dominant side. Furthermore, it has also been shown that women who suffer a Colles' fracture during middle age have a significantly higher-than-normal risk of fracture of the femoral neck in later life.

3. Middle-aged women who fit the typical profile described in the previous chapter—Caucasian, slight build, with sedentary occupation and interests, whose diet includes a high proportion of proteins, and who has smoked moderately to heavily over a long period of her life.

The physician may have recognized that pronounced osteoporosis is likely to occur at a future time in a patient who presently displays no symptoms. Such patients may be specifically referred to the physical therapist for advice and counseling with regard to the importance of activity, both to maintain and improve general physical capacity, and to reduce the progressive bone loss to a minimum.

More frequently, patients are referred for physical therapy to deal with some other designated medical condition, and the existence of, or a predisposition to, osteoporosis is discovered by the therapist during the assessment.

ADVICE AND COUNSEL ON INCREASING PHYSICAL ACTIVITY

If no cardiovascular or respiratory problems exist, the patient should be made aware of the possibility of problems that may arise later from osteoporosis, advised of the importance of general physical activity in reducing this possibility, and counseled on suitable alternative activity programs available in the area.

SELECTION OF APPROPRIATE ACTIVITY PROGRAM

In general, the greater the amount of weight-bearing physical activity performed over a period of time, the greater the effect on the bone density. Jogging, tennis and other racquet sports, aerobic classes, and dancing have all been shown to be beneficial, and undoubtedly, skating and cross-country skiing would be equally helpful. Some progressive pre-activity training program is often advisable to reduce the possibility of strain or injury from these activities. For less active individuals, the benefits of regular walking and stair climbing should not be underestimated.

One of the most important points concerning an activity program is that it should be enjoyable. If you are successful in persuading a patient to include an increased amount of activity in her lifestyle, and to enroll in a suitable program, you have made a start. Unless she finds the program enjoyable, she will soon drop out. The attrition rate from adult activity classes is high, yet if attendance is not continued the risk of later problems from advanced osteoporosis increases.

PRE-ACTIVITY EXERCISE PROGRAM

The therapist devises a pre-activity program of exercises to increase the strength and speed of contraction of the paravertebral muscles and the muscles around the hip in order to give greater hydraulic support to the weight-bearing bones in these areas, which are at particular risk of fracture during activity.

When osteoporosis is extensive or severe, care should be taken to select a program in which the mechanical forces developed in the weight-bearing bones during the prescribed activities is not likely to cause fracture.

In young, fit individuals there is a close relationship between maximum voluntary contraction, which can be generated in a muscle, and the speed with which force is developed by the contraction. This relationship is often absent in older persons, especially in those suffering from a variety of medical problems. In addition to exercises designed to increase the strength of isometric and isotonic contractions, it is advisable to include specific speed-training exercises in this program.

The therapist also needs to bear in mind that, because these patients are middle-aged or elderly, greater attention needs to be given to the proper performance of stretching exercises for all the major muscle groups prior to strength training in order to avoid muscle injuries.

CHANGES IN BONE DENSITY EXPECTED FROM ACTIVITY PROGRAM

Although varied results have been reported in the literature concerning changes in bone density that result from regular participation in activity programs, a number of generalizations may be made, including the following:

1. In almost all cases the patient's previous rate of bone loss is reduced;
2. In many cases the patient's rate of bone loss is reduced to the average for their age group;
3. In some cases bone loss may be halted completely;
4. In some cases the bone density may be increased;
5. The intensity of exercises included in the activity program, the frequency of attendance, and the duration of the program all appear to be strongly and positively correlated with beneficial changes to the bone density;
6. Considerable improvement is noted in both general physical capacity and in the speed and contraction of the muscles well in advance of any detectable changes in bone density.

The clinical significance of changes in bone density, which may accompany or follow any program of treatment for osteoporosis, should be assessed with caution. Increases in total bone density are mostly caused by an increase in cortical thickness through bone deposition on the endosteal surfaces. Although, in most cases, an increase in density and cortical thickness is associated with an increase in bone strength, this relationship does not always occur. In addition, some drug management programs for osteoporosis have shown that, although the bone density may have increased, the bone tissue is abnormal in composition, and is more brittle than usual.

In other studies, increases of cortical bone have been accompanied by reduction in the trabecular bone content. Whether this produces an overall increase or decrease in the strength of the bone appears open to question.

It should be understood that, whereas the cortex retains its capacity to repair or replace bone throughout life, trabecular bone is more limited in this ability. Loss of trabecular bone involves both a reduction in the thickness of some trabeculae and a complete loss of others (particularly the horizontal ones). Improvement is limited to adding further bone to those trabecular bridges that remain intact; those that have been completely eroded are not replaced. Loss of trabeculae followed by restoration of normal bone density does not restore normal mechanical strength to the bone.

Although various approaches to the treatment of osteoporosis, including physical activity, have been shown to have a beneficial effect on bone density, no treatment has yet been directly shown to reduce the risk of later clinically significant fractures.

Patients with osteoporosis are treated medically with various drugs. Low dosage of estrogen—even when continued for long periods—is now considered to be safe by many physicians. Fluoride has been shown to be helpful in increasing bone density in many cases. Dietary supplements of calcium and vitamin D are regularly prescribed. To date, no specific interactive effects have been reported between the use of these drugs, either singly or in combination, and specific exercise routines or general activity programs. In the not too distant future more detailed information on such interactive effects should become available.

SUGGESTED READING

Aloia JF et al. Prevention of involutional bone loss by exercise. Ann Intern Med 1978; 89:356–358.

Chow RK et al. The effect of exercise on bone mass of osteoporotic patients on fluoride treatment. Clin Invest Med 1987; 10:59–63.

Krolner B et al. Physical exercise as a prophylactic against involutional bone loss—a controlled trial. Clin Sci 1983; 64:541–546.

Sinaki M, Mikkelsen BA. Postmenopausal spinal osteoporosis—flexion versus extension exercises. Arch Phys Med Rehab 1984; 65:583–586.

Smith EL. Exercise for prevention of osteoporosis—a review. Physician Sports Med 1982; 10:72–83.

ROLE OF THE PHYSICAL THERAPIST IN THE MANAGEMENT OF OSTEOPOROTIC FRACTURES

BARRIE PICKLES, B.P.T., M.S.

In women with advanced osteoporosis, an acute compression fracture often occurs during some ordinary physical activity, such as bending forwards to put on a shoe, rising from a chair, picking up an object from the floor, coughing, or sneezing. Alternatively, fractures may result from a minor slip or twist, or as the result of a fall, which under ordinary circumstances would be unlikely to cause a fracture. These fractures most often occur in the vertebral bodies of the lower thoracic and upper lumbar vertebrae; their incidence is lower in the upper end of the femur, in the bones of the forearm, and elsewhere in the body. This chapter only reviews the physical therapist's role in the management of spinal compression fractures. However, the same principles of treatment may be applied to the management of osteoporotic fractures in other bones.

VERTEBRAL COMPRESSION FRACTURES

Vertebral compression fractures may be divided into two groups—fractures that do not result in wedging of the vertebral body, and those that do.

FRACTURES WITHOUT WEDGING

Where no wedging of the vertebral body occurs, careful examination of the x-ray film may reveal evidence of microtrauma in some part of the trabecular pattern. These microfractures are seen as small, localized condensations within the trabecular network, most often as short, horizontal, pencil-line-thick marks that interrupt the normal regular honeycomb pattern. The bone cortex remains intact, and no displacement occurs. The patient may complain of some minor discomfort at the site of the injury or from reactive spasm of the deep paravertebral muscles in the area.

Unless other injuries are present, most of these patients respond well to a program of bed rest and analgesics for 1 or 2 days after injury, followed by immediate resumption of their normal activities. It is important to reduce the period of bed rest to a minimum to avoid unnecessary bone mineral loss from recumbency and loss of muscle function from disuse.

If the patient has been hospitalized as a precautionary measure, the therapist may have an opportunity during the few days normally required to reactivate the patient, to reeducate postural control; to teach the patient the importance of regular performance of exercises to improve the strength and speed of contraction of the back extensor muscles; to emphasize the importance of safe procedures while bending and lifting; to stress the desirability of increased amounts of planned physical activity once the immediate problems have been dealt with; and to arrange for follow-up by the therapist as a bridging link with continuing activity programs.

FRACTURES WITH WEDGING

When compression forces are applied to a vertebra, damage to the horizontal trabeculae occurs first, being followed, in sequence, by damage to the oblique and vertical trabeculae, and finally by fracture of the bone cortex. Fracture of the cortex, usually at the anterior or anterolateral aspects of the vertebral body, results in wedging of the bone. Wedging of more than one vertebral body may result from a single accident.

If anterior or anterolateral wedging occurs in a vertebral body, the ligaments of the apophyseal joints, the ligamenta flava and the supraspinous ligaments in the area, and the paravertebral muscles at that level are all stretched. An increased mechanical strain is thrown on spinal segments above and below the site of the fracture and possibly also on the sacroiliac joints. Wedge fractures are always accompanied by extensive soft tissue damage and subsequent degeneration. Occasionally, there may also be stretching or compression of one or more nerve roots, or adhesions forming around these, thereby giving rise to problems of referred pain and tenderness.

The Pre-Ambulatory Period

A 2-week period of bed rest is usually needed to allow severe pain a chance to subside, and for healing of the damaged tissues to be well underway, before mobilization is attempted. Most patients require medication for their discomfort throughout this period. Unless some chest or heart condition renders it inadvisable, the patient should lie flat with only a single pillow under her head during this time.

If the wedge fracture affects L1 or L2, there may

be some upset to the sympathetic nervous system. This upset may create two problems. For a few days after the injury a paralytic ileus may occur, but this almost always resolves itself without treatment. The second problem, orthostatic hypotension, may present some difficulty to the therapist when mobilization of the patient begins.

Orthostatic hypotension often occurs—partly as the result of being confined to bed for a 2-week period, partly due to inactivity during this time, partly associated with digestive difficulties, and partly caused by upset to the working of the celiac sympathetic ganglion. Before making any attempt to have the patient stand, the therapist should make use of the tilt table to check the patient's reaction to being placed in an increasingly vertical position, after being fully recumbent for some time.

At first, any change in angle from the horizontal should be made slowly and almost imperceptibly and the patient allowed to adjust for a short period at each 10-degree increase in the angle of tilt before progressing to a more vertical position. The patient should be able to remain in the vertical position for at least 5 minutes, without becoming faint or developing feelings of nausea, before weight bearing is attempted.

Some form of brace needs to be worn by the patient until the fracture is healed. Most patients find the rigid type of brace too heavy, too cumbersome, and too uncomfortable. A semi-rigid corset, with plastic supporting stays, porous cloth material and Velcro fastenings is more easily tolerated; a brace with shoulder harness straps appears to be just as effective as the rigid type, yet has the added advantages of being able to be worn under the patient's normal clothing, and in being readily washable. The patient must clearly understand that the support needs to be applied on every occasion before weight bearing is attempted, until the fracture is healed. The support will also be worn during the tilt table sessions.

Another aspect of the pre-ambulatory program should be a progressive program of exercises to ensure that normal movements are possible to all joints of the limbs; to mobilize any adhesions that may have formed during the period of recumbency; to teach safe procedures for rolling over in bed and for transfers to the tilt table; and to increase the strength and speed of contraction in the back extensor muscles. These muscles are particularly weakened as a result of the injury. Whereas the density of the wedged vertebra has been increased, as the immediate effect of its compression, and is therefore at reduced risk of further fracture once the present injury has healed, the previously unfractured bones *are* at increased risk of later fracture if the hydraulic support mechanism cannot be improved.

The risk of spinal fracture at a later time is also increased significantly if flexion exercises are incorporated into the exercise treatment program. Trunk flexion exercises should therefore be avoided.

Ambulatory Period

Once the patient is able to be vertical for 5 minutes or more on the tilt table, she is usually allowed to sit out of bed for short periods of time for increasing long intervals. For a start, 15 minutes is long enough, and the patient is often glad to get back into bed after only this short time. Although placing greater demands on the nursing and physical therapy staff, the patient benefits more, and improves more rapidly, from a number of short periods out of bed than from a single longer session. Four to six sessions a day should be aimed for.

Each period out of bed should be progressively increased until the patient is able to sit out for most of the day. A continuing watch must be kept to monitor the patient's orthostatic state. If the patient should begin to feel faint at any time while sitting out, she should be returned to bed to recover for a little while. It is important, however, to get the patient out of bed again a short time later, not allowing the faintness to be used as an excuse for not continuing to progress in the rehabilitation program.

Pain should be monitored while the patient is sitting out of bed. A high proportion of the frail elderly ladies who suffer wedge fracture injury complain of a variety of aches and pains once mobilization begins. Many aches result from muscle fatigue, others are caused by stretching of ligaments or by pressure from the support. In the long run it will be more profitable to heed a patient's complaints of aching and stiffness and to allow frequent breaks and rest periods, rather than insisting that she continue to sit out for a little while longer and put up with the pain.

Patients who are able to sit out of bed are also able to commence standing and balance programs. The therapist needs to check the fitting of the support carefully once the patient can stand upright. Slack straps and incorrect application of the support can unnecessarily prejudice the effectiveness of the whole rehabilitation program. The height of any walking frame, which is used to help support the patient, needs to be properly adjusted; if the walking frame is too small, the patient will be forced to bend forwards and in doing so will place unnecessary strains on her body, as well as making her balance more difficult. Attention to a large number of these apparently small and insignificant points makes all the difference between success and failure in the achievement of independence.

Subsequent emphasis needs to be turned to increasing endurance capacity (the distance the patient can walk, the time she can remain on her feet, the number of stairs she can manage) and her physical work capacity (the ability to walk a given distance, or climb a given number of stairs in a particular period of time).

One final item for the therapist to bear in mind is that some severely affected osteoporotic patients suffer fractures of the lower thoracic vertebrae, thereby producing the typical "dowager's hump" deformity and its accompanying respiratory problems. It is advisable in any treatment program for osteoporotic patients to include exercises to maintain thoracic expansion as much as possible and to improve control of breathing.

This chapter is limited to a consideration of the place of exercises and activity in the management of patients with osteoporotic fractures. The physical therapist may need to use other modalities to deal with particular problems as they arise—ultrasonic therapy to help soften some of the adhesions that may develop, inductive heating by short wave diathermy or microwave to ease muscle discomfort, transcutaneous electrical nerve stimulation to relieve some of the localized pain—but these are given in order to increase the amount of exercise and activity the patient can tolerate, rather than having any direct effect on the osteoporosis.

The plea is made to physical therapists to recognize the high incidence of osteoporosis in middle-aged and elderly women, the disability and death that are directly attributable to this condition, and the fact that through the use of therapeutic exercise and health counseling, physical therapy can offer considerable hope for improvement to those who suffer from osteoporosis.

SUGGESTED READING

Frost HM. Clinical management of the symptomatic osteoporotic patient. Orthop Clin N Am 1981; 12:671–681.

Johnston CC et al. Heterogeneity of fracture syndromes in post-menopausal women. J Clin Endocrinol Metab 1985; 61:551–556.

Larson KA, Shannon SC. Decreasing the incidence of osteoporosis-related injuries through diet and exercise. Pub Health Rep 1984; 99:809–813.

Sinaki M. Postmenopausal spinal osteoporosis—physical therapy and rehabilitation principles. Mayo Clin Proc 1982; 57:699–703.

PHYSICAL THERAPY IN HEMOPHILIA

JENNIFER INGLIS ELLIS, Dip. P.T., M.A.P.A., M.C.P.A.

Hemophilia is a hereditary blood clotting disorder. Hemophilia A or classic hemophilia affects the Factor VIII gene; hemophilia B or Christmas disease affects the Factor IX gene. Both are sex-linked recessive disorders affecting males, and both manifest similar bleeding disorders, mostly into muscles and joints.

Von Willebrand's bleeding disorder is inherited in either an autosomal dominant or recessive pattern, affecting males and females. These patients tend to bruise easily and bleed mainly into mucosal membranes rather than joints and muscles.

Persons born with severe hemophilia, i.e., less than 1 percent of clotting factor, remain severe throughout their lifetime, and the moderate (1 to 5 percent clotting factor) remain moderate. The level of clotting factor may vary with von Willebrand's disease.

MANAGEMENT OF HEMOPHILIA

Medical management aims to prevent or to control acute bleeding episodes. Persons with severe hemophilia are usually on a home infusion program of Factor VIII or Factor IX concentrate replacement. They either treat themselves with a prophylactic dose, or with each bleeding episode. Prompt, early treatment prevents joint or muscle damage.

The medical management should be long term as the person's problem will be life long. A comprehensive team of specialists is needed to care for the person with hemophilia. The team should include a nurse-coordinator, a hematologist, an orthopaedic surgeon, a rheumatologist, a dentist, a social worker, and a physical therapist. Each member of the team is directly involved in regular clinical evaluation and treatment recommendations, as well as acting as a consultant to the hemophiliac, the family, or others involved in the case. Adults should be evaluated at least once a year; children, twice a year. Consistency of evaluating personnel is of utmost importance for comparison at subsequent evaluations.

PHYSIOTHERAPY

Prevention should be the prime aim of every physical therapist. Research has shown that those persons with hemophilia who are physically active and fit bleed less and require less factor replacement. Strong muscles surrounding a joint protect it; this is the best possible joint protection.

Many people with hemophilia have grown up in an overprotective environment at home and at school, and have sedentary lifestyles. It is of the utmost importance to educate these people in the importance of being physically active and in maintaining a regular recreational exercise program. As well as educating the person with hemophilia, others must also be advised: the family needs to be told of the need for regular exercise. Advice can be given on the use of protective equipment, such as a helmet for skating, and a padded seat for bike riding. The school teacher and gym teacher should be visited at least once a year. Work personnel often need advice. The therapist must act as a resource person for other health care personnel and promote workshops or seminars for staff in smaller outlying areas.

The physiotherapist evaluates and treats the individual with hemophilia at regular clinic sessions and also in scheduled treatment sessions.

Evaluation

Consistency of personnel is of utmost importance for comparison at subsequent evaluations.

Subjectively, the physical therapist must listen for symptoms of an acute bleed and record the time of onset; note the length of morning stiffness and the amount of pain; record the number of bleeds per joint since the last assessment; enquire about specific problems of activities of daily living (ADL); record the patient's job and days missed because of bleeds; and enquire about recreational or physical pursuits.

Objectively, the physical therapist must measure the circumference of an acute joint or muscle and compare it to the other side and to previous measurements; examine the joints for chronic "boggy" hemarthroses, for crepitus, and for ligamentous laxity; measure joint range of motion; measure muscle bulk above and below affected joints; record muscle strength, including grip strength if there is elbow or hand involvement; check for leg length discrepancies; look at posture and for a scoliosis, which may result from leg length difference; and carry out a functional inquiry that should include gait analysis, use of cane, crutches or wheelchair, stair climbing ability, and any difficulties with self-infusion, lifting, or carrying heavy objects. The therapist must keep in mind that an over-vigorous examination may cause a bleed.

Treatment

The joints commonly affected are the ankles, knees, and elbows, less commonly hips, shoulders, and wrists. The commonly affected muscle groups are the calf, forearm, and iliopsoas.

The therapist and the patient must remember that there is no such thing as a minor bleed. All bleeds must be taken seriously and treated promptly.

Acute Hemarthrosis or Muscle Bleed

The first treatment is infusion of clotting factor. If infusion is delayed or if bleeding is not controlled, painful swelling occurs in the joint or muscle, thus leading to the limb being held in a flexed position.

Splinting of the joint or limb in a functional resting position may be necessary to prevent or decrease deformity.

Rest, ice, elevation, compression, and immobilization all help to control the bleeding. Avoidance of weight bearing may be necessary with leg involvement. Daily circumference measurements should be recorded.

Subacute Hemarthrosis or Muscle Bleed

When pain subsides and daily circumference measurements indicate that hemostasis is achieved, gentle isometric contractions and range of motion exercises should commence. Splints may be left off during the day, but worn at night. Hydrotherapy is an ideal way to commence exercising.

Exercises should progress gradually to resisted concentric and eccentric muscle work. Careful stretching by splinting is helpful to reduce contractures, but the therapist must keep in mind that too much splinting causes muscle wasting. Faradism, biofeedback, manually-resisted exercises, balance, and other facilitation techniques all may be used. Transcutaneous nerve stimulation (TNS) is helpful to control pain during treatment.

Many knees strengthen well on a controlled Cybex, Orthotron type strengthening program, but not all joints tolerate this. Weights through range are not recommended, rather manual resistance controlled through range is preferable. Stretching should be avoided or tried with extreme caution. Strengthening of the opposing muscle group has a stretching effect.

Chronic Joint

The chronic hemophilia joint presents with a thickened synovium caused by continual irritation from unresolved bleeds. There are adhesions within the joint, and the articular cartilage is rough and irregular. There may be loss of range of motion, ligamentous laxity, deformity, and muscle weakness.

Treatment aims are directed towards mainte-

nance of joint function and advice concerning assistive devices and ADLs. Splinting may help protect joints and prevent contractions. However, too much splinting quickly leads to muscle wasting. Manual therapy has a place in treatments aimed at maintaining and increasing joint range. Administration of clotting factor prior to treatment prevents bleeding. The maintenance of a daily exercise program should be stressed. Exercises are for range of motion, strength, and endurance.

Recreational activities, as well as general fitness, should be stressed. Children should participate in school physical education. The specific problems of individual hemophiliacs should be taken into account when deciding upon an appropriate recreational activity. For example, a person with an affected ankle should not play soccer. Generally, noncontact sports, such as swimming, golf, tennis, cycling, and running should be encouraged. Contact sports, such as ice hockey, boxing, or football, are not recommended.

Advice on activities of daily living and on assistive devices includes suggestions of a raised toilet seat for knee problems, raise in a shoe for leg length discrepancy, insoles or metatarsal bars for feet, protective high-cut boots for ankle problems; cane or crutches may be necessary to reduce stress on a knee or ankle, as may be recommendations for referrals to an occupational therapist.

Treatment of Specific Joints

Ankle. This is the most commonly affected joint and one of the hardest to manage. The talofibular and talotibial joints are usually affected.

The acute hemarthrosis may need no weight bearing, a resting splint, or taping for several days. Taping is especially effective in settling the joint. As the swelling subsides, a light canvas ankle support with high-cut boots or running shoes protects the joint. This protection may be necessary for more vigorous activities, following the resolution of the hemarthrosis.

In the chronic ankle, dorsiflexion is lost first. The toe extensors tend to compensate for the lack of dorsiflexion; this compensation results in a claw toes-dropped metatarsal heads deformity.

Use of the toe extensors must be discouraged and proper heel-toe gait monitored. Balance-board exercises and stationary bicycling are good for strengthening joints. Mobilizations help to regain some dorsiflexion. Footwear should be assessed in detail.

Knee. The person with an affected knee often has an affected ankle on the opposite side. This is a common problem and a very disabling one.

With an acute hemarthrosis, the joint becomes flexed. A resting splint without weight bearing may be necessary. As the swelling subsides, isometric exercises at various ranges are helpful, as is hydrotherapy

The chronic joint presents with a chronically thickened synovium, and one leg may be longer than the other, owing to hemarthroses stimulating quicker growth of the epiphyses. The patellofemoral joint is usually involved and may become fixed. Quadriceps weakness and flexion deformity are common. The physical therapist must strengthen the quadriceps and reduce contraction with a variety of techniques, including Faradism, a Cybex machine (in some instances), manually-resisted knee extension through range, a stationary bicycle, a treadmill, and swimming. Hip extension should be maintained to prevent hip flexion contracture.

Elbow. Resumption of active movement (e.g., prolonged writing), too soon after an acute hemarthrosis may cause further bleeding.

In the chronic joint, bony overgrowth and premature closing of the epiphyses occur, thereby limiting all movements. Marked improvement in range is seldom gained by exercise, so emphasis should be on strengthening.

Stretching is contraindicated because of the danger of myositis ossificans.

Hip. Bleeding in and around the hip may be dangerous as a common site is the iliopsoas bursa, where swelling could compress the femoral nerve.

Two tests to differentiate hip and iliopsoas involvement are (1) iliopsoas involvement is indicated when an active sit-up or resisted hip flexion causes pain; and (2) pain on passive hip rotation indicates a hip problem. The joint assumes a flexed position. Traction in hospital may be necessary.

The patient should be nonweight bearing until pain subsides. Hydrotherapy is helpful to regain hip movement.

The chronic damaged hip may be replaced with an artificial joint.

Hemorrhage into Soft Tissues. Common areas of hemorrhage are thighs, calves, and forearms. Recurrence is especially common in the legs. Muscle bleeds notoriously take a long time to resolve—up to 6 weeks or longer.

Calf. Bleeding occurs into the gastrocnemius-soleus muscles. The ankle is plantar flexed, the knee flexed, and the person is able to walk on tiptoe. A resting splint may be necessary, with nonweight bearing.

Exercising should be commenced as early as possible, because of the danger of the development of contractures from the hematoma. Exercise in a cool whirlpool (90° F) is helpful.

The use of ultrasonography to resolve hematomas is controversial. If given, it should be only after all bleeding has ceased for several days, and, in children, the growth plates should be avoided.

Iliopsoas. A bleed here is potentially life threatening as it is often diagnosed late and a lot of blood may be lost. Groin pain is severe, and the hip is flexed. Resisted hip flexion or active sit-ups cause pain. Femoral nerve compression may produce sensory and motor deficits.

Despite rest, hospitalization and the administration of large doses of clotting factor, recurrence is common when walking resumes.

Exercise should be commenced only when pain has subsided and movement is more tolerable.

Forearm Hematoma. This may compress the ulnar or median nerve branches, producing sensory or motor loss in the hand. The wrist assumes a flexed position. Early active hand and finger exercises are essential to ensure complete recovery, as severe loss of function can occur. Volkmans ischemic contracture may occur without exercise treatment.

The physical therapist has become a vitally important member of the hemophilia team. The therapist must ensure that those people with hemophilia under his or her care, keep as physically active and fit as possible, thereby reducing the number of bleeding episodes, with resultant better quality of life.

SUGGESTED READING

Boone DC, ed. Comprehensive management of hemophilia. Philadelphia: FA Davis, 1976.

Greene WB, Mostrom E. Use of modified isokinetic strengthening program in patients with severe hemophilia (abstract) Dev Med Child Neurol 1982; 24:236.

Hemophilia and sports. The National Hemophilia Foundation 1985.

Hilgartner MD, Montgomery R. Understanding von Willebrand's disease. The National Hemophilia Foundation, 1985.

Koch B. Cohen S, Luban NC, Eng G. Hemophiliac knee: rehabilitation techniques. Arch Phys Med Rehabil 1982; 63:379–385.

Physical therapy in hemophilia. The National Hemophilia Foundation. The Canadian Hemophilia Society, 1986.

Rizza CR. Effect of exercise on level of antihaemophilic globulin in human blood. J Physiol 1961; 156:128–135.

Strickler EM, Greene WB. Isokinetic torque levels in hemophiliac knee musculature. Arch Phys Med Rehabil 1984; Vol. 65.

PHYSICAL THERAPY IN PATIENTS WITH ACQUIRED IMMUNODEFICIENCY SYNDROME

RANDALL GEE, B.A., P.T.
DONNA L. KASABIAN, P.T.

As the number of people diagnosed with acquired immunodeficiency syndrome (AIDS), continues to grow, so does the importance for each medical discipline to develop a comprehensive treatment approach to deal with people with AIDS. A physical therapy approach should be realistic, practical, and functionally oriented. The A.I.M.S. (assessment, instruction, mobility, and support) approach to people with AIDS is such an approach.

Diagnosis of AIDS is based on the presence of a disease that at least is moderately indicative of an underlying immunodeficiency.* The diagnosis can be confirmed in several different ways: the disease as noted above is matched with a positive HIV antibody test; the disease itself is definitively diagnosed (as outlined by the CDC); a definitive diagnosis of an above noted disease prior to the onset of another, plus the presence of a T-helper lymphocyte count of less than 400 per cubic millimeter. If there is evidence of another source of immunodeficiency, a diagnosis of AIDS can be ruled out.

Clinically, patients with AIDS present with a wide variety of symptoms and manifestations of the numerous diseases. These symptoms include generalized weakness, hemiparesis, paraparesis, pulmonary compromise, ataxia, tremor, and altered mental status. Patients with secondary cancers often complain of pain over the sites of lesions. Decreased range of motion is commonly noted in weak patients secondary to prolonged positioning and a decreased level of activity. Severe generalized muscle atrophy is a major symptom of HIV wasting syndrome, which is one of the new syndromes added to the CDC's list of AIDS diseases. In children, the HIV encephalopathy may be manifested by motor and cognitive dysfunction, as well as by loss of behavioral developmental milestones. Besides the physical signs and symptoms that often occur with AIDS, there are many psychological, social, and emotional problems that need to be considered when working with the AIDS patient. Fear, anger, isolation, embarrassment, and rejection are issues that the patient encounters and, depending on how they are dealt with, may have an effect on the outcome of physical therapy goals.

THE A.I.M.S. APPROACH

The A.I.M.S. approach to patients with AIDS is based on the types of patients and treatments we worked on in our facility within our health care system. It is a broad-based approach with flexibility for individual health facility policy, departmental procedures, and individual therapist's feelings. The CDC has published a document entitled "Recommendations for Prevention of HIV Transmission in Health-Care Settings" and it should be available in all departments planning to treat AIDS patients.

A—Assessment

The key to any successful patient intervention is a thorough and practical assessment. Physical therapists routinely assess the musculoskeletal, neuromuscular, and cardiopulmonary systems of most patients; however, in the AIDS patient, the emphasis of the evaluation needs to be the status of functional mobility. How mobile was the patient prior to admission? What is the current mobility status? If the patient is not functioning at his preadmission level, why not? What are mobility needs at home, at work, socially? What resources are available after discharge i.e., home physical therapy, outpatient physical therapy, visiting nurse?

Based on the findings from the assessment, the physical therapist needs to answer the following questions: will the patient benefit from physical therapy intervention?; is physical therapy appropriate for this patient?

In setting treatment goals for patients with AIDS, the emphasis is on increasing independence in functional mobility skills; improving the quality of life through preventive therapeutic intervention; and

---

* A partial list of Centers for Disease Control (CDC) diseases that are indicative of a moderate underlying immunodeficiency: *Pneumocystis carinii* pneumonia, chronic cryptosporidiosis, toxoplasmosis, extraintestinal strongyloidiasis, isosporiasis, candidiasis (esophageal, bronchial, or pulmonary), cryptococcosis, histoplasmosis, mycobacterial infection with *Mycobacterium avium* complex or *Microbacterium kansasii,* cytomegalovirus infection, chronic mucocutaneous or disseminated herpes simplex virus infection, progressive multifocal leukoencephalopathy, Subgroup D—Secondary cancers—i.e., Kaposi's sarcoma, nonHodgkin's lymphoma, primary lymphoma of the brain, HIV encephalopathy; HIV wasting syndrome.

facilitating and assisting with hospital discharge planning.

I—Instruction

In keeping with the guidelines for setting treatment goals, the attainment of the stated goals can be facilitated by instructing the patient, his family or significant other, and other supportive health care workers in appropriate topics.

For the bed-bound patient, immediate instruction begins with the importance of changing positions on a regular schedule to prevent skin breakdown and to facilitate increasing mobility. When the patient is able to get out of bed, the importance of increasing "up time," or time out of bed, is stressed. Improved functional skills, better morale, and improved digestive and respiratory functioning are the rewards the patient notices by following through with your instructions. Because of the decreased level of activity that most AIDS patients experience at some point during their illness, instruction in a self range of motion exercise program is begun in order to prevent joint and muscle tightness, pain, and eventual disability if left unmoved.

Besides the patient, family, friends, and nursing personnel are included in the instruction process. The emphasis should be on how to assist the patient rather than in how to do it for him or her. Instruction includes preventive measures for skin breakdown and pulmonary toilet, in addition to possible transfer techniques, guarding during ambulation, and active-assisted or passive range of motion.

M—Mobility

The primary goal of physical therapy is to help the patient attain the highest level of independence in functional mobility. Towards this end, the treatment plan is geared to initiate progressive mobility from current status to maximum potential or discharge. Techniques used vary with the level of strength, range of motion, pulmonary function, and mental status. Treatment plans and goals change with progress or deterioration. A step by step progression may start with working on bed mobility and move on to progressive weight bearing and ultimately towards ambulation. Techniques used include passive modalities such as a tilt table, or Nelson bed to facilitate weight bearing, as well as active programs such as trunk control exercises in sitting, partial standing from elevated surfaces, and posture and balance exercises while sitting and standing. Strengthening and passive range of motion exercises are geared to increasing the mobility level, not to achieving a maximum progression of resistance or joint function.

S—Support

The care and treatment of AIDS patients is best performed in a multidisciplinary team setting. Physical therapists are vital members of the team in the successful management of AIDS patients. However, going beyond the actual treatment techniques that we have to offer, we as physical therapists represent, to the patient, the family, and other health care workers, the hope of rehabilitation, increasing function, and eventual discharge. To some, we fill the role of rehabilitation therapist, to others we may show the truth about how debilitated and disabled a patient really is, but to all, we show that physical therapists are willing to share the joys and sorrows, successes and failures, triumphs and defeats in working with AIDS patients.

The physical therapy approach to patients with AIDS includes a functionally based assessment; an instructional component geared towards the prevention of decreasing function and dependence; treatment goals that are focused on increasing functional mobility; and emotional and physical support for the patient, family, and the rest of the health care team.

SUGGESTED READING

Centers for Disease Control. Recommendations for prevention of HIV transmission in health-care settings. MMWR 1987; 36 (suppl 2S): 3S–18S.
Centers for Disease Control. Revision of the CDC surveillance case definition for acquired immunodeficiency syndrome. MMWR 1987; 36 (suppl 1S): 4S–6S.
Herron M. Living with AIDS. Whole Earth Rev 1985; 34.
Various Authors. The abc of AIDS. Br Med J 1987; 294:1083–1085, 1145–1147, 1214–1218, 1274–1277, 1334–1337, 1399–1401, 1474–1476, 1536–1538, 1671–1673; 295: 33–35, 104–106, 200–203, 256–257, 320–321, 373–376.

PHYSICAL THERAPY IN A PSYCHIATRIC HOSPITAL

CAROL STUART-BUTTLE, M.S., P.T.

Physical therapists have functioned traditionally within a medical setting such as the acute care or rehabilitation hospital. Their role has been primarily to provide direct service in the restoration of physical capabilities following illness or injury. Physical therapists have long been in a psychiatric setting, providing restoration of function impaired by mental illness. However, only recently with wider attention, has physical therapy in a psychiatric setting become recognized as another area of specialization.

Psychiatric hospitals have two types of patient wards: "locked" units and "open" units. Locked units house patients who require close supervision. The patients are able to acquire activity privileges, which permit progressively less supervision, until perhaps transfer to an open unit. Adult psychiatric hospitals have patients ranging from about 15 years of age to geriatric. The hospital often is organized into programs, which address the needs of a particular group such as adolescents or those with eating disorders. Many hospitals offer a Drug and Alcohol Rehabilitation program.

An "Activity Therapy" Department is present in most hospitals. The size of the department and type of therapists vary with each facility, but may include staff with expertise in music, art, movement, dance, drama, occupational and recreational therapy. These disciplines provide a medium for psychiatric treatment.

Indications

Conditions treated by the physical therapist are similar to the neuromusculoskeletal complaints seen in a typical outpatient department. In the psychiatric population there are physically handicapped individuals who are wheelchair bound. Physical conditions that relate to a psychiatric disorder include deconditioning secondary to depression, self-inflicted injuries, psychosomatic musculoskeletal complaints, sympathetic reflex dystrophy, Volkmann's ischemic contractures secondary to drug abuse, cerebellar dysfunctions and neuropathies secondary to substance abuse, anxiety conditions requiring relaxation, and postural dysfunctions.

Interdisciplinary Roles

Psychiatrists are the main source of referral, although the nursing staff usually is responsible for noticing a physical or functional problem. Patients themselves sometimes request therapy, having heard about it from fellow patients. As in any setting, physical therapists need to develop a good rapport with their referral source. Involvement in the treatment team helps establish such communication.

The concept of a treatment team is spoken of in many settings, but more than lip-service is necessary for effective physical therapy in a psychiatric hospital. Full-time physical therapy service provides the opportunity for an integrated contribution to the therapeutic team and milieu. Therefore both the mind and body are addressed in the treatment of psychiatric conditions. The treatment team comprises nursing, activity therapy, social services, physicians, psychologists, and physical therapy. Written and spoken communication is of prime importance. The patient chart is a source for a physical and psychiatric history. Summaries from psychological testing give a profile of the cognitive and developmental state and IQ, as well as an indication of organic versus non-organic mental processes.

Usually the medical physician remains apart from the team concept but is a useful contact for the physical therapist. The internist (who is responsible for physical wellbeing) may refer patients but also should be consulted if a medical question arises. Some facilities may hold "medical rounds," especially with a geriatric population. Attendance at such meetings can be helpful for keeping abreast of medical issues. Discussion with the psychiatrist aids the therapist in deciding the extent a patient may need defocusing from a physical ailment. Occasionally, deferrment of treatment for a physical problem is beneficial to the patient, if current psychiatric issues are especially dominant.

Nursing staff of the team are an excellent source from whom to determine the implications of the psychiatric diagnosis and status, and the privilege level of the patient. Activity therapists are able to provide an activity history including the patient's compliance to a program. Communication with social services becomes important with impending discharge, and also when family meetings and family education are indicated.

Team communication is maintained effectively through progress notes in the patient charts and attendance at staff and patient meetings. Meetings in psychiatric settings are frequent and often therapeutic in nature. Since the physical therapist is not involved in psychiatric treatment per se, attendance at meetings may be less often than for other team members. Such meetings, however, can provide useful insight in a case, and assist in developing an optimal approach to the patient to attain effective physical therapy treatment.

ROLE OF PHYSICAL THERAPY

In the psychiatric hospital, the physical therapist is one of the few individuals whose prime concern is somatic complaints. Therefore, the physical therapist has the role of consultant, therapist (treating physical problems closely interrelated with psychiatric conditions, problems with little psychiatric component, and psychosomatic disorders), and teacher (of relaxation, exercises, body mechanics, and posture), as well as instructor to family members. In hospitals with few activity therapists, the physical therapists may be more involved in body awareness and sensory integration. More time may also be dedicated to relaxation techniques and biofeedback. An especially close rapport may develop with physically handicapped patients, because the patient knows a therapist accepts and understands the handicap. Typically, other staff members are not familiar with the physical limitations, and are less adept at assisting with transfers and daily care. The therapist can provide education of the staff on such matters. Promotion of independence with activities of daily living is a large psychological contribution, for which the physical therapist primarily is responsible.

There are some general comments to be made about a physical therapist's approach to the treatment of psychiatric patients. The comments are concerned with the danger of stepping out of the professional bounds of a physical therapist, and the essential aims to motivate and to progress the patient.

There are times when the physical therapist may inadvertently "play" psychiatrist or counselor especially when a rapport exists between the therapist and patient. Unless the physical therapist has further qualifications, caution must be taken to avoid treating outside of the role of physical therapy. However, the psychiatric goals should be reinforced by the physical therapist, as should the physical goals by the other staff of the hospital. Team meetings help clarify the goals, and provide information on the psychiatric status of the patient. The therapist should be aware of these issues, which can contribute to a patient's mood.

Patients' active participation in their treatment programs is especially important in the psychiatric setting. Even if treatments are passive, such as hot packs, the treatment program must require the patient's participation and responsibility to prevent a dependent relationship. Responsibility may be promoted, for example, by enforcing timely arrival for appointments. The therapist often needs to motivate the patients. Motivation is a large problem with depression in the geriatric population.

A general approach of physical therapy is to progress a patient to a higher level of comfort or function. This approach is important particularly with psychiatric patients because progress is slower and harder to achieve, and so there is a greater risk of ineffective, "stagnant" treatments. Progress may be assisted by introducing exercises early in a treatment program and, minimizing the passive form of treatments. Patients also may be progressed to participate in hospital activities such as those offered by movement and recreational therapists.

A patient may have a very short attention span and poor concentration, which rapidly demand creative alternatives from the therapist as well as one-on-one supervision. Other psychiatric conditions may render a patient incapable of following an exercise program but the therapist can implement a functional treatment approach.

Psychiatric patients require feedback on their physical progress just as other patients. Statements need to be sincere, consistent, and reassuring. This reassurance of improving physical health in a psychosomatic patient can be especially helpful. However, somatization is a form of expression, or symptom. If one form is removed, another means of expression, or alternative somatizing will occur until the root of the problem improves. That is not to say there is no benefit from treatment of psychosomatic complaints. Simultaneous treatment of mind and body during a hospital admission can be very effective. In circumstances where the patient has some self awareness, a physical therapist may be influential in helping the patient develop mental control over physical problems. Muscle tension, which patients can potentially control, is an example. Biofeedback, for control of the autonomic system including for example, heart rate and peripheral body temperature, teaches a patient about the potential for mentally controlling the body.

Treatment sessions often take longer with psychiatric than with nonpsychiatric patients, and frequently one-on-one is necessary. The patients commonly have a history of rejection, which is why many demand attention. During the hospital stay, patients are encouraged to talk and analyze their problems. The therapist needs to be a good listener and handle termination and interruptions of conversations with tact and greater sensitivity than normally is required within other physical therapy settings. Some patients lack understanding of social nuances and the necessity for divided attention.

Touch

Treatments appear to be much more effective when "hands on" approaches are adopted, such as massage. Physical contact gives an element of therapeutic touch, with intimacy and caring which promotes relaxation. Patients who have physically withdrawn, with an abhorrence of touch, may be helped by the "legitimate" touch of the therapist. Massage as a tool is time consuming but effective, yet it is a "passive" treatment. Its use should be frequent but prudent. Using massage inconsistently, or alternating it with other modalities, may prevent a patient from developing a dependency. Because of the enjoyment of massage, a patient can become manipulative and demand treatments when they are beyond being beneficial. "Weaning" a patient from massage is not always easy. One method is to reassure the patient that other modalities are now appropriate. Compromises or contracts can be made, such as rewarding a patient's increased activity, by an occasional massage. Rewards and contracts require careful handling on the part of the therapist. A patient must be encouraged to see the physical benefit of participation in therapy, not participation for the sole reward of a massage or hot pack.

Psychiatric patients generally are being assisted with resolving personal issues. Sexuality is a common issue. As mentioned before, our profession has a license to touch and we may become casual about close physical contact. Be aware how your approach may be affecting your patient.

Relaxation

Relaxation often should be addressed as part of a treatment. Patients from a substance abuse program should also be considered for relaxation training, because their days are spent in intensive, emotional meetings, which create immense tension as personal issues are resolved. Tapes for relaxation to sleep are usually available for patients. Activity therapists may contribute with imagery methods. Often, those patients manifesting muscular tension respond well to contract-relax techniques, and this approach sometimes is offered only by physical therapy. Biofeedback techniques are also effective treatment approaches to relaxation.

Alternative Modalities

Hydrotherapy is used in a conventional way for wounds or heat treatment. More emphasis also is given for relaxation purposes, especially with catatonic cases. Therapy in the swimming pool provides a useful medium to encourage further exercise and a sensory experience for those with a touching phobia.

Mention should be made of less widely used treatment approaches, such as myofascial release, somatosensory release, acupressure treatments, Feldenkrais and Alexander techniques. There is potential for those with expertise in these methods to apply them in the psychiatric setting and assess their effectiveness. The psychiatric patient is not typically a trusting one, which may negatively influence the outcome of the myofascial and somatosensory release methods.

Cautions

Behavioral requirements of the therapist and some treatment techniques have been discussed so far. There are several "cautions" which should be mentioned also. The therapist must not become a victim of manipulation. Awareness of being manipulated by patients prevents the patient dominating the situation in an adverse way. Bear in mind that patients view physical therapists as separate from their psychiatric staff. Often the patients will behave differently in physical therapy, with less tendency to "act out."

Adverse patient behavior requires a tolerant and patient therapist. Psychiatric conditions can render people with socially inappropriate behavior, rude, abusive, and physically violent. Some patients have difficulty organizing or planning small daily events, and making decisions. More than one activity or demand on the patient can cause the person to overreact, as they cannot cope with the level of stress. Being able to control emotions or to express them appropriately, includes a patient's ability to express affection for the therapist. Such expression can come in indirect ways. The physical therapist should contribute to psychiatric goals by helping guide and teach the patient to organize and integrate tasks. Above all, the therapist must be a consistent element in the lives of the patients. Consistency and patience helps a therapist survive some of the rigorous "testing" by patients who often misbehave until they develop a relationship and trust. Psychotic patients are those who confuse reality with unreality. Reality always should be reinforced.

Some patients in an addiction program have addictive personalities. Physical therapy is no exception and such patients are difficult to progress through treatment. Instigating as independent a program as possible, can help prevent a passive dependence. Similarly, the addictive patient group is prone to use transcutaneous electrical nerve stimulation on a long-term basis.

When "nothing works" in a nonpsychiatric facility, the therapist discharges the patient or refers them to someone who may help. In a psychiatric hospital, there is greater possibility of continuing treatment long after the patient has reached a plateau, often because of manipulative undercurrents. To reiterate, always attempt to progress the patient or else discharge them, albeit for a short time.

Precautions should be taken against displaying any solutions which may abet suicide, such as Betadine. Some patients recovering from alcohol abuse are given a drug called Antabuse, which provokes an adverse physical reaction when in contact with alcohol. The therapist must remember not to use alcohol to remove oil after a massage, with such patients. Many antidepressive drugs have a hypotension side-effect, which can interfere with therapy.

Electroshock therapy (EST) is still used, although it is not as popular a treatment as it used to be. A side effect of the treatments is temporary loss of memory, which returns over a few weeks post cessation of the therapy course. This may be frustrating from a physical therapist's standpoint and necessitates allowing for it and being flexible in treatment approaches.

An older population usually has multiple medical problems. Worthy of particular mention is the increase in cardiac instability, such as arrhythmias and tachycardia, with depression and, or increased anxiety. Caution with exercise is necessary, but reassuring the patient can help decrease anxiety. The therapist also may assist the patient in determining safe functional levels.

Psychiatric crises usually are forewarned by subtle signs to which the nursing staff are atuned. Therefore, an unstable patient either comes to the department supervised, or physical therapy treatments are postponed. However, prudence dictates that two people should be in the department when patients are present.

SUGGESTED READING

Diagnostic and statistical manual of mental disorders. 3rd ed. American Psychiatric Association, 1984.

Green SA. Mind and body, the psychology of illness. American Psychiatric Press Inc. 1985.

Haber J et al. Comprehensive psychiatric nursing. 3rd ed. New York: McGraw Hill, 1987.

Kiev A, ed. Somatic manifestations of depressive disorders. New York: American Elsevier, 1974.

Sargant W, Slater E. An introduction to physical methods of treatment in psychiatry. 5th ed. New York: Science House, 1972.

Schroder PJ. Recognizing transference and countertransference. J Psychosoc Nurs 1985; 23:21–26.

MANAGEMENT OF SUBSTANCE ABUSE

LORNA SAGORSKY, B.Sc.
JOYCE CONATY, B.Sc.

It is estimated that between 20 and 30 percent of patients admitted to general hospitals have addiction problems and perhaps 1 percent are diagnosed during their stay. An awareness of this very relevant health factor should be appreciated and the problem identified by all members of a health team. Physical therapists, who often have close continuing contact with their patients, can be valuable members of this team.

The World Health Organization defines alcoholics as "those excessive drinkers whose dependence on alcohol has attained such a degree that it shows a noticeable mental disturbance or an interference with bodily and mental health, interpersonal relations, and smooth social and economic functioning, or who show the prodromal signs of such developments. They, therefore, require treatment."

The following treatment approaches were developed by and are currently practiced in the OT/PT/RT Department Addiction Research Foundation (ARF) of Ontario. The Clinical Institute is a hospital setting where individuals with chemical dependencies including alcoholism are treated both in medical and in psychosocial settings. As a teaching hospital, it is fully affiliated with the University of Toronto.

Clients in the Clinical Institute are either self-referred or are coerced into treatment via the legal system or as a result of medical or psychosocial problems. The Clinical Institute offers a wide spectrum of treatment services that can be divided as follows:

Medical Services—These include a twenty bed hospital ward, an emergency department, and outpatient clinics.

Psychosocial Services—These include both inpatient and outpatient components. Outpatients either attend group day programs or individual counseling. The day programs last 3 or 4 weeks and run from 9 AM to 5 PM. There are three Day Programs at the Clinical Institute. These are the Young Drug Users Program (YDUP) for those aged from 16 to 30, the Abstinent Lifestyle Treatment Program (ALTP) for those aged from 25 and over, and the Program For the Employed (PFE) where the employer is directly involved. Physical therapists provide stress management and relaxation training in the first two programs.

Patients who require an inpatient status while attending a day program are offered residential facilities. All residential patients are screened for drugs in order to maintain a drug free environment

In the Clinical Institute, physical therapy has been offered for 10 years, and we as physical therapists see an average of 800 clients a year. Clients fall into all social and economic categories—from the business executive to the homeless street youth—ranging in ages from 12 to 80. All these clients have one common denominator—all have a presumed drug or alcohol problem. Their addictions also run the gamut from cocaine to alcohol to contact cement thinner. Most substance use is treated in the same way; there is no hierarchy of "better" and "worse" drugs at ARF. From the behavioral viewpoint, these substances have, at times, succeeded in creating an environment for the user that is temporarily preferable to the reality of his or her life.

Physical therapy is offered in both the medical and the psychosocial services of the Clinical Institute. In the day treatment programs, clients are treated through group counseling, using a behavioral approach. Groups last 3 or 4 weeks and relaxation sessions are offered 2 or 3 times a week. Individual outpatient counseling is attended for as long as clients and therapists see it as appropriate.

The Medical Unit is also served by the Physical Therapy department. Patients in this setting have medical problems resulting from their use, which has necessitated medical and nursing care.

RELAXATION THERAPY AS USED IN TREATING DEPENDENCIES

Theory*

The use of relaxation therapy and stress management in the sociobehavioral treatment programs is based on the functional-analytic approach to the treatment of substance abuse. This therapeutic intervention identifies the specific factors in an individual's life that occur either immediately before excess drinking begins (the "antecedents") or soon after it has been initiated (the "consequences"). These are referred to as the maintaining factors of drinking, and they in turn refer to the ongoing daily pattern. The functional analysis is appropriately integrated into the treatment of stress. Stress situations that have been "relieved"

---

* Theory derived from Miller P, Mastria M. Alternatives to alcohol abuse. Champaign, IL: Research Press, 1977

by substance use in the past are identified and alternative behaviors (usually including relaxation) are offered as substitutes. The derived changes are slower and possibly less dramatic than those attained by drugs, but they can serve as coping alternatives for the client in the stressful situation.

The behavior replacement is applied both to the antecedent and to the consequence of drug use. For example, "feeling scared about talking to the boss" could be an antecedent to, and "feeling relaxed and confident" could be a consequence of, a drinking episode. Treatment here would focus on how to feel less intimidated by the employer and how to feel relaxed and confident without drugs. In other words, presenting alternative behaviors can increase the clients' repertoire of response in stressful situations.

Antecedents

Some general categories of antecedents to the drinking episode that we frequently deal with are unpleasant *emotional, physiological,* or *cognitive* states. Alternative ways of dealing with these states are presented through stress management and relaxation training.* (See footnote on p 271).

Emotional Factors. The relationship between stress and drug use is very complex. An important connection between unpleasant emotional states (anxiety and stress) and excess substance abuse has been noted for a long time. According to this theory, alcohol can serve to reduce negative feelings, thereby resulting in a more positive emotional state, or at least cessation of the negative state. Investigations have also found that relapse to many addictive behaviors occurs frequently in negative emotional states or situations.

It has also been clinically observed that a generalized increased level of emotion can also result in excessive drinking. This may be the reason that some alcoholics report drinking when feeling excessively positive. Alternative ways to deal with this arousal must be explored.

In general, because of the complexity of this issue, stress as a maintaining factor of excessive consumption must be assessed *individually* for the optimum exploitation of the stress management intervention. This assessment is done through the functional analysis. The nature of specific stress-producing situations must be determined for each individual.

Physiological Factors. Drinking and other drug use can be seen as an attempt to decrease physical discomfort and pain. In our groups, problem drinkers do report use of alcohol or drugs to decrease backaches and headaches, etc. With this in mind, such conditions are investigated and treated while clients are in treatment.

Cognitive Factors. Clinically, many alcoholics report that thoughts that precede drinking are neg-

ative self-statements, retaliatory thoughts, rejection of responsibility ("I don't care"), or thoughts directly related to guilt and past misdemeanors. Clients report that excess drinking may function to block out some of these thoughts temporarily.

TREATMENT: ESSENTIAL CHARACTERISTICS OF THE APPROACH

Group Relaxation and Stress Management

Following are the components of the group treatments as administered by the authors in Day Treatment Programs.

It should be emphasized that this group treatment is part of a *broad spectrum* treatment approach. Clients also attend many other structured group activities led by social workers, occupational therapists, recreation therapists, and nurses. These groups include social skills training, vocational counseling, leisure counseling, recreation, and task-oriented small group therapy. These are all aimed at making a meaningful change in the clients' lifestyle. The skills attained in the stress management and relaxation groups are incorporated as part of the overall plan of treatment. Stress is "managed" in order to help clients function more effectively and to enable clients to use all the skills and strategies that they acquire in the treatment program.

Exclusion criteria could include marked hearing loss, resulting in an inability to hear the instructions, frank organic brain damage, or current major withdrawal from drugs or alcohol (i.e., clients must be physically stable).

Treatment Sessions

Assessment

Patients are assessed in terms of physical and cognitive symptoms and ability to cope with varying stress-producing situations. This information is gathered by the use of the Personal Tension Profile (Fig. 1). The Coping and Relaxation Assignment (Fig. 2) looks at areas such as sleep problems, confrontation and conflict, ability to problem solve, patience, and assertiveness. The assessment forms help the therapist and the treatment team to pinpoint specific areas to be addressed in treatment.

As physical therapists, we are very sensitive to the physical symptoms identified by the clients. Muscle tension is identified on at least half the tension profiles, and we can help deal with that through appropriate exercise, postural correction, and other physical means. Clients with sleeping difficulty are identified, and the amount of caffeine consumed is noted.

NAME:_____   DATE:_____

Do you experience any of the following symptoms? If so, how often?

	Check One: Never	Daily	Weekly	Monthly
Headaches, (migraine, sinus, tension)				
Difficulty falling asleep				
Stomach pain or problem (tightness, "butterflies," gas, heartburn)				
Difficulty concentrating				
Easily irritated				
Uncomfortable breathing (shallow, rapid)				
Sweating excessively				

How much of your alcohol/drug use is a way of dealing with stressful feelings (being uptight, afraid, frustrated or "down"). Circle the appropriate number:

none   one-quarter   one-half   three-quarters   all

What other ways do you have of dealing with stressful feelings? Please list:

_____

_____

Have you had any previous experience with relaxation techniques, yoga or meditation? Yes ( ) No ( )
If yes, please explain: _____

How many hours do you sleep a night?_____ hours.
How many caffeine drinks (coffee, tea, cola) do you drink a day?_____ cups.
Do you often feel very tired?   Yes ( )   No ( )
How many cigarettes do you smoke a day?_____ packs.

   Have you ever had ulcers?   Yes ( )   No ( )
           low back pain?   Yes ( )   No ( )
             asthma?   Yes ( )   No ( )

Rate the way you feel now on this 10 point scale.

1	2	3	4	5	6	7	8	9	10
Totally relaxed				Moderately tense			Extremely tense (the most uncomfortable you can be)		

What do you think could change these feelings (for better or for worse)?

_____

_____

Addiction Research Foundation
November 1986 OT/PT Dept.

Figure 1 Personal tension profile.

Group sessions are composed of educational, training, and practice components and are of 1-hour duration. These sessions are a departure from groups traditionally offered by physical therapists. As facilitators, we try to keep the sessions client centered and present didactic material as simply as possible. The agenda is kept fluid, always responsive to client needs, and the general topics are based on the functional analysis related to client situations.

Educational Component

The first half hour of each session is devoted to discussion focusing on a relevant topic. Clients are encouraged to share information and experiences and to give feedback to others on a regular basis. Feedback of a personal nature is especially encouraged. Clients discuss how they have managed a similar situation, or they "normalize" the problem by sharing that they too have this problem. The role of the group leader (i.e., the physical therapist) is to facilitate discussion to keep topics relevant to the designated subject matter and to focus on problems.

The following are the topics discussed in group sessions:

The Concept of Stress—an understanding of stress as an adaptation to change
The Alarm Response—physiology and normalizing the body's response to stress

---

Here are some examples of tension situations. In the space provided, write all the ways you know to decrease tension feelings and become more relaxed in each situation.

1. You are in the middle of a very emotional argument. Your face is flushed, your speech is becoming less controlled and you are very upset.

2. You can't fall asleep. You toss and turn restlessly, worrying about all the sleep you are missing. You can't keep your thoughts from racing over the day's happenings.

3. You've had a busy, hectic day. You arrive home very wound up, feeling restless and unable to sit still for long.

4. You have been looking foward to meeting a friend for a long time. It's already 20 minutes after the time you arranged to meet and he/she still has not arrived.

5. You've been invited with others to meet a group of people. You enter the room and hear the noise of people laughing and talking but you know no one to turn to.

6. The person who works next to you has been putting you down constantly over the past few months. As you enter your workplace you see him looking at you and giggling to another worker.

Figure 2   Coping and relaxation assignment.

Coping Patterns—basic ways of dealing with stressful situations
Sleep—a basic understanding of normal sleep, and ways to induce sleep naturally
Emotions—an understanding and acceptance of feelings and how to deal with them
Negative Thinking Patterns—an understanding of some of the cognitions that can cause stress
Backache and Headache—an understanding of the mechanisms of pain, and drug-free ways to deal with these conditions
Breathing Techniques—the use of breathing to control stress
Social Stress—techniques to promote feeling comfortable in social situations
Problem-Solving Techniques—a basic 7-step problem-solving strategy
Revision of Tension Diary—Once a week, the clients are given a Tension Diary (Fig. 3) in which to monitor the amount and the effects of stress during the preceding week. They are also asked to monitor use of stress reduction strategies. The efficacy of these strategies is evaluated and discussed.

Training Component (Relaxation Techniques)

The techniques currently used are progressive muscular, autogenic, and Benson's meditation. Initially, most people find it easier to relax in a lying position because the body is totally supported. It is thought to be especially important that clients not leave the program with the impression relaxation can only be achieved in lying; thus, a progression to sitting is part of all relaxation techniques. It is desirable to be able to control stress in all situations and positions. Owing to confusion between the states of sleep and relaxation, there is a need to differentiate between the two. We have found that clients who simply fall asleep in a session have not necessarily acquired any skill in relaxing because they don't learn the techniques.

For training in lying, the crook-lying position is used with pillows supporting the knees and head. We have observed that the lying position can be uncomfortable for some clients because they may experience feelings of vulnerability.

In sitting, once again, maximum body support is demonstrated. Clients are instructed to sit with their lower backs up against a chair. A small pillow can be used for extra back support, and the knees should be at least level with the hips with feet flat on the floor. Arms are rested on the sides of the chair or on pillows on the laps.

NAME: DUE DATE:

What did you do to decrease your stress/tension level? or *What made you feel good today.*	*What increased your stress/tension level?*
Day 1	
Day 2	
Day 3	
Day 4	
Day 5	
Day 6	
Day 7	

Record average stress/tension level during the day (using scale provided). Use space below to note briefly tension level and tension control during each day.

Stress/ Tension Level	DAY 1	DAY 2	DAY 3	DAY 4	DAY 5	DAY 6	DAY 7
5							
4							
3							
2							
1							
0							

Addiction Research Foundation
OT/PT/RT Discipline
January 1987

Figure 3 Tension Diary

Progressive Muscular Relaxation. This technique was first described by Dr. Edmund Jacobson whose research in the 1930s showed that by directly relaxing the skeletal muscles, the central nervous system relaxes along with the autonomic system. The technique involves alternatively tensing and relaxing muscle groups, while the client is in a relaxed position. The isometric contractions last about 5 to 10 seconds, and then the tension is released for about 20 seconds with attention given to the sensation of relaxation. The sessions usually last about 20 to 25 minutes. A very important component of the training is the teaching of diaphragmatic breathing, which increases the feeling of relaxation. It accompanies, and is incorporated into, the tense-relax cycle.

In our experience, progressive muscle relaxation is a good introductory technique, which is familiar to most physical therapists. It helps individuals develop an awareness of their muscles, where their muscles are, and how they relax. We have often noted decreased body awareness among our clients. Furthermore, learning to relax muscles can help quiet emotions and thinking and can help control breathing. Most clients derive some benefit from an increased body awareness—especially those who tend to somaticize their tension.

Benson's Meditation. This relaxation technique was introduced in the 1950s by Dr. Herbert Benson, who used it primarily to relax patients in order to reduce their blood pressure. It is based on the Eastern forms of meditation where emphasis is placed both on somatic and cognitive relaxation. The goal is to induce a state of consciousness that involves deep relaxation, passivity, and detachment from surroundings.

The four components that evoke what Benson called the "Relaxation Response" are a quiet environment, a mental device, a passive attitude, and a comfortable position. The mental device is the repetition of a word, sound, or phrase paired with normal expiration. This technique is taught in sitting with eyes closed. Sessions last 10 to 15 minutes. In addition to the use of the mental device, definite suggestion, focusing on relaxing certain muscle groups, is given by the therapist.

Benson's technique is used frequently in our groups. We have found this technique particularly appropriate for younger clients. Some of those who obtain instant gratification from the pharmacologic effect of drugs may find Benson's technique a reasonable alternative. Benson's seems to work quickly, and the use of the mental device is an excellent way to replace the racing, incessant thoughts plague many clients.

Autogenic Techniques

Autogenic training is a system of psychosomatic self-regulation that was developed in Germany in the early part of the century. Using this method, a gradual acquisition of autonomic control is acquired by passive concentration. The focal point of concentration is on self-directed mental images. This concentration results in a relaxed state. Sessions last about 20 minutes. Diaphragmatic breathing is also included as part of the training regimen.

Autogenic techniques are used sparingly. They seem more appropriate for older clients. The passive repetition of feeling phrases can be dull and even seen as humorous by the younger clients. In our experience, those who have found the use of imagery to be relaxing, do better with these techniques. Clients who have a negative response to progressive muscle relaxation are candidates for autogenic techniques.

Practice Component

Clients are usually given exposure to all three techniques. Because relaxation is such an individual experience, they should find the technique that suits them best. Autogenic techniques or Benson's meditation are natural progressions to progressive muscular relaxation as clients can now begin to learn to relax their muscles with minimal tensing.

Following each session, clients are asked to report any physical or mental changes to reinforce utilization of the techniques. At this stage, any problems would be discussed. The physical therapist gives feedback from observations of posture, breathing, and muscle tension. Clients do not always report achieving a state of deep relaxation, but most seem to derive some positive benefit. They report feelings of calmness, clear mindedness, a natural high, floating, tingling, warmth, an awareness of breathing, decreased headaches, and loose muscles.

Clients who benefit from these techniques are those that are prepared to release their natural "guard" in order eventually to feel more comfortable. This release particularly appeals to some drug users. They are told "you can let go and your body will keep functioning." However, this can sometimes lead to increased feelings of vulnerability. Taking this risk for possible long-term gain is not always something that clients (especially the younger ones) are prepared to do.

Clients are led to understand that relaxation is a skill (it is likened to learning to ride a bicycle) and that, in order to attain any skill, practice is a vital component. To attain any effect, daily practice is encouraged. In addition, clients are encouraged to incorporate their increased ability to recognize stress and body awareness into daily coping.

Although the practice of the techniques lasts from 10 to 25 minutes, the eventual aim is for the client to be able to use "relaxation recall." That is the final feeling of relaxation that was achieved at the end of the session can be recalled and achieved in a very short time. This can be attained by recalling the feeling or by using some sort of cue (which could be visual or verbal in nature).

Relaxing can also be practiced by listening to cassette tapes. Although tapes are occasionally used at the Clinical Institute, their use is not encouraged during treatment. Verbal instructions allow for more flexibility in pacing the exercises and in responding to the needs of the group. Clients can buy tapes to practice at home but sole dependence on the tape in order to relax must be prevented. We believe that simply listening to a tape is not relaxation therapy. We feel that all three components (i.e., education, training, and practice) must be included for therapy to be complete.

STRESS MANAGEMENT AND RELAXATION THERAPY

Outpatient Individual Treatment

There certainly exists the need for individual (one-on-one) counseling in the area of stress management and relaxation. Clients often request individual treatment because being in a group causes them much discomfort, or because they feel that their issues are particularly sensitive and require confidentiality.

Clients referred for outpatient relaxation and stress management counseling have either identified, or it has been identified by their primary care worker, that stress or insomnia is a problem to them. They have also agreed to attend relaxation sessions in order to manage their stress and help deal with their addiction. The number of treatment sessions depends on the needs, but clients usually attend from 2 to 8 sessions.

A strong collaboration exists between the stress management therapist and the outpatient counselor. Mutual concerns are frequently discussed and treatment is coordinated both in content and timing so that the client can derive maximum benefit.

Treatment Outline of Individual Sessions

Assessment

Once again, the assessment forms previously described are utilized. Further information attained during the initial interview with the client is very valuable. Body language, description of a typical day, description of particularly stressful events, and the former use of drugs to alleviate stress are all taken into account when planning treatment.

Treatment Sessions

The individual sessions differ from the group sessions in that the individual's needs are even more precisely and accurately met. Didactic material is focused more directly on areas that the client and therapist have mutually deemed to be problematic. This results in tailor-made treatment, both in levels of conceptualization and in focus of attention. Special emphasis is placed on skills and deficits in dealing with stressful or potentially stressful situations.

A very useful treatment tool is the "stress diary." Clients monitor significant events that have caused them to feel stressed or have caused cravings to use drugs. These diaries are reviewed and processed in each session and help to focus treatment to the current needs (form 3 [see Figure 3] or a more detailed version of this can be used).

A common behavioral technique that may be appropriate in individual counseling is the use of role playing. Interpersonal situations that are difficult to perform are role played (i.e., practiced) with the therapist or with a neutral party, in order to make the actual performance easier.

In this situation, the physical therapist is especially observant and sensitive to physical areas. Pain and physical discomfort are often identified as ongoing antecedents to feeling "down" and depressed.

Instead of taking these factors as unchangeable, we deal with them. We treat what we can and refer out those problems that we are unable to treat here. Clients have been referred to pain clinics, for orthopaedic consultants, for vocational assessment, and to other physical therapy settings when appropriate.

Relaxation training remains an integral part of the treatment. The concept of being able to perform more comfortably with a relaxed body and mind is always emphasized.

TREATMENT SESSION OUTCOMES

In the Clinical Institute, we do not directly measure physical correlates of relaxation. We have, at times, taken pulses before and after the techniques, and this has often shown that decreased physical arousal has occurred. At this time, our judgment of the efficacy of our treatment is based upon our clients' reports.

Many clients use the techniques to help them fall asleep at night. In fact, these techniques are an extremely valuable component in any pre-bedtime regimen for clients with insomnia.

Clients generally report using the breathing techniques, more than the whole relaxation routine. They seem to remember to use the breathing when they feel stressed (i.e., dealing with conflict, socializing, and drug refusal). Those that have practiced the techniques do find that even using the breathing in stressful situations is much more effective.

A factor that helps clients to try these techniques effectively is their ability or decision to take control over environmental situations. Treatment sessions help the client to move from an external locus (i.e., drugs) to an internal locus.

A useful way to present the whole concept of relaxation and stress management is as an experiential episode. "Let's see if you *can* make yourself feel different on your own." This challenge is often acceptable to clients entering treatment, and they are often surprised as to how much change they can effect. It also adds to self-esteem, which is often a problem with substance abusers.

MEDICAL UNIT

Currently, alcohol-related problems represent over 50 percent of admissions to the 20-bed medical unit. The remainder involves other substances, such as benzodiazepines, barbiturates, narcotics, and cocaine. Referrals for physical therapy services in the Medical Unit include requests for medical physical therapy and relaxation training. The latter comprises the bulk of the referrals. Of the medical referrals, a 2-year survey, 1985–86, indicated that referrals for trauma and orthopaedic conditions were most numerous—outnumbering neurologic and repiratory conditions by a ratio of 4 to 1.

Patients in the Medical Unit present with complex psychosocial problems. These problems are discussed and incorporated into treatment plans at weekly multidisciplinary psychosocial conferences, where the physical therapist is an integral team member.

Alcohol Withdrawal

The role of the physical therapist in the Medical Unit is not unlike the role in a general hospital setting. However, in addition to the usual expectations of sensitivity and understanding, there needs to be an understanding of the patient with alcohol and drug problems and the management of withdrawal symptoms.

Symptoms of alcohol withdrawal include anxiety, tremor, anorexia, and insomnia. In addition, there can be diaphoresis, tachycardia, hypertension, and agitation. Seizures (e.g., confusion, disorientation) or poor physical state can mask underlying injuries. The more critical state of delirium tremens is seen infrequently owing to the aggressive treatment of early withdrawal with diazepam.

Physical therapy can be requested during the early withdrawal period to assess and treat some neurologic problems, e.g., an inability to walk when early mobilization could help general recovery. Often neurologic problems, such as ataxia, tend to resolve rapidly following recovery from withdrawal.

Symptoms of withdrawal can last up to 5 days. Physical therapy might be requested for respiratory problems during the withdrawal period; referred patients tend to be heavy smokers. A prolonged period of intoxication can depress respiration and the cough reflex. Standard treatments are utilized for anyone diagnosed with pneumonia or chronic obstructive lung disease.

Trauma and Orthopaedic Conditions

Patients referred for physical therapy on the Medical Unit may have ongoing orthopaedic problems, may have injured themselves while intoxicated, or may have become dependent on drugs (physician prescribed or self-medication) or alcohol as the result of an injury. The most common diagnoses are fractures, back problems, and soft tissue injuries. These injuries are treated in much the same way as in a general hospital setting. However, the addiction would be actively treated in the Medical Unit.

Those who have become dependent on substances while attempting to manage pain come to the Medical Unit to withdraw from these substances. While the patient is in the Medical Unit, pain management and the abuse of addictive medications are the focus of treatment. The physical therapist's role is to provide alternate ways to prevent or deal with pain and disability. For example, treatments could include back education, posture correction, exercise, heat and cold applications. It has been our experience that tolerance of pain is unpredictable when looking at the underlying injury. Prolonged physiologic and psychological dependence on chemicals seems to have a direct affect on individual's ability to deal with pain; this must be taken into consideration when planning treatment. When ongoing pain management is a problem, it is dealt with by referral to a pain clinic.

A brief case example illustrates how physical therapy is integrated into the complete treatment approach on the Medical Unit.

The case involves a 20-year-old female admitted for investigation of an alcohol withdrawal seizure. Medical problems included moderate back pain. Psychosocial problems included alcohol abuse, a suicide attempt, unemployment, illiteracy, and a problematic living situation.

The assessment and treatment in this case is much the same as in other medical settings, but there are several important differences. First, abstinence is enforced in the Medical Unit through a process of drug and alcohol testing. This allows assessment of the severity of back pain while the patient is drug free. In this case, the patient reported back pain of 7-months duration, but she had been able to ignore it during this period because of her drinking. She attributed the pain to her previous occupation as a punch press operator. She also had a history of scoliosis surgery.

Treatment with this patient included back education, heat, and back and abdominal strengthening exercises. These are the usual treatments, but the physical therapist has an opportunity to try them while the patient is drug and alcohol free. This could likely improve the effectiveness of treatment by increasing understanding and compliance with a program of back education and exercises.

Another characteristic of the assessment and treatment approach of the Medical Unit is that the therapist functions as part of a team with the medical and nursing staff. The team approach is a holistic one and particularly supports nondrug interventions, such as physical therapy. The team reviews a variety of lifestyle factors that reinforce drug and alcohol abuse. In the above case, taking into account the patient's illiteracy, no written material was given. The therapist is able to have valuable input regarding vocational plans and direction. The problem of alcohol abuse is dealt with in outpatient counseling.

This example illustrates how the therapist is given leverage in terms of treatment, through the guarantee of a drug- and alcohol-free environment and through a holistic team approach. In another setting, the therapist working with such a patient may be aware of the abuse of alcohol or drugs, but because the patient or the therapist is reluctant to confront it, nothing is done about it. In addition, substance abuse may interfere with the effect of the physical therapy interventions. In the Medical Unit, alcohol abuse is not seen as just a nuisance factor, but as the focus of an active treatment goal.

Neurologic Conditions

Neurologic impairment can arise from the direct consequences of alcohol abuse and, much less frequently, from drug abuse. Alcohol destroys central nervous system cells and causes axonal degeneration of peripheral nerves, which results in either temporary or permanent effects. As previously mentioned, the neurologic recovery following withdrawal from alcohol can be dramatic as compared to other conditions presenting with similar symptoms. Physical therapists can benefit from the knowledge of the possible connection between surprisingly rapid neurologic recovery and alcohol withdrawal.

The most commonly seen conditions are polyneuropathy, myopathy, encephalopathy (Wernicke's and Korsakoff's), and dementia. In addition, patients with these conditions are frequently in poor physical condition, ataxic, malnourished, weak, anemic, emaciated, and have a variety of other problems including cardiac and gastrointestinal conditions.

Again, physical therapy treatments are as in a general hospital setting, involving heat or cold to decrease pain, muscle reeducation, active exercises, and gait training. Depending on the assessment, referrals can be made to Home Care.

Anxiety, Stress-Related Conditions

Other patients seen by physical therapy or the Medical Unit are those with anxiety- and stress-related conditions. These patients are often admitted as a result of a psychosocial or medical crisis in their lives. Treatment initially includes medical management of withdrawal from drugs and alcohol. Their current symptoms frequently include somatic complaints and difficulty with sleeping. Many identify that drugs or alcohol have helped them cope with these symptoms in the past. Relaxation techniques are offered as one form of nonchemical intervention. When successfully practiced, these techniques can allow patients an alternative way to help get to sleep, to deal with the physical and emotional effect of withdrawal, and to

"survive" in the unit. The technique most frequently used with this population is progressive muscle relaxation as it is simple and requires less concentration than other techniques.

POSTSCRIPT

The physical therapist comes to the field with a "medical model" that complements any psychosocial treatment strategy. This can be extremely helpful in identifying and priorizing essential issues requiring attention. It also helps other team members understand medical issues and take these into account when planning treatment.

A good understanding of body mechanics, kinesiology, and orthopaedics adds to the efficient teaching of relaxation techniques. No physical therapist can logically request that a patient relax if the body is not fully supported or if any antigravity muscles are working. The understanding of the musculoskeletal system and its concommitant pathology (including the normal aging process) is also useful in dealing with many clients, especially those whose drug use initially arose from a legitimate need for pain medication, i.e., as a result of trauma or illness. Explanations of the underlying condition (sometimes the first time the client may have heard this) and effective coping strategies to deal with current disability (e.g., sleeping positions) have been shown to be extremely important in continued patient care.

Physical therapy is playing an important and certainly an interesting role in the treatment of addictions in the Clinical Institute of the Addiction Research Foundation. The medical and observational skills of the physical therapists, allied with the pychosocial/behavioral components of treatment programs, results in a treatment modality which deals uniquely with the varying and complex problems of a needy population group.

The views expressed in this publication are those of the authors and do not necessarily reflect those of the Addiction Research Foundation.

SUGGESTED READING

Benson H. The relaxation response. New York: Avon, 1975.
Davis M, Eshelman ER. McKay M. The relaxation and stress reduction workbook. California: New Harbinger, 1982.
Madders J. Stress and relaxation. Toronto: Prentice-Hall, 1979.
Miller P, Mastria MA. Alternatives to alcohol abuse. Champaign, IL: Research Press, 1977.
Woofolk RL, Lehrer PM. Principles and practice of stress management. New York: Guilford Press, 1984.

PHYSICAL THERAPY IN HOSPICE

JANE TOOT, Ph.D., P.T.

THE NATURE OF HOSPICE

Hospice, a concept of care for dying patients, focuses on providing comfort measures rather than aggressively searching for a cure. Dame Cicely Saunders promoted this concept in England in the late 1960s. Her contention was that the health care system should provide an option for patients to seek palliative as well as aggressive care in the last stages of life:

You matter because you are. You matter to the
last moment of your life, and we will do all we
can not only to help you die peacefully but
also to live until you die.

–Cicely Saunders

Hospice addresses symptom control from a wholistic view under the direction of an interdisciplinary team. As a basis for discussion of the practical and philosophical aspects of providing physical therapy to hospice patients, Table 1 presents a review of care approaches in traditional settings and in hospice.

The overall direction of hospice can be best summarized through the Dying Person's Bill of Rights, which is provided in Table 2.

PHYSICAL THERAPY

Physical therapy certainly fits with many of the tenets of hospice, such as the interdisciplinary team, inclusion of the patient and family as the care unit, provision of treatment in various in- and outpatient settings, and attention to the comfort of the patient. Why then would hospice be considered as a nontraditional setting for physical therapy? The answer to that question might come through considerations of physical therapy as it is typically pictured.

Physical therapists generally think in terms of improving the physical and/or functional level of their patients. It is believed and expected that the patient will be habilitated or rehabilitated and will get better, due in great part to physical therapy. At worst, even if the patient's condition does not improve, his ability to perform daily activities will. On the other hand,

the patient with a last-stage life-threatening illness presents a much different challenge to a therapist. As with other patients, the therapist expects that therapy will bring an improvement. However, in these instances the therapist knows that improvement will be circumscribed by the relentless progression of the disease process. Accordingly, the physical therapist must not only evaluate his patient very carefully but also himself. With many of our patients we consider the psychological aspects of disability. As we develop treatment plans, we try to take into account the effects of diminished function, body image, and self-worth. However, the components of a life philosophy may only exist as several separate pieces. The composite product, not having received enough attention from introspection and review of life experiences, may not be an integral part of our treatment approach. No other group of patients requires the depth of self-appraisal that is demanded when treating patients in the final days of life. In order to work effectively with patients who are dying, one must have developed a coherent set of values about living. This is not an easy task, nor one that is usually initiated unless circumstances demand such activity:

There are three things extremely hard: steel, a
diamond, and to know oneself.

—Megiddo Message

Once the therapist recognizes his own attitudes regarding this patient population and realizes the goals of hospice intervention, he or she can approach the patient or family care unit with appropriate, and often effective, treatment plans.

Specific Activities of Physical Therapy in Hospice

Certainly various modalities can provide relief from discomfort encountered as a result of prolonged bed rest, decreased muscle mass, poor positioning and general debilitation secondary to disease processes. The judicious use of heat, cold, and gentle massage singly or in combination may ease aching muscles, loosen tightness in tendons, and assist circulation. Utilization of transcutaneous electrical nerve stimulation (TENS) has been successful with some cases of chronic pain, particularly with patients who are cognizant and who demonstrate highly localized problems. For example, TENS has been used effectively with cancer patients who demonstrate bone metastases.

Exercises ranging from active resistive to passive

Physical Therapy in Hospice / 281

TABLE I Philosophical Differences

Traditional Care	Hospice Care
Approach to patients is that only cure is worthwhile and that aggressive measures will be followed regardless of prognosis. Care is usually confined to physical aspects of disease process.	Recognition by patient and physician that cure is not likely but much can be done for the patient's comfort and sense of well-being. Therefore symptomatic treatment is administered addressing all sources of discomfort—physical, psychological, social, spiritual.
Physician directs all decisions regarding care of patient. Will contact other professionals as he/she believes is indicated.	Professional/volunteer team determines needs to be addressed. A "circle of care" is established with equal interaction among caregivers (see Fig. 1).
The patient is seen as a disease entity. The disease is the focus of care.	The patient/family is the care unit. The interaction of their needs dictates care focus. The patient is a contributing member of the team.
Pain medication is given on a limited PRN basis. Fear of addiction prevents controlling pain in many instances. The patient is placed in an anxiety-producing situation which can exacerbate pain.	Pain treated through titration of medication according to patient pain cycle and metabolism. Goal is to eliminate pain while maintaining normal affect. Once pain cycle is established, medications are administered to anticipate pain rather than to react to it.
Symptoms are treated in isolation. One medication can diminish or even counteract effects of others.	Symptom control is orchestrated to enhance effects of medications.
Patient is usually housed in acute care facility. Protocols and procedures follow those dictated by institution regarding meal times, visitors, use of own belongings.	Patient may be treated at home or in-patient facility. Efforts concentrate on facilitation of home care. However, if an in-patient facility is used, individual schedules are considered, visitors are welcome at any time, and use of personal belongings is encouraged.
Use of professional health caregivers to provide attention within area of expertise. Can result in gaps in service and attention. While patient may be overloaded and confused by inconsistent use of many disciplines, family is shunted aside.	Inclusion of family members and trained volunteers as valued members of care team. Attention tends to be consistent over a 24-hour day/7-day-per-week basis. A core-team is utilized with ancillary members coming in as needed.
Care limited to stay in institution while treating disease. Rarely establish contact with survivors after death.	Bereavement care is an integral part of care plan. Can continue up to a year following patient's death. Seen as proactive intervention for survivors.

can help to prevent contractures, and even maintain a level of functional strength for patients who are essentially confined to bed. Learning how to use assistive devices such as wheelchairs, lightweight splints, walkers, and activity aids may all assist the patient in completing activities of daily living (ADLs) and contribute to feelings of self-worth. Not to be forgotten is that these same activities make provision of care easier for the family member and/or home health aide

Another significant role which can be filled by physical therapy is that of an educator. Educational intervention would include teaching appropriate body mechanics to be utilized during transfers and completion of ADLs. Targeted for such instruction would be

TABLE 2 The Dying Person's Bill of Rights

I have the right to be treated as a living human being until I die

I have the right to maintain a sense of hopefulness, however changing its focus may be

I have the right to be cared for by those who can maintain a sense of hopefulness, however changing this might be

I have a right to express my feelings and emotions about my approaching death in my own way

I have the right to participate in decisions concerning my care

I have the right to expect continuing medical and nursing attention even though "cure" goals must be changed to "comfort" goals

I have the right not to die alone

I have the right to be free from pain

I have the right to have my questions answered honestly

I have the right not to be deceived

I have the right to have help from and for my family in accepting my death

I have the right to die in peace and dignity

I have the right to retain my individuality and not be judged for my decisions which may be contrary to beliefs of others

I have the right to discuss and enlarge my religious and/or spiritual experiences, whatever these may mean to others

I have the right to expect that the sanctity of the human body will be respected after death

I have the right to be cared for by caring, sensitive, knowledgeable people who will attempt to understand my needs and will be able to gain some satisfaction in helping me face my death

This Bill of Rights was created at a workshop on "The Terminally Ill Patient and the Helping Person" in Lansing, Michigan, sponsored by the Southwestern Michigan Inservice Education Council and conducted by Amelia J. Barbus, Associate Professor of Nursing, Wayne State University, Detroit, Michigan. From Whitman H, Lukes SJ. Behavior modification for terminally ill patients. Am J Nurs 1975; 75:99.

the patient or family care unit and other team members, including professionals and volunteers. Safety issues are of prime importance because of patient weakness and fragility.

As hospice endeavors to facilitate the patient returning to his own home for care, accurate evaluation of the home environment for equipment—needs, type, and placement, is necessary. While this function may be completed by nursing, it could be the responsibility of physical therapy. Home evaluations of this nature may be done as a direct service by physical therapy. However, physical therapy, as a service on an interdisciplinary team, may elect to present a mini-series of inservices for team members clarifying components of environmental evaluation. In this way, whoever is involved with the initial home visit will be able to gather the necessary information.

Finally, physical therapists may be involved with bereavement services. Hospice offers programs for survivors of patients, which range from simple monitoring through phone calls, all the way through elaborate group seminars dealing with physical and psychosocial health. With the latter, physical therapy may very well present proactive programs of exercise to the survivor, a high-risk population for stress-related illnesses.

Preparation of Therapists for Work in Hospice

The above activities are not out of the ordinary for physical therapy. Several courses in anatomy, neurology, physiology, and kinesiology provide a basis for later presentations in modalities and therapeutic exercise with indications and contraindications for use in all areas of disability. However, the educational preparation of physical therapists does have serious gaps in psychosocial issues of disability, values clarification, lifespan development, learning styles, and educational methodology. These subjects may be covered in physical therapy curricula, but often as afterthoughts, and they usually are not an integral part of other course materials. However, these topics are the areas in which therapists need to have sound knowledge in order to work successfully with hospice patients. Indeed, awareness and understanding of these subjects would assist therapists to be more effective with all patient groups.

Another area that should be included in physical therapy curricula is the concept of interdisciplinary teams—difficulties and advantages in their formation, development, and use. Many care settings use a multidisciplinary approach, and physical therapy educators regularly inform students about other professions that may work on a case with physical therapy. Rarely, however, are the procedures, environments, and communication skills necessary for team building adequately addressed. Figure 1 depicts the "circle of care," which provides services for the patient or family care unit and demonstrates the intricacies of the interdisciplinary approach.

The inner circle shows the recipient of care who interacts on a regular, on-going basis with the next circle, or the core team. This group of individuals is consistently involved with the care unit and rarely contains more than six people. The broken circle represents individuals who are called upon for information and service. However, they are considered as ancillary members of the team and step back when they are no longer needed. The individuals on the ancillary team may also step to the other circle and act as liaisons to the outer circle or community in organizing services, obtaining equipment, providing education, and recruiting volunteers. The support provided by the outermost circle is of a secondary nature to the care unit, but often is crucial for the morale of the two caregiver circles.

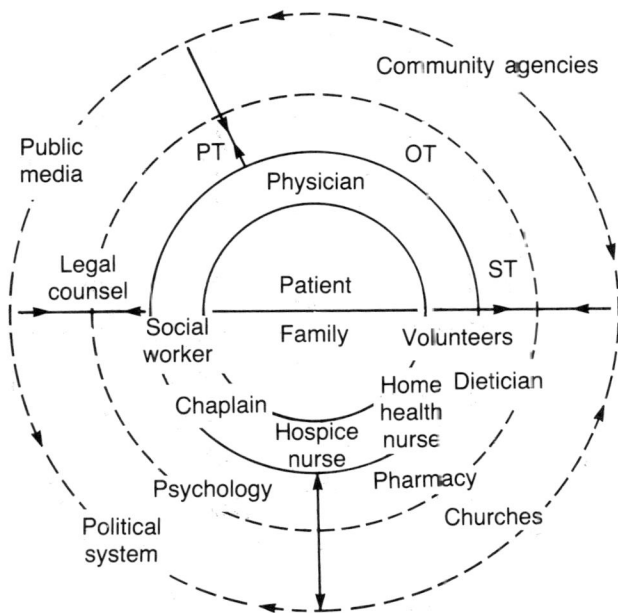

Figure 1 A circle of care.

tients in growing numbers will also bring a more intensive use of hospice. Second, physical therapy educators are beginning to recognize the need for psychosocial and medicolegal issues to be incorporated throughout the curriculum as awareness of the needs and expectations encountered by those patients and families dealing with chronic and life-threatening illnesses builds in the health professions. A logical assumption would then follow that graduates would be more comfortable with these populations and understand the viability of physical therapy interventions. Third, the rising use of home care will incorporate numbers of interdisciplinary teams in creative programming to maximize professional input in time-effective intervention.

In conclusion, physical therapy has a definite role to fill in hospice. It is a position that demands not only clinical and academic knowledge but a strong sense of self and of personal values system. It is this last requirement coupled with understanding and acceptance of the strengths and weaknesses of the human condition that presents the greatest challenge to the health professions—including physical therapy.

The healer has to keep striving for...the space...in which healer and patient can reach out to each other as travelers sharing the same broken human condition.

—Henri JM Nouwen, *Reaching out*

Such an encircling system denotes several important concepts. They include the following:

1. The center of the circle is the care unit
2. No care unit is "dropped through the cracks"
3. Cooperation and communication among all members is crucial
4. The typical medical pyramid is not in evidence. Everyone shares responsibility on an equal basis.

The concept implied with this diagram is the abilities of the several team members, which must mesh in hospice.

FUTURE ROLES

In the future, the role of physical therapy in a hospice setting will become more familiar both to providers and consumers. Many factors will bring about this increased involvement. First, hospice will be a more frequently chosen care alternative as populations of elderly increase. The presence of AIDS pa-

SUGGESTED READING

Cohen K. Hospice prescription for terminal care. Germantown, MD: Aspen, 1979.

Graham J. In the company of others. New York: Harcourt Brace Jovanovich, 1982.

Kastenbaum RJ. Death society and human experience. St. Louis: CV Mosby, 1977.

Mount B. Challenges in palliative care. Am J Hospice Care 1985; 2(6):22–29.

Nelson R, Currier D. Clinical electrotherapy. Norwalk, CT: Appleton & Lange, 1987.

Nouwen HJM. Reaching out. New York: Doubleday, 1975.

Stoddard S. The hospice movement. New York: Vintage Books, 1978.

Pitzele SK. We are not alone: learning to live with chronic illness. Minneapolis: Thompson, 1985.